volume is one of the Cardiothoracic Surgery Series,
Edited by Joe R. Utley

Thi

Periopera
Cardiac
Dysfuncti

Volume II

Perioperative Cardiac Dysfunction

Volume III

Editor

Joe R. Utley, M.D.

Cardiothoracic Surgeon
Spartanburg General Hospital
Spartanburg, South Carolina
Clinical Professor of Surgery
Medical University of South Carolina

Editorial Associate

Rosanne Betleski, B.A.

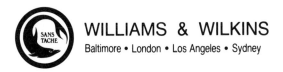

WILLIAMS & WILKINS
Baltimore • London • Los Angeles • Sydney

Editor: John N. Gardner
Associate Editor: Victoria M. Vaughn
Copy Editor: Shelley Potler
Design: Bert Smith
Illustration Planning: Reginald R. Stanley
Production: Raymond E. Reter

Copyright ©, 1985
Williams & Wilkins
428 East Preston Street
Baltimore, MD 21202, U.S.A.

Accurate indications, adverse reactions, and dosage schedules for drugs are provided
in this book, but it is possible that they may change. The reader is urged to review
the package information data of the manufacturers of the medications mentioned.

Printed in the United States of America

Library of Congress Cataloging in Publication Data

Perioperative cardiac dysfunction.

(Cardiothoracic surgery series)
"The topics presented in this monograph were discussed at two symposia conducted
in San Diego in November 1982 and December 1983"—Pref.
Includes index.
1. Heart—Diseases—Congresses. 2. Heart—Surgery—Complications and sequelae—Congresses. I. Utley, Joe R. II. Betleski, Rosanne. III. Series. [DNLM: 1. Heart
Diseases—complications—congresses. 2. Intraoperative Complications—Congresses. 3. Postoperative Complications—Congresses. WG 200 P445 1982–83]

RC681.A2P44 1985   617'.01   84-19529
ISBN 0-683-08503-4

Composed and printed at the   85 86 87 88 89
Waverly Press, Inc.   10 9 8 7 6 5 4 3 2 1

Series Editor's Foreword

Volumes I and II of the Cardiothoracic Surgery Series dealt with topics related principally to cardiopulmonary bypass. In Volume III we address topics closely related to cardiopulmonary bypass, but dealing primarily with events in the perioperative period which may cause the heart to perform poorly. This is obviously of great importance to cardiac surgeons, cardiac anesthesiologists, intensivists, and nurses dealing with the cardiac surgery patient, but there are also many principles presented here applicable to any patient with heart disease undergoing operative therapy for noncardiac disease. The preoperative, intraoperative, and postoperative use of drugs to control the ischemic syndromes in patients with coronary disease is an area applicable to patients undergoing noncardiac surgery. In this monograph we have attempted to review the current status of the use of various forms of augmentation devices to improve pump function postoperatively. The use of various inotropic drugs as well as vasodilators are reviewed. The very important areas of cardiac arrhythmias and pacing are explored. A very exciting chapter on the effect of reflexes on cardiac function is included, and the important influences of pericardial function, the dilated ventricle, diastolic function, afterload mismatch, and pulmonary hypertension are explored.

The material in this monograph clearly illustrates the importance of the contribution of nonsurgeons, particularly cardiologists and anesthesiologists, in the perioperative care of the surgical patient. It is the goal of this series to increase the knowledge, capabilities, standards of practice, and performance of the reader. We have attempted to cover a broad series of topics and to present current knowledge and understanding of the important issues related to cardiac function in the surgical patient.

—Joe R. Utley, M.D.

Preface

The topics presented in this monograph were discussed at two symposia conducted in San Diego in November 1982 and December 1983. During these symposia, a wide variety of physicians dealing with cardiac dysfunction in the surgical patients presented current views related to preoperative, interoperative, and postoperative alterations in cardiac function. The information presented in these chapters is often quite basic, but in each instance has a direct applicability to the clinical setting.

—Joe R. Utley, M.D.

Contributors

John R. Brazier, M.D., Northridge, California

David Bregman, M.D., Chair, Department of Surgery and Director, Thoracic and Cardiovascular Surgery, St. Joseph's Hospital and Medical Center, Patterson, New Jersey

Gerald D. Buckberg, M.D., F.A.C.S., Professor of Surgery, University of California Los Angeles, Los Angeles, California

D.C. Chung, M.D., Associate Professor of Anesthesiology, University of Western Ontario, London, Ontario, Canada

Thomas Conahan, III, M.D., Associate Professor of Anesthesiology, The Hospital of the University of Pennsylvania, Philadelphia, Pennsylvania

Jack D. Copeland, M.D., Professor of Chief, Section of Cardiovascular and Thoracic Surgery, University of Arizona Health Sciences Center, Tucson, Arizona

Pat O. Daily, M.D., Clinical Professor of Surgery and Chief, Division of Cardiothoracic Surgery, University of California San Diego, San Diego, California

Walter P. Dembitsky, M.D., Associate Clinical Professor of Surgery, University of California San Diego, San Diego, California

Donald C. Finlayson, M.D., Professor of Anesthesiology, Emory University School of Medicine, and Director, Critical Care Medicine, Emory Hospital, Atlanta, Georgia

Victor F. Froelicher, M.D., Professor of Medicine, University of California, Irvine and Chief, Cardiology Section, Long Beach Veterans Administration Medical Center, Long Beach, California

Renee S. Hartz, M.D. Associate Professor of Surgery, Northwestern University Medical School, Chicago, Illinois

Ellis L. Jones, M.D., Professor at Surgery, Emory University School of Medicine, Atlanta, Georgia

Martin M. LeWinter, M.D., Associate Professor of Medicine, University of California, San Diego and Director, Non-Invasive Cardiac Graphics, San Diego Veterans Administration Medical Center, San Diego, California

John C. Longhurst, M.D., Ph.D., Associate Professor of Medicine, University of California San Diego, San Diego, California

Douglas H. McConnell, M.D., Clinical Instructor in Surgery, University of California, Los Angeles School of Medicine and Memorial Medical Center of Long Beach, California

Lawrence L. Michaelis, M.D., Professor of Surgery and Chair, Division of Cardiothoracic Surgery, Northwestern University Medical School, Chicago, Illinois

Richard Michalik, M.D., Associate in Surgery, Cardiothoracic Surgery, Emory University School of Medicine, Atlanta, Georgia

William S. Pierce, M.D., Professor of Surgery, The College of Medicine, Pennsylvania State University, Hershey, Pennsylvania

Aidan A. Raney, Associate Clinical Professor of Surgery, University of California San Diego, San Diego, California

Laurence S. Reisner, M.D., Clinical Professor of Anesthesiology and Reproductive Medicine, University of California San Diego, San Diego, California

Wayne E. Richenbacher, M.D., Resident in Surgery, The College of Medicine, Pennsylvania State University, Hershey, Pennsylvania

Arthur J. Roberts, M.D., Professor of Surgery and Chair, Cardiothoracic Surgery, Boston University School of Medicine, Boston, Massachusetts

John M. Robertson, M.D., Medical Resident, University of California Los Angeles, Los Angeles, California

Francis Robicsek, M.D., Clinical Professor of Surgery, University of North Carolina and Chair, Department of Thoracic and Cardiovascular Surgery, Charlotte Memorial Hospital and Medical Center, Charlotte, North Carolina

Gene Robinson, M.D., Medical Student, University of California San Diego, San Diego, California

John J. Ross, Jr., M.D., Professor of Medicine and Head, Division of Cardiology, University of California San Diego, San Diego, California

Ralph Shabetai, M.D., Professor of Medicine, University of California, San Diego and Chief, Cardiology Division, San Diego Veterans Administration Medical Center, San Diego, California

Julie A. Swain, M.D., Assistant Professor of Surgery and Head, Division of Cardiothoracic Surgery, University of Louisiana, Shreveport, Louisiana

Albert L. Waldo, M.D., Professor of Medicine and Senior Scientist, Cardiovascular Research and Training Center, University of Alabama School of Medicine, Birmingham, Alabama

James D. Wisheart, B.Sc., M.Ch., F.R.C.S., Cardiothoracic Surgery, British Royal Infirmary and Royal Bristol Hospital for Sick Children, Bristol, England

Contents

Series Editor's Foreword v
Preface vii
Contributors ix

Chapter 1   The Pericardium as a Source of Cardiac Dysfunction

Ralph Shabetai, M.D. 1

Chapter 2   Cardiac Dysfunction: Special Considerations During Pregnancy

Laurence S. Reisner, M.D. 15

Chapter 3   Arterial Baroreceptors and Cardiac Receptors, Their Physiology and Pathophysiology

John C. Longhurst, M.D., Ph.D. 30

Chapter 4   Recent Advances in Balloon Counterpulsation

David Bregman, M.D. 51

Chapter 5   Temporary Extracorporeal Postoperative Circulatory Support Using the Roller of Rotor Impeller Pump

Walter P. Dembitsky, M.D., Aidan A. Raney, M.D., and Pat O. Daily, M.D. 63

Chapter 6   Ventricular Assist Devices

Wayne E. Richenbacher, M.D., and William S. Pierce, M.D. 74

Chapter 7   Anesthetic Consideration in Coronary Artery Disease

Thomas J. Conahan, III, M.D. 89

Chapter 8   Intraoperative Protection of the Myocardium

Renee S. Hartz, M.D., and Lawrence L. Michaelis, M.D. 97

Chapter 9   Perioperative Myocardial Infarction in Open Heart Surgery

Arthur J. Roberts, M.D. 107

Chapter 10   Reanimation of the Heart

Francis Robicsek, M.D. 122

Chapter 11   Perioperative Coronary Spasm

Donald C. Finlayson, M.D. 131

Chapter 12   Determinants of Myocardial Performance and the Adequacy of Subendocardial Blood Flow

Gerald D. Buckberg, M.D., F.A.C.S., John M. Robertson, M.D., Douglas H. McConnell, M.D., and John R. Brazier, M.D.   139

Chapter 13   Afterload Mismatch in the Perioperative Period

John J. Ross, Jr., M.D.   159

Chapter 14   Coronary Bypass Soon after Myocardial Infarction

Elis L. Jones, M.D., and Richard Michalik, M.D.   170

Chapter 15   Perioperative Arrhythmias—Use of Epicardial Wire Electrodes for Diagnosis and Treatment

Albert L. Waldo, M.D.   180

Chapter 16   Diastolic Function and the Hypertrophied Ventricle

Martin M. LeWinter, M.D.   200

Chapter 17   Coronary Artery Disease in Noncardiac Surgery

Julie A. Swain, M.D.   213

Chapter 18   Perioperative Vasodilator Therapy

James D. Wisheart, B.Sc., M.Ch., F.R.C.S.   217

Chapter 19   Perioperative Uses of Inotropic Drugs

Jack D. Copeland, M.D.   230

Chapter 20   Digitalis and Digitalis Toxicity

D. C. Chung, M.D.   241

Chapter 21   Perioperative Cardiac Rehabilitation

Gene Robinson, M.D., and Victor F. Froelicher, Jr., M.D.   254

Appendix   271

Index   279

CHAPTER 1

THE PERICARDIUM AS A SOURCE OF CARDIAC DYSFUNCTION

RALPH SHABETAI, M.D.

The pericardium influences cardiac function, especially diastolic function by acting as an external restraint that under appropriate circumstances, can limit filling of the cardiac chambers and reinforces interaction between them. Before considering the specific perioperative syndromes attributable to the pericardium, it is appropriate to review briefly the relevant aspects of normal pericardial physiology. At once, it becomes apparent that the pericardium presents an enigma to the physiologist: it has been shown repeatedly from the early part of the century[1,2] to the present time[3] that under appropriate circumstances, the pericardium is responsible for elevations of left ventricular diastolic pressure, limitation of left ventricular volume, and alterations in the shapes of the left and right ventricles with subsequent modification of their diastolic compliances and of their performances in systole.[4] On the other hand, the pericardium can be subtotally or partially removed, or individuals may be born with all or substantial parts of the pericardium missing, yet in both these circumstances, no harmful effects from deficiency or absence of the pericardium can be demonstrated. Life is neither threatened nor shortened, symptoms do not appear, and cardiac dysfunction cannot be documented even using modern sophisticated techniques.

The pericardium fits the heart quite snugly, leaving a small space, the *pericardial reserve volume*, to allow the heart to expand in response to changes in blood volume and in response to respiration, changes in posture, and straining. The pericardium can stretch when the straining forces are prolonged as in normal growth, or when the heart is chronically dilated, but it is highly resistant to any attempt to stretch abruptly to a size larger than its residual volume permits. The histological basis for this resistance to acute stretching is a collagen which is present in large bundles of wavey fibers.[5] When the waves are straightened out the pericardium is almost infinitely stiff, thus, the pericardium forcefully resists acute dilation of the cardiac chambers. The response to chronic stretch obviously has to be different, otherwise pericardial constriction would be the inevitable outcome of normal growth and of cardiomegaly owing to congestive heart failure.

ACUTE DILATION

When the heart is presented with an acute large volume load, dilation of its chambers is restrained by the pericardium because of its inability to deform rapidly. When the heart is exposed to an insult prompting acute dilation, especially dilation of all four cardiac chambers, intrapericardial pressure rises dramatically, reflecting the restraining force of the pericardium. If the heart becomes acutely dilated in the course of cardiac surgery when the pericardium is opened, it is a common observation that it is impossible to close the pericardium without a dramatic rise in venous pressure and fall in arterial blood pressure and cardiac output.

It has been shown by numerous investigators[6] and in this laboratory[3] that when a large volume of fluid is rapidly infused in dogs, intrapericardial pressure rises from its normal subatmospheric level to positive values, frequently in the range of 7 to 10 mm Hg. These infusions are well known to cause the filling pressures on the two sides of the heart to rise substantially, but when the cardiac filling pressures are measured *transmurally*, that is, when intrapericardial pressure is subtracted from intracardiac pressure, the rise is considerably smaller. This indicates that a substantial proportion of the increase in intracardiac filling pressure is in fact borne by the taut pericardium. A fascinating example of this phenomenon was published by Bartle and Hermann[7] in 1968. These workers reported on the hemodynamic findings in four patients undergoing operation for acute mitral regurgitation secondary to rupture of chordae tendineae. The patients were studied in a matter of hours or days after the rupture. Intrapericardial pressure, unfortunately, was not measured, but in addition to the expected findings of severe pulmonary hypertension and extremely tall spiking systolic pressure waves in the left atrial or pulmonary wedge pressure tracings, an unexpected, hitherto unreported observation was made, namely, that left and right ventricular diastolic pressures were equal to each other and equal to the left and right atrial pressures during atrial diastole. This observation was correctly interpreted to mean that the pericardium was actively resisting acute dilation of the left atrium and left ventricle causing the hemodynamic findings of hyper-acute mitral regurgitation to resemble those of constrictive pericarditis (Figure 1.1).

In general, it has been easier to demonstrate pericardial restraint upon cardiac fill-

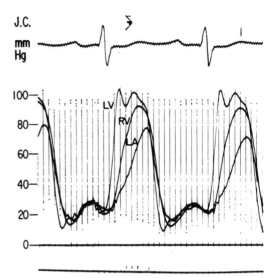

Figure 1.1. Left ventricular, right ventricular, and left atrial pressures are recorded in a case of acute mitral incompetence. Note that the pressures from these sites are equal during diastole. The left atrial pressure pulse is characterized by a tall, narrow systolic wave characteristic of acute mitral valve incompetence. (From Bartle SH, Hermann HJ: Acute mitral regurgitation in man. Hemodynamic evidence and observations indicating an early role for the pericardium. *Circulation* 36:839–851, 1967. By permission of the American Heart Association, Inc.)

ing and dilation when the heart is faced with an acute volume overload compared with a pressure overload. Thus, pericardial restraint is usually difficult and often impossible to demonstrate following occlusion of the pulmonary artery or aorta.[8,9] This difference is explicable because volume overload produces greater cardiac dilation than pressure overload and because volume overload dilates all four cardiac chambers, whereas pressure overload primarily influences the dimenions of one or two cardiac chambers.

It is now well known that the volume and pressure existing in a cardiac chamber influence the pressure, volume, and geometry of the remaining cardiac chambers.[10] This interaction is in part due to muscle fibers shared by both ventricles, and changes in the position and radius of curvature of the interventricular septum which change the diastolic properties of the ventricles, producing in their turn alterations in the systolic performance of the heart, as measured for instance, by the pressure that the ventricles can develop.[4] In this context, it is important to point out that ventricular interaction, as would be anticipated, is much stronger in the presence of the pericardium.[11, 12]

From the foregoing, it should be apparent that there are important implications for the clinical surgeon. Measurement of intracardiac and pulmonary wedge pressures in the intra- and perioperative period must take into account the possible influence of the pericardium, or when the pericardium has been left open, of the mediastinum which can rapidly substitute for the pericardium as an effective external restraint upon the heart. Indeed, among pulmonologists, it has become fashionable to refer to "the cardiac fossa," implying that the lungs rather than the pericardium provide the external pressure against which the heart must fill. It should also be apparent that if, in the perioperative period, the pericardium is thicker and tougher than normal, or if fluids accumulate in the pericardial or mediastinal space, that external restraint becomes proportionately more important and can, in fact, dominate the clinical picture.

POSTOPERATIVE CONSTRICTIVE PERICARDITIS

The last several years have witnessed changes in the etiology of constrictive pericarditis. Less tuberculous cases, and less cases with heavy calcification of the pericardium are now encountered. Cases are less chronic, with subacute constrictive pericarditis or subacute effusive constrictive pericarditis[13] now being common causes of pericardial constriction. Among these causes of constrictive pericarditis, perioperative pericarditis, and particularly postoperative pericarditis now loom large on the horizon of the cardiac surgeon.

It has been recognized that postoperative "pericarditis" although usually a benign and inevitable accompaniment of cardiac surgery can, perhaps in 0.2% of cases,[14] give rise to hemodynamically significant constriction. The constriction, although occasionally severe, is usually more modest than that which is encountered in classical chronic constrictive pericarditis. Sometimes constriction is so mild that it cannot be diagnosed without recourse to provocative testing, usually fluid challenge.

The single most important factor in arriving at the correct diagnosis is to keep the possibility of postoperative constrictive pericarditis in mind when evaluating any patient who is not doing well in the weeks or months following a cardiac operation. Thus, in addition to the usual considerations such as a poorly functioning prosthesis, a missed hemodynamic lesion, failure to preserve the integrity of the myocardium during operation, the prior existence of irreversible myocardial damage, and the toxic effect of drugs, the surgeon must consider the possibility that the patient's difficulties stem from pericardial constriction.

Clinical Signs

By far the single most important physical sign is abnormality of the jugular venous pressure (Fig. 1.2). In all cases, except when the constriction is "occult," a subject which will be referred to later, the venous pressure is elevated. Furthermore, its contour is abnormal, showing abnormally deep and abnormally rapid y descents. Frequently, the x descent is also unduly prominent. Another abnormal characteristic of constriction by the pericardium is the absence of the normal respiratory variation in jugular venous pressure. Thus, the venous pressure fails to drop during inspiration. In many cases, abnormalities of the venous pressure may be the only clinical findings, but in some patients there will be, in addition, fatigue, ankle swelling, and perhaps enlargement of the liver.

Since this is a subacute disease, it should not be surprising that the clinical manifestations differ from those of classical constrictive pericarditis. Anasarca and cardiac cachexia, the hallmarks of chronic tuberculous pericarditis, are almost always absent.

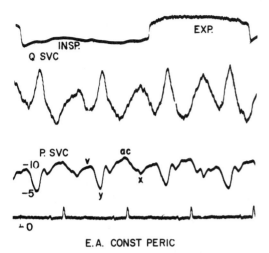

Figure 1.2. This pressure tracing was obtained from the lower reaches of the superior vena cava in the same patient illustrated in Figure 1.4 and 1.5. In this patient with mild constrictive pericarditis, the right atrial pressure is moderately elevated. Respiratory variation is absent. Note the very prominent Y descent. Above the pressure tracing is a tracing of blood flow velocity in the superior vena cava. Notice that this too is not influenced by respiration. Blood flow is bimodal, corresponding with the X and Y descents. The sharpest acceleration occurs simultaneously with the Y descent of pressure, which is more profound than the X descent. (From Shabetai R: *The Pericardium*, Grune & Stratton, New York, 1981.)

Indeed, ascites is usually absent, and even edema is uncommon, especially in patients receiving diuretics in the postoperative period, as most are. Atrial fibrillation is common in chronic constrictive pericarditis, but when atrial fibrillation is found in postoperative cases, it is usually caused by some other factor such as chronic rheumatic heart disease, or ischemia.

If patients have complaints, they are usually those of general malaise, or a feeling that they have not recovered as rapidly as they had anticipated from the cardiac operation. Some of the patients will complain of ankle swelling and of an increase in weight.

The clinical examination is directed first to finding the common causes of these complaints such as malfunction of a prosthetic or heterograft valve, myocardial infarction, fluid and electrolyte imbalance, and myocardial dysfunction. Murmurs, gallopsounds, and palpable evidence of ventricular dyskinesia are important in this connection. Laboratory studies, such as echocardiography and measurement of the ejection fraction, can be important aids in this differential diagnosis, when it is not obvious on clinical grounds.

In patients whose only problem is postoperative constrictive pericarditis, no unusual or unexpected cardiac murmurs should be detected, the blood pressure and pulse should be close to normal, and there should be no signs of prosthetic dysfunction. However, the venous pressure is usually found to be moderately or definitely elevated. Inspection of the jugular venous pulse shows a rapid inward motion (the y descent) that can easily be recognized at the bedside because it is asynchronous with the carotid pulse. When a prominent y descent is found, the differential diagnosis often narrows down to tricuspid regurgitation versus constrictive pericarditis. This differentiation can be extremely difficult, and sometimes cannot be made without hemodynamic studies.

Laboratory Findings

In patients who have the appropriate symptoms and abnormalities of the venous pressure, postoperative constrictive pericarditis is a reasonable initial diagnosis. Echocardiography may confirm that the ventricles fill only in the first period of diastole but show very little subsequent expansion in dimensions during the second half of diastole. The echocardiogram may also show notching of the intraventricular septum, and in some cases, thickening of the pericardium can be detected both by M-mode and two-dimensional echocardiography. The observation that the ventricles appear to fill only in the first third of diastole is sometimes made from M-mode echocardiography, but often is most dramatically demonstrated by two-dimensional echocardiography which allows the observer to sit and watch the time course of filling and emptying of the two ventricles on a fluorescent screen. However, it should be noted that echocardiography which has been such an enormous boon in the diagnosis of pericardial effusion, is considerably less useful in the diagnosis of constrictive pericarditis. This deficiency of echocardiography, not surprisingly, is most evident when constriction is mild or subtle, and when the pericardium has sustained a loss of compliance without substantial thickening, the very circumstances that are frequently associated with postoperative constrictive pericarditis.

Recently, it has been shown that computerized tomography is an excellent tool for visualizing the thickness of the pericardium[15] (Fig. 1.3). Contrast enhancement is usually employed, although it is

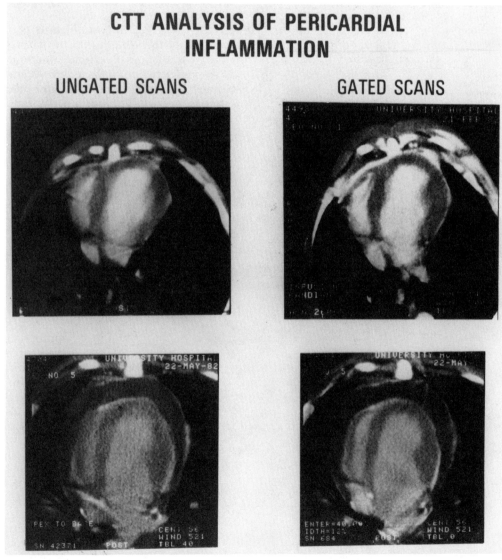

CTT ANALYSIS OF PERICARDIAL INFLAMMATION

UNGATED SCANS   **GATED SCANS**

Figure 1.3. Computerized tomogram of the heart demonstrates thickening of the pericardium. The thickened pericardium (along with an effusion in the lower panels) can be brought out by contrast enhancement, and seen with or without gating (CTT = computerized transmission tomography).

frequently possible to demonstrate the pericardium satisfactorily without the use of contrast material. Visualization of the pericardium does not necessarily require gating. Computerized tomography can be useful when postoperative constrictive pericarditis is suspected, but it must be remembered once again, that the pericardium in these cases will not be nearly so thick and dramatically abnormal as it is in classical chronic tuberculous constrictive pericarditis. Furthermore, we have been shown by computerized tomography, that a "pseudopericardium" may form around the heart in cases in which the pericardium has been left open.

Cardiac Catheterization

When the diagnosis of postoperative pericarditis is seriously suspected, cardiac catheterization should be performed. It is important to measure left and right ventricular pressure simultaneously, or else to measure simultaneously left ventricular and right atrial pressures because, in many cases, the waveform will be that of the early diastolic dip and plateau, and the left and right heart filling pressures will be found to be equal to each other (Figs. 1.4 and 1.5). Meticulous

technique is essential when dealing with venous pressure and cardiac filling pressures, since a difference of only 3 to 5 mm Hg may make, confirm, or refute the diagnosis. Special attention must therefore be paid to exact "zero" levels (atmospheric) of the transducers and to ascertain that the recording systems are absolutely equisensitive. Great care must also be taken with the damping characteristics by selection of appropriate catheters, needles, connecting tubing, stopcocks, and transducers. This is because the so called "dip and plateau phenomenon" or the "square root sign" is a frequent paraphenomenon associated with suboptimum damping characteristics.[16] This is frequently observed when left ventricular pressure is measured through a pigtail catheter that is being employed for left ventriculography.

Occult Constrictive Pericarditis

This entity was first proposed by Bush and his colleagues from Columbus, Ohio.[17] As its name implies, this is a syndrome of constrictive pericarditis that is so mild that it is not clinically evident, requiring a provocative maneuver for its disclosure. The maneuver that Bush et al. elected was a

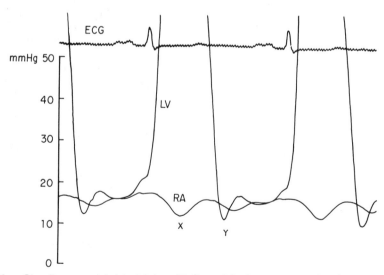

Figure 1.4. Simultaneous right atrial and left ventricular pressure tracings are from a case of postoperative constrictive pericarditis. Note the elevated right atrial and left ventricular filling pressure and prominent x and y descent of atrial pressure pulse.

Post-Op constriction

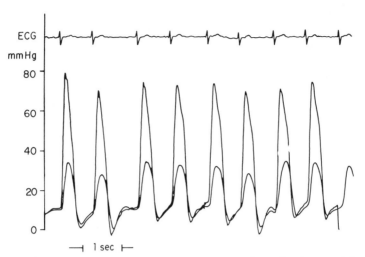

Figure 1.5. Simultaneously recorded pressures are from both ventricles in a case of postoperative constrictive pericarditis. Note the equal diastolic pressures and the dip of early diastolic pressure. The plateau is abbreviated by tachycardia.

rapid infusion of normal saline, usually around 1 liter in about 10 minutes. The patients studied were complaining of obscure chest pain and many of them gave a history of earlier acute pericarditis. When studied under basal conditions, hemodynamics were normal. Specifically, left ventricular filling pressure was higher than right, systemic and pulmonary venous pressures were normal and unequal, and the systemic venous pressure fell during inspiration. Following the fluid challenge, the hemodynamic abnormalities that characterize constrictive pericarditis made their appearance. Respiratory variation disappeared from the systemic venous pressure, which became equal to the pulmonary wedge pressure. Both pressures displayed prominent x and y descents and both were substantially elevated. The ventricular diastolic dip and plateau phenomenon, absent in the basal state, appeared in both ventricles after fluid loading. That these patients were in fact suffering from an occult form of constrictive pericarditis was confirmed when the patients were referred for pericardiectomy. At thoracotomy, the operating surgeons observed limitation of cardiac motion, and that

the pericardium was abnormally thickened. The resected pericardial tissue showed fibrosis and chronic inflammation when it was examined histologically.

These observations created a considerable stir in the cardiological community, but surprisingly few cases have been reported by other investigators who have employed the fluid challenge technique to diagnose occult constrictive pericarditis. Nevertheless, patients who have undergone recent cardiac surgery would seem to be logical candidates; therefore fluid challenge has been used in postoperative patients with unexplained persistence of systemic or pulmonary venous congestion. Thus far, however, fluid challenge has not proved particularly useful in the assessment of patients after cardiac operations.

Intravenous fluid challenges have been used for many clinical indications in the past, but surprisingly, the detailed normal responses of intracardiac pressures to volume loading have not been properly established. While it is known that rapid infusion causes an increase in right and left atrial pressures in normal subjects, alterations in pressure-wave contours, respiratory variation in systemic venous pressure, and the difference between pulmonary and systemic venous pressure have not been established. Thus, it is imperative that the normal responses to rapid fluid infusion be accurately described. Furthermore, interpretation of the hemodynamic response to fluid challenge in patients who have recently undergone cardiac surgery is fraught with hazard because neither the normal hemodynamic responses to fluid challenge, nor how these changes may be modified by cardiac surgery and pericardiotomy is known. For this reason, we are currently undertaking studies in our cardiac catheterization laboratory to determine the normal hemodynamic changes that occur after a 1000-ml intravenous saline challenge, and to learn how this response may be modified by cardiac surgery and pericardiotomy. From this study, we also hope to learn whether patients develop occult constrictive pericardial disease as a result of cardiac surgery.

OVERT POSTOPERATIVE CONSTRICTIVE PERICARDIAL DISEASE

A number of reports of constrictive pericardial disease complicating cardiac surgery have appeared over the last several years.[14, 18-25] However, according to a recent review,[14] only about 0.2% of patients undergoing cardiac operations subsequently develop this complication. In some of the cases, there is a history of unusually severe pericarditis or pericardial effusion in the first postoperative days, or operation was complicated by the postpericardiotomy syndrome. In a majority of cases, however, there are no clues that postoperative constrictive pericarditis is going to develop. The causes are unknown, although it has been suggested that extrinsic factors[14] such as talc, povidone-iodine solution,[26] or hypothermic solutions[27] may be implicated. I think it more likely that this is an immune response to pericardial injury, similar perhaps to the postpericardiotomy syndrome, although proof of this hypothesis is lacking.

Patients with the severe overt syndrome are very ill. They clearly are not doing well

weeks or months following what should have been a satisfactory cardiac operation. Control of fluid retention requires ever increasing doses of potent diuretics, and despite them, the venous pressure shows the abnormalities that characterize constrictive pericardial disease. When the heart is auscultated, there may be a third heart sound in the early part of diastole, the "pericardial knock," but by this time, pericardial friction rub and pericardial effusion, if they were present earlier, will have disappeared.

The electrocardiogram is not really helpful, but the changes of chronic pericarditis, namely widespread T-wave inversions, may be present. However, identical abnormalities are found in a number of postoperative patients who do not have constrictive pericardial disease. Likewise, abnormalities detected by the chest radiogram are nonspecific, and in some cases, the radiogram remains entirely normal. Radionucleotide studies are not particularly helpful. In the absence of complicating hemodynamic factors, the ejection fraction at rest and during exercise should be normal, or at any rate, uninfluenced by the constricting process. In rare cases where the pericardium is grossly thickened, or a pericardial effusion persists, these abnormalities may be detected at the time of radionucleotide study. The role of echocardiography in this diagnosis has been described in earlier paragraphs; here I would summarize by stating that the abnormalities are reasonably specific, but not at all sensitive in making this diagnosis. As mentioned earlier, computerized tomography is a promising new technique, but experience is limited and we still have to learn the specificity and sensitivity of this test in the diagnosis of postoperative constrictive pericardial disease.

Differential Diagnosis

The principal disorders to be kept in mind in the differential diagnosis of postoperative constrictive pericardial disease have been enumerated in the introductory paragraphs. I will limit this section to a discussion of tricuspid incompetence and restrictive myocardial disease, the two conditions that often remain to be ruled out after a systematic evaluation of patients who are not doing as well as would have been anticipated following cardiac operations has been carried out.

TRICUSPID VALVE INCOMPETENCE

Tricuspid valve incompetence and constrictive pericardial disease have so many features in common that distinguishing between them may be difficult even for the experienced hemodynamicist. In both, systemic venous congestion may dominate the clinical picture, so that peripheral edema, and a raised jugular venous pressure are common to both. In severe cases of both conditions, enlargement of the liver and peritoneal or pleural effusions may be found. Characteristically, a pansystolic murmur that increases in intensity during inspiration can be detected between the lower left sternal edge and the cardiac apex in patients with tricuspid incompetence. Unfortunately, however, this murmur may be soft and difficult to appreciate, and in many cases of hemodynamically documented tricuspid incompetence, the murmur has been absent. Likewise, the characteristic abnormalities of the venous pulse in tricuspid incompetence are a tall systolic wave and a deep and rapidly inscribed y wave. However, in many cases of tricuspid incompetence in which the right atrium is greatly enlarged, this chamber may become abnormally compliant and therefore able to absorb a large regurgitant volume without generating a significant systolic (v) wave. When this occurs, the prominent and rapid y descent persists and therefore the abnormalities of the jugular venous pulse become impossible or difficult to distinguish from those of constrictive pericardial disease. It is when the systolic murmur and jugular pulsation are both absent that the differential diagnosis is so formidable a challenge.

The clues pointing to the tricuspid valve are enlargement of the right ventricle and right atrium, and severe pulmonary hypertension. Paradoxical motion of the interventricular septum, observed echocardiographically, is a good clue to the presence of tricuspid incompetence, but frequently is found postoperatively in patients who have neither tricuspid incompetence nor constrictive pericardial disease. Atrial fibrillation and the presence of severe rheumatic mitral valve disease favor tricuspid incompetence, but certainly do not rule out constrictive pericardial disease. Right ventricular enlargement can sometimes be suspected clinically because of a parasternal heave, but is more readily detected by two-dimensional echocardiography. Assessment of right ventricular size by M-mode echocardiography is unreliable except in extreme cases. The electrocardiogram usually fails to disclose enlargement of the right ventricle unless there is considerable pulmonary hypertension. Right atrial enlargement may be disclosed by a tall pointed P wave in leads II and V_1, and may be seen by two-dimensional echocardiography. The M-mode echocardiogram is virtually useless in detecting right atrial enlargement. Right-sided enlargement can often be suspected from a plain chest radiogram, but then it is difficult to distinguish between right atrial and right ventricular enlargement.

Cardiac Catheterization and Angiocardiography

The solution to this difficult problem will almost always require hemodynamic studies. In the more stubborn cases, inspection of the right atrial pressure tracing does not add to the information that can be gleaned by an astute clinician after inspection of the neck veins. If there is *organic* tricuspid valve disease, there may be tricuspid stenosis as well as incompetence. This can best be assessed by obtaining the simultaneous pressure tracings at high sensitivity from the right ventricle and right atrium to observe a diastolic pressure gradient, especially during inspiration. Functional tricuspid regurgitation is frequently associated with severe pulmonary arterial hypertension and dilatation of the right heart chambers. The latter can usually be appreciated during catheterization of the pulmonary artery, and the former may be documented by recording systolic pressure above 60 mm Hg in the pulmonary artery. The most important test, however, is right ventriculography which will document and quantify tricuspid regurgitation. Severe tricuspid regurgitation is characterized by *may look like constriction*

dense opacification of the right atrium and the venae cavae following injection of contrast medium into the right ventricle.

RESTRICTIVE CARDIOMYOPATHY

⊛ When the picture of restriction to cardiac filling develops after heart surgery, the most common cause is constrictive pericardial disease. On occasion, however, the disease may involve the myocardium rather than the pericardium. The symptoms and clinical findings are the same as those associated with pericardial constriction. The hemodynamic findings also are very similar. Unfortunately, it is sometimes impossible to distinguish between constriction by the pericardium and restriction by the myocardium, even after exhaustive noninvasive and hemodynamic studies. One observation that has proved useful in many instances is that in constrictive pericardial disease, the left and right heart filling pressures are equal to one another, whereas in restrictive myocardial disease, the left ventricular filling pressure exceeds the right.[28] If uncertainty exists, endomyocardial biopsy should be undertaken before subjecting the patient to pericardiectomy. However, it should be appreciated that although endomyocardial biopsy is of proven value in the differentiation between constrictive pericarditis and myocardial diseases of other etiology,[29] there is little if any published information regarding its value in the differential diagnosis in postoperative cases.

Treatment

Treatment of postoperative constrictive pericardial disease is pericardiectomy which should be as complete as possible, and should include visceral as well as parietal pericardium. It has been suggested that some cases respond to treatment with steroids or nonsteroidal anti-inflammatory agents combined with diuretics.[14] However, nothing short of pericardiectomy is likely to succeed once true constriction is established. In some cases, pericardiectomy does not always result in cure, because the disease process may extend into the myocardium.

Right Ventricular Infarction

Massive infarction of the right ventricle occurring postoperatively, can result in elevation of the jugular venous pressure, and abnormalities of left and right ventricular diastolic pressures that closely simulate the abnormalities of constrictive pericardial disease.[30] The filling pressures of the two ventricles are often equal or nearly so, presumably owing to the acutely dilated right ventricle which stretches the pericardium over the whole heart. This is another example of acute chamber dilation enhancing the restraining function of the pericardium. Isolated right ventricular infarction is unusual, so that there will frequently also be electrocardiographic evidence of myocardial infarction, usually of the inferior or posterior wall. Radionuclide scans of the heart may reveal the right ventricular infarction.

ACUTE PERICARDITIS

Pericardial injury is an inevitable consequence of cardiac surgery, and therefore, in the first few postoperative days, pericarditis exists. Symptoms and signs may or may not be present, depending upon the extent of associated epicardial injury. Furthermore, the symptoms and signs of pericardial disease may be overwhelmed by those of heart disease, pulmonary disease, and artificial ventilation. Pericardial friction rubs are almost invariable at some time in the early days after a heart operation, but may be obscured by mediastinal crunch, surgical emphysema, and the general hubbub of an intensive care unit. Some degree of T-wave alteration is a frequent sequel of cardiac operations, but is less common after saphenous vein bypass grafting than after operations that involve large incisions into, and substantial resections of myocardium. The changes can seldom be distinguished with certainty from those of ischemia, drug effects, and electrolyte changes. Similarly, it is next to impossible to pick out pericardial pain from other sources of postoperative pain and discomfort. There have not been many routine echocardiographic studies of postoperative patients, but the available evidence suggests that some degree of pericardial effusion is common. Highly satisfactory echocardiographic studies are difficult to obtain in the early postoperative period.

THE POSTPERICARDIOTOMY SYNDROME

Pericarditis in the early days after cardiac surgery is almost universal, therefore the postpericardiotomy syndrome is defined as the appearance or persistence of pericardial disease 1 week or longer after any operation in which the pericardium was opened. The symptoms are chest pain, which may be pleuritic or crushing in nature, and is sometimes confused with postoperative chest wall pain, the general malaise associated with pyrexia and, when effusions are large, dyspnea. The usual differential diagnosis includes heart failure, myocardial ischemia, the mononucleosis-like syndrome with splenomegaly that may appear after cardiopulmonary bypass, and incisional pain.

The postpericardiotomy syndrome is characterized by the appearance of pericarditis after the local causes of postoperative inflammation have died away. Frequently, there is associated pleurisy, and sometimes a parenchymal pulmonary infiltrate.

The constitutional findings include moderate fever and leukocytosis, and a pericardial friction rub can usually be heard at some stage. Untreated, the syndrome may persist for many weeks and, even when treated, is subject to recurrences. Electrocardiograms may show the reappearance of ST-segment and T-wave changes consistent with pericarditis, and almost always, the echocardiogram documents pericardial effusion, often substantial in quantity. Evidence of pleural effusion can be elicited both by clinical and radiological examination. Rarely, the syndrome leads to cardiac tamponade, and cases with frequent recurrences may even develop constrictive pericardial disease.

Etiology

The cause of the postpericardiotomy syndrome is not known, but has been exten-

sively studied by Engle and associates[31-35] who have established a number of facts which shed light on the etiology of this disturbing syndrome. These workers have presented evidence that strongly suggest that the postpericardiotomy syndrome is triggered by a combination of an autoimmune reaction to injury coupled with viral infection. The basis for this unexpected dual etiology is the strong association of the postpericardiotomy syndrome with the development of antiheart antibodies together with antiviral antibodies in the postoperative period. The injury component is surgical trauma to pericardial cells and the appearance of blood in the pericardial cavity, thus linking the pericardiotomy syndrome to the allied syndromes that may follow blunt[36] or sharp[37] injury of the chest or may complicate myocardial infarction (Dressler's Syndrome).[38] Whether a viral infection is acquired in the hospital from personnel and other patients, or whether it is introduced from the air in the operating room has not yet been determined. Of interest from the immunological point of view, the syndrome is exceedingly rare in infants and very young children who have not developed immunological competency.[36] The postpericardiotomy syndrome may complicate any type of heart surgery, belying the earlier concept that it was associated with rheumatic heart disease, and may occur after the pericardium has been opened during the course of any thoracic operation, including noncardiac operations.

Treatment

The postpericardiotomy syndrome, being in large part an autoimmune reaction, responds well to treatment with anti-inflammatory agents. Steroids should be avoided whenever possible by giving a thorough trial with other anti-inflammatory drugs such as indomethacin and Motrin. Large doses are appropriate when the process is active, but as soon as clinical manifestations have disappeared, the drug that has been selected should be progressively reduced until the dose that just suppresses the clinical manifestations is found. Because of the recurrent nature of the disorder, it is wise to continue this dose for several weeks before finally discontinuing it. When recourse to steroids is necessary because of persistence of the syndrome and severe symptoms in spite of treatment with other anti-inflammatory agents, prednisone, 80 mg daily, should be given. Once again, the dose must be tapered as rapidly as possible. Whenever possible, alternate-day treatment is preferred. The dose of steroid required and the danger of steroid dependency may be reduced by combining prednisone with a nonsteroidal agent.

CARDIAC TAMPONADE

Postoperative bleeding into the pericardial space, or (when the pericardium has been left widely open) into the mediastinum is an important cause of hypotension during the postoperative period. Most of the instances occur in the first postoperative hours or day, under which circumstances it is usually promptly recognized and treated. Cardiac tamponade complicates on the average of 4% of cardiac operations and is associated with the postoperative use of anticoagulants. Less commonly, tamponade is delayed by several days.[40–54] This so-called delayed postoperative cardiac tamponade is most apt to be atypical and the possibility of cardiac tamponade may not be uppermost in the mind of physicians seeing patients who have already been discharged, if not from the hospital, at least from the intensive care unit.

Classical Cardiac Tamponade

The syndrome of classical cardiac tamponade is well known to the readers of this book, therefore, I will not elaborate upon it, but simply summarize the major findings. The symptoms vary from mild dyspnea and discomfort in the chest or throat, through extreme fatigue and respiratory distress to stupor and coma. The jugular venous pressure is grossly elevated and shows a characteristic abnormality that distinguishes it from heart failure or constrictive pericarditis. In cardiac tamponade, the y descent is absent, the only negative wave being a sharp x descent which can be recognized at the bedside because it is exactly synchronous with the carotid pulse. Inspiratory decline in jugular or central venous pressure is, in contradistinction to constrictive pericardial disease, preserved in cardiac tamponade. In mild cases, the blood pressure is normal, but in the more severe and acute cases, likely to be encountered in the early postoperative setting, some degree of hypotension is usual, and in many cases severe. Pulsus paradoxus is usually present. The echocardiogram shows a pericardial effusion which, while it frequently surrounds the whole heart, may be confined to the back of the heart.[39] The echocardiogram may also show swinging of the heart and exaggerated respiratory variation in the left and right ventricular dimensions as well as other abnormalities,[55] but it should be emphasized that cardiac tamponade is above all a clinical diagnosis. Hemodynamic studies confirm elevation of the central venous pressure and absence of its y descent. Left and right heart filling pressures are found to be equal to each other, often most conveniently documented by recording simultaneously at equal sensitivity left ventricular and right atrial pressures.

Atypical Features Associated with the PostOperative Patients

Several features combine to thwart the correct diagnosis of cardiac tamponade in postoperative patients, especially when tamponade is delayed.[39] A variety of factors other than cardiac tamponade may account for an increase in venous pressure and a decrease in cardiac output and blood pressure. Changes in cardiac size may not be appreciated from portable chest radiograms in which there is parenchymal or pleural disease. Pulsus paradoxus is difficult or impossible to evaluate in patients who are severely dyspneic from other causes or who are being ventilated artificially. Echocardiography, relied upon so heavily to make the diagnosis of pericardial effusion upon which the diagnosis of cardiac tamponade depends, is less satisfactory in postoperative patients, because technical failures are common. Left ventricular disease characterized by low compliance and a high left ventricular diastolic pressure as may be found in a number of postoperative patients, may prevent the development of pulsus paradoxus when it would otherwise occur. Left pleural effusion, common in postoperative patients, may obfuscate the echocardiographic diagnosis of pericardial effusion.

The diagnosis is particularly difficult when tamponade is caused by a blood clot rather than fluid and when compression of the heart is not generalized but localized either by loculation, or because a clot is compressing only one or two of the cardiac chambers. When the left-sided chambers are compressed, right atrial pressure although elevated, does not rise sufficiently high to equal the left ventricular filling pressure. These cases, therefore simulate left ventricular failure because they are, in fact, due to severe extrinsic obstruction to left ventricular filling. The jugular venous pressure may be difficult to evaluate in postoperative patients, especially when respirations are labored, when an endotracheal tube is in place, or after surgical emphysema has developed.

The chief ingredient in arriving at the correct diagnosis in spite of so many atypical features, is to consider seriously the possibility of cardiac tamponade in any patient who deteriorates either in the immediate postoperative period, or unexpectedly several days to a week or two later. Great pains must be taken to obtain satisfactory echocardiograms in spite of the technical difficulties, and these are less in the case of two-dimensional echocardiography. In other cases, contrast-enhanced computerized tomography will demonstrate the pericardial effusion and the condition of the pericardium when echocardiography fails to do so satisfactorily. When a pericardial effusion, localized or generalized, or a pericardial clot is demonstrated in the patient who is not doing well for unexplained reasons, the pericardium should be evacuated. This may be done surgically, either by reopening the incision, or if one is confident of the diagnosis, through the subxyphoid approach, but in many instances pericardiocentesis has proven to be satisfactory.[54]

References

1. Barnard HL: The functions of the pericardium. *J Physiol (Lond)* 22:43, 1898.
2. Kuno Y: The significance of the pericardium. *J Physiol* 50:1, 1915.
3. Shirato K, Shabetai R, Bhargava V, et al: Alteration of left ventricular diastolic pressure-segment length relation produced by the epicardium. Effects of cardiac distension and afterload reduction in conscious dogs. *Circulation* 57:1191, 1978.
4. Janiki JS, Weber KT: The pericardium and ventricular interaction, distensibility and function. *Am J Physiol* 238:H494, 1980.
5. Rabkin SW, Ping Hwa Hu: Mathematical and mechanical modeling of stress strain relationship of pericardium. *Am J Physiol* 229:896, 1975.
6. Holt JP, Rhode EA, Kines H: Pericardial and ventricular pressure. *Circ Res* 8:1171, 1960.
7. Bartle SH, Hermann HJ: Acute mitral regurgitation in man. Hemodynamic evidence and observations indicating an early role for the pericardium. *Circulation* 36:839, 1968.
8. Prindle KH, Gold HK, Beiser GD, et al: Influence of pericardiectomy on cat right ventricular function after pulmonary arterial constriction. *Am J Cardiol* 31:260, 1973.
9. Kenner HM, Wood EH: Intrapericardial, intrapleural and intracardiac pressures during acute heart failure in dogs studied without thoracotomy. *Circ Res* 19:1071, 1966.
10. Taylor RR, Covell JW, Sonnenblick EH, et al: Dependence of ventricular distensibility on filling of the opposite ventricle. *Am J Physiol* 213:711, 1967.
11. Stokland O, Miller MM, Lekven J, et al: The significance of the intact pericardium for cardiac performance in the dog. *Circ Res* 47:27, 1980.
12. Glantz SA, Misbach GA, Moores WY, et al: The pericardium substantially affects the left ventricular diastolic pressure-volume relationship in the dog. *Circ Res* 42:433, 1978.
13. Hancock EW: Subacute effusive constrictive pericarditis. *Circulation* 43:183, 1971.
14. Kutcher MA, King SB, Alimburg BN, et al: Constrictive pericarditis as a complication of cardiac surgery: Recognition of an entity. *Circulation* 50:742, 1982.
15. Isner JM, Carter BL, Bankoff MS, et al: Computerized tomography in the diagnosis of pericardial heart disease. *Ann Intern Med* 97:473, 1982.
16. Shabetai R: *The Pericardium*. Grune & Stratton, 1981, New York.
17. Bush CA, Stang JM, Wooley CF, et al: Occult constrictive pericardial disease. Diagnosis by rapid volume expansion and correction by pericardiectomy. *Circulation* 56:924, 1977.
18. Marsa R, Mehta S, Willis W, et al: Constrictive pericarditis after myocardial revascularization: Report of three cases. *Am J Cardiol* 44:177, 1979.
19. Cohen MV, Greenberg MA: Constrictive pericarditis: Early and late complication of cardiac surgery. *Am J Cardiol* 43:657, 1979.
20. Lorell B, Leinbach RC, Pohost GM, et al: Right

ventricular infarction: Clinical diagnosis and differentiation from cardiac tamponade and pericardial constriction. *Am J Cardiol* 43:465, 1979.

21. Rice PL, Pifarre R, Montoya A: Constrictive pericarditis following cardiac surgery. *Ann Thorac Surg* 31:450, 1980.

22. Peters W, Scheinman M, Raskin S, et al: Unusual complications of thoracic pacemakers. *Am J Cardiol* 45:1088, 1980.

23. Kendall ME, Rhodes GF, Wolfe W: Cardiac constriction following aorta to coronary bypass surgery. *J Thorac Cardiovasc Surg* 64:142, 1972.

24. Brown DF, Older T: Pericardial constriction as a late complication of coronary bypass surgery. *J Thorac Cardiovasc Surg* 74:61, 1977.

25. Rubio PA, Farrell EM, Goens RW: Severe adhesive-constrictive pericarditis after coronary artery bypass. *South Med J* 73:90, 1980.

26. Feldman RW, Mozersky DJ, Hagood CO: The use of povidone-iodine in vascular surgery. *J Thorac Cardiovasc Surg* 69:972, 1975.

27. Speicher CE, Ferrigan L, Wolfson SK et al: Cold injury of pericardium and myocardium in cardiac hypothermia. *Surg Gynecol Obstet* 114:659, 1962.

28. Meany E, Shabetai R, Bhargava M, et al: Cardiac amyloidosis, constrictive pericarditis and restrictive cardiomyopathy. *Am J Cardiol* 38:547, 1976.

29. Swanton RH, Brooksby IAB, Davies MJ, et al: Systolic and diastolic ventricular function in cardiac amyloidosis. Studies in six cases diagnosed with endomyocardial biopsy. *Am J Cardiol* 39:658, 1977.

30. Jensen DP, Goolsby JP, Oliva PH: Hemodynamic pattern resembling pericardial constriction after acute inferior myocardial infarction with right ventricular infarction. *Am J Cardiol* 42:858, 1978.

31. Engle MA, Zabriskie JB, Senterfit LB, et al: Viral illness and the postpericardiotomy syndrome. A prospective study in children. *Circulation* 62:1151, 1980.

32. Ito T, Engle MA, Goldberg HP: Post-pericardiotomy syndrome following surgery for non-rheumatic heart disease. *Circulation* 17:549, 1958.

33. Engle MA, Ito T: The post-pericardiotomy syndrome. *Am J Cardiol* 7:73, 1961.

34. Engle MA, Gay WA Jr, Kaminsky ME, et al: The post-pericardiotomy syndrome then and now. In: *Current Problems in Cardiology*, Vol. 3, no. 2, Chicago, Year Book Medical Publishers, 1978.

35. Engle MA, Zabriskie JB, Senterfit LB, et al: Immunologic and virologic studies in the post-pericardiotomy syndrome. *J Pediatr* 87:1103, 1975.

36. Sbokos CG, Karyannacos PE, Kotaxis A, et al: Traumatic hemopericardium and chronic constrictive pericarditis. *Ann Thorac Surg* 23:225, 1977.

37. Goldsteins S, Yu PN: Constrictive pericarditis after blunt chest trauma. *Am Heart J* 69:544, 1965.

38. Dressler W: The post myocardial infarction syndrome. A report on 66 cases. *Arch Intern Med* 103:28, 1959.

39. Jones MR, Vine DL, Attas M, et al: Late isolated left ventricular tamponade. *J Thorac Cardiovasc Surg* 77:142, 1979.

40. Engelman RM, Spencer FC, Reed GE, et al: Cardiac tamponade following open-heart surgery. *Circulation* 41, 42:(Suppl 2):165, 1970.

41. Radley-Smith R, Gonzalez-Lavin L, Somerville J: Pericardial effusion with tamponade following anastomosis of the ascending aorta to the right pulmonary artery (Waterston's operation). *J Thorac Cardiovasc Surg* 60:565, 1970.

42. Nelson RM, Jenson CB, Smoot WM: Pericardial tamponade following open-heart surgery. *J Thorac Cardiovasc Surg* 58:510, 1969.

43. Craddock DR, Logan A, Fadali A: Reoperation for hemorrhage following cardiopulmonary bypass. *Br J Surg* 55:17, 1968.

44. Merrill W, Donahoo JS, Brawley RK, et al: Late cardiac tamponade. A potentially lethal complication of open-heart surgery. *J Thorac Cardiovasc Surg* 72:929, 1976.

45. Fernando HA, Friedman HS, Lejam F, et al: Late cardiac tamponade following open-heart surgery. Detection by echocardiography. *Ann Thorac Surg* 24:174, 1977.

46. Hill JD, Johnson DC, Miller GE, et al: Latent mediastinal tamponade after open-heart surgery. *Arch Surg* 99:808, 1969.

47. Somerville J, Yacoub M, Ross DN, et al: Aorta to right pulmonary artery anastomosis (Waterston's operation) for cyanotic heart disease. *Circulation* 39:593, 1969.

48. Fraser DG, Ullyot DJ: Mediastinal tamponade after open-heart surgery. *J Thorac Cardiovasc Surg* 66:629, 1973.

49. Berger RL, Loveless G, Warner O: Delayed and latent postcardiotomy tamponade. *Ann Thorac Surg* 12:22, 1971.

50. Prewitt TA, Rackley CE, Wilcox BR, et al: Cardiac tamponade as a late complication of open-heart surgery. *Am Heart J* 76:139, 1968.

51. Scott RAP, Drew CE: Delayed pericardial effusion with tamponade after cardiac surgery. *Br Heart J* 35:1304, 1973.

52. Ellison LH, Kirsh MM: Delayed mediastinal tamponade after open heart surgery. *Chest* 65:64, 1974.

53. Borken AM, Schaff HV, Gardner TJ, et al: Diagnosis and management of post operative pericardial effusions and late cardiac tamponade following open heart surgery. *Ann Thorac Surg* 31:512, 1981.

54. D'Cruz IA, Cohen HC, Prabhu R, et al: Diagnosis of cardiac tamponade by echocardiography. Changes in mitral valve motion and ventricular dimensions, with special reference to paradoxical pulse. *Circulation* 52:460, 1975.

55. Reddy PS, Curtiss EI, O'Toole JD, et al: Cardiac tamponade: Hemodynamic observations in man. *Circulation* 58:265, 1978.

CHAPTER 2

CARDIAC DYSFUNCTION: SPECIAL CONSIDERATIONS DURING PREGNANCY

LAURENCE S. REISNER, M.D.

The incidence of cardiac disease during pregnancy has declined during the last four decades. While cardiac disease was present in 3.6% of all pregnancies in the 1940s, the current rate is approximately 1.5%.[1] The primary etiology of cardiac problems during pregnancy is rheumatic fever, with mitral stenosis being the predominant lesion. However, the proportion of patients with rheumatic heart disease is diminishing, and as a result of improvements in medical and surgical therapy, the number of patients with congenital heart disease has increased. The most commonly observed congenital lesions are atrial septal defect, patent ductus arteriosus, and ventricular septal defect. Another type of cardiac disease which is occurring with increasing frequency in urban areas is acute bacterial endocarditis induced by intravenous drug abuse.[2] This may require valve replacement during pregnancy or the patient may present with pregnancy subsequent to a prosthetic valve insertion while on anticoagulant therapy. The number of patients with asymetric septal hypertrophy (idiopathic hypertrophic subaortic stenosis) also appears to be increasing, probably as a result of better diagnosis.[3]

Maternal mortality from heart disease during pregnancy varies widely depending on the type of lesion and the patient's New York Heart Association (NYHA) functional classification. For instance, the patient with asymptomatic heart disease has only a 0.05% chance of dying from heart disease while a parturient with significant mitral stenosis and atrial fibrillation has a mortality rate approaching 20%.[4-6] The average mortality for NYHA Class I and II patients is 0.25%; for Class III and IV patients it is 5.5%, with an overall average of about 0.5%.[5,6] In reviewing the literature one encounters difficulty in assessing the potential mortality risk accurately because the majority of the published figures are from long-term studies. Many of the maternal deaths had occurred in earlier years, and some of the authors reported a very low mortality, even for patients who were seriously ill in the more recent years of their study.[1]

THE CARDIOVASCULAR ALTERATIONS OF PREGNANCY

The physiological effects of pregnancy on the cardiovascular system must be understood. These changes may profoundly affect the hemodynamic performance of the pregnant cardiac patient. In addition, some of the hemodynamic alterations that occur during gestation result in physical changes that may confuse the examiner attempting to assess the status of the patient. Some of the changes of pregnancy resemble the findings of cardiac decompensation and others may mask previously existing signs.

Anatomical Changes

The heart is displaced upward anteriorly, and to the left during pregnancy. This is caused by the enlarging uterus and becomes most evident in the third trimester of pregnancy. The electrocardiographic changes include left axis deviation and nonspecific ST-T wave depression. A Q wave may be seen in lead III or AVR and inverted T waves may appear in leads III or V_1 through V_3.[7]

Vascular Volume Alterations

The total blood volume is increased during pregnancy. This increase begins early in gestation and reaches its maximum during the second trimester between 24 and 32 weeks.[8] The magnitude of this increase varies widely, but is 30 to 50% with a single pregnancy and somewhat larger with twin gestation. There is an increase in both plasma volume and red cell mass, although the plasma volume expansion is greater, resulting in the apparent anemia of pregnancy. In the normal population, however, this should result in only a slight decline in hemoglobin concentration, especially if treated prophylactically with oral iron.[6] After reaching its peak, the blood volume remains at this level until after parturition and then declines as a result of blood loss at delivery and postpartum diuresis (Fig. 2.1). The blood volume returns to normal, nonpregnant levels by 6 to 8 weeks postpartum. The physiological mechanisms responsible for this hypervolemia of pregnancy are believed to be due to the hormonal changes of gestation. The hypervolemia acts as a buffer against the maternal blood loss experience at delivery. The mean decrease in blood volume observed after vaginal delivery is 0.61 liters, and 1.03 liters 1 hour postpartum cesarean section.[9]

Hemodynamic Alterations

Cardiac output is also increased during pregnancy in synchrony with blood volume. It begins to rise at about 8 to 10 weeks of gestation and reaches its maximum at 28 to 32 weeks. The magnitude of this increase is also 30 to 50%, and it persists until the time of parturition. The elevation in cardiac output is the net result of a 10 to 15% increase in heart rate and a 30 to 35% increase in stroke volume.[10] There may be further increases in cardiac output during labor. This is mediated by the catecholamine release in response to pain and by the increase in circulating blood volume brought about by uterine contractions. The Valsalva maneuver often utilized during the delivery process adds an additional cardiac afterload.[11]

Systemic vascular resistance gradually decreases and reaches its lowest levels during the second trimester. Systemic vascular resistance decreases 15% from pregnancy levels and rises slightly as term pregnancy approaches. This results in a decrease in mean arterial blood pressure and diastolic pressure and a slight decrease in systolic pressure. Venous capacitance increases, but central venous pressure remains in the normal range. Blood flow to the kidneys, breasts, and skeletal muscle increases, and

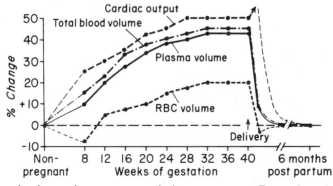

Figure 2.1. Blood volume changes occur during pregnancy. Reproduced with permission from J. J. Bonica (61).

uterine blood is elevated from 1% of the cardiac output in the nonpregnant state to 10–15% of the cardiac output at term (Figs. 2.1 and 2.2).

All of these hemodynamic alterations are due partly to the effect of high estrogen levels. There is an arteriovenous fistula effect in the uteroplacental vascular bed contributing to the overall decrease in systemic vascular resistance. The cardiovascular changes of pregnancy have been reproduced in the nonpregnant ewe by the infusion of estrogen, producing levels similar to those during gestation.[11, 13] Decreased sensitivity to angiotensin and the cardiac dilat-

ing effect of the increased blood volume as well as other undefined humoral factors may well be involved.[10]

Vena caval compression occurs in the pregnant woman at approximately the 20th to 24th week of gestation. The enlarging gravid uterus compresses the vena cava against the lumbar spine at the point of maximum lordosis, effectively diminishing cardiac return, particularly in the supine position. Fortunately, there is usually sufficient collateral venous return via the vertebral plexus which directs blood back to the heart through the azygous system (Fig. 2.3). If the pregnant patient lies on her back for

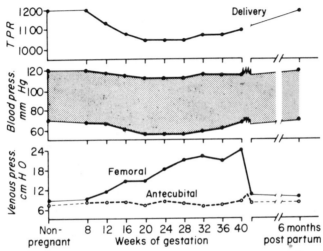

Figure 2.2. Vascular pressure changes occur during pregnancy. Reproduced with permission from J. J. Bonica (61).

SITES OF OBSTRUCTION

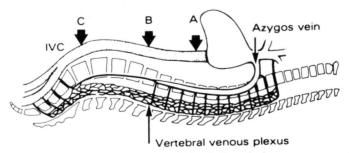

Figure 2.3. The vena cava and its collateral circulation during pregnancy are shown. The usual sites of compression are: (A) suprahepatic in lordotic position; (B) uterus at term; (C) pressure at pelvic brim. Reproduced with permission from P. R. Bromage (62).

very long, compensatory mechanisms must be called into action or hypotension sufficient to cause unconsciousness may result. This supine hypotensive syndrome occurs in 10 to 20% of gravidas. No pregnant patient should be kept in the supine position, especially patients with cardiac disease. Measures of cardiac performance and blood volume will also be affected by inferior vena caval occlusion. This factor led early investigators to believe that both cardiac output and blood volume decreased as term pregnancy approached![14,15] Obstruction of the aorta may also occur by the same mechanical process, and uteroplacental blood flow may be compromised.

Clinical Findings

There are several clinical findings in pregnancy which alter the cardiovascular examination and make the diagnosis of cardiac disease and cardiac decompensation more difficult. The first heart sound may have a wider split than normal. The second heart sound may present with an accentuated pulmonic component, and a third heart sound is present in 88% of parturients. A soft (grade 1–2/6) systolic flow murmur is present in virtually all pregnant women. A fourth heart sound or a diastolic murmur may rarely be heard.[16] Murmur-like hums may be heard over the chest as a result of increased flow through the mammary arteries and veins. As a result of the decrease in peripheral vascular resistance, the murmurs of aortic or mitral insufficiency may become softer or inaudible due to improved forward flow. Edema of the lower extremities occurs in virtually every woman during pregnancy as a result of the vena caval obstruction, and should not be confused with the edema of cardiac failure. The chest X-ray during pregnancy often shows a pattern consistent with mild pulmonary vascular congestion as a manifestation of the increased blood volume and the cardiothoracic ratio is increased, presumably because of the elevation of the diaphragm and displacement of the heart.[7] If the chest film is properly taken, e.g., upright and at full inspiration, these changes do not occur.[17] The azygous vein is frequently visible due to the increased blood flow through this system.

The respiratory changes of pregnancy may also confuse the examiner. Both respiratory rate and tidal volume increase early in pregnancy and maintain alveolar ventilation 50% greater than normal. This is brought about by the rise in serum progesterone.[18] Residual volume and functional residual capacity are decreased by the elevated diaphragm to about 20% of nonpregnant values. These changes result in a compensated respiratory alkalosis, a mild hyperoxia, and subjective feelings of shortness of breath late in pregnancy.

Diagnostic Features

The diagnosis of cardiac disease during pregnancy or of decompensation in a patient with a known pre-existing lesion may be difficult. Those features which appear to be most reliable are: (1) a pulse rate greater than 100 before labor or greater than 110 between contractions while in labor; (2) a marked increase in cardiac silhouette on chest X-ray; (3) a clearly audible diastolic murmur; (4) a systolic murmur equal to grade 3 out of 6 or greater; and (5) the presence of arrhythmias. This latter finding is more difficult to interpret as it is not uncommon for normal pregnant women to have premature atrial contractions or periods of supraventricular tachycardia. Premature ventricular contractions also are occasionally observed. The onset of arrhythmias, particularly tachyarrhythmias, however, may be a manifestation of, or lead to decompensation in a patient with, pre-existing disease such as tight mitral stenosis.

THE STRESSES OF LABOR AND DELIVERY

The events surrounding labor and delivery, either by the vaginal route or cesarean section, add additional stress to the parturient afflicted with cardiac disease. Pain during labor and its associated catecholamine release may increase cardiac output as much as 85% above the nonlaboring values.[11] The magnitude of increased cardiac output experienced by a patient with significant cardiac impairment may be less, based upon exercise studies in these types of patients.[19] Cardiac output increases even in the absence of pain because the uterus expels as much as 500 cc of blood into central circulation with each contraction. Aortocaval compression may occur if care is not exercised to avoid the supine position, and intravenous fluid administration may cause difficulty from under- and overadministration. In the second stage of labor, the patient will bear down and perform the Valsalva maneuver. This results in wide swings of venous and arterial pressure and has been shown to cause acute decompensation. This should be avoided in patients with significant cardiac lesions.[20] The lithotomy position may also produce an unnecessarily acute increase in circulating blood volume, and should be avoided when possible. Immediately after delivery, the uterus contracts and expels from 500 to 700 cc of blood into central circulation. Therefore, even though there is a net decrease in total blood volume, central circulating blood volume is temporarily increased. The immediate postdelivery period is indeed a time of rapid hemodynamic adjustments.

Pharmacological challenges may also be imposed during the labor and delivery sequence. Drugs used for obstetric purposes may have significant effects on the cardiovascular system. Oxytocin, utilized to augment uterine contractions in labor, or more frequently, to decrease postpartum bleeding, has a direct vasodilator effect when given as a bolus of greater than 2 units. This causes a fall in mean arterial blood pressure and a compensatory elevation in pulse rate and cardiac output.[21,22] This drug should only be administered as a dilute infusion to avoid these hemodynamic effects. Ergot preparations are also occasionally administered to induce a sustained increase in uterine tone as a measure to control postpartum bleeding. These compounds cause a generalized vasoconstriction and have been shown to elevate peripheral vascular resistance as much as 48%.[23] Their use should be extremely limited, particularly for the parturient with cardiac disease. Magnesium sulfate is the therapeutic agent of choice for the prevention of seizures in patients with pre-eclampsia. While the normal therapeutic levels of 4 to 8 mEg/L of magnesium do not have any significant cardiovascular ef-

fects, it must be remembered that this drug is a mild, direct-acting vasodilator and that at higher levels it depresses both conduction and myocardial contractility.[24] The cardiovascular consequences of the various analgesic and anesthetic techniques employed during parturition have been reviewed quite adequately elsewhere.[25,26] They must, however, be carefully considered with respect to each individual patient's obstetric and cardiac situation.

The Major Risk Periods

Four time periods are of critical importance in the pregnant patient with cardiac disease. Each of these periods is a time for careful reassessment of therapeutic goals and treatment plans. Consultation is frequently required to ensure optimum management.

THE FIRST RISK PERIOD

The first major challenge occurs during the second trimester, i.e., 14 to 28 weeks of gestation. Both cardiac output and blood volume have reached their maximum, although the peaks are not achieved simultaneously. The fact that a patient with cardiac disease tolerates this portion of her gestation without apparent distress is reassuring, but is not an indicator of her ability to experience the additional stresses placed upon her during labor and delivery.

THE SECOND RISK PERIOD

When the patient enters the first stage of labor, new and additional strain may be placed on the cardiovascular system. Pain-induced elevations in plasma catecholamine levels and changes in central blood volume with uterine contractions contribute to the increased demands on the heart. Other potential problems are those associated with supine positioning, intravenous fluid administration, and the use of analgesic techniques. Invasive hemodynamic monitoring is indicated for those patients in functional Class III and IV. Although patients in functional Classes I and II rarely require pulmonary artery catheters or arterial lines, there are some exceptions. Patients with coarctation of the aorta, aortic aneurysm, aortic stenosis, right-to-left shunts, and primary pulmonary hypertension are all candidates for aggressive monitoring as their hemodynamic status is subject to sudden and profound change.

THE THIRD RISK PERIOD

During the second stage of labor, in addition to the Valsalva maneuver, the patient may be exposed to the lithotomy position, additional fluids, blood loss, and anesthesia. Consultation between the obstetrician, the cardiologist, and the anesthesiologist should be carried out prior to the actual delivery in order to arrive at an optimum management plan. The second stage of labor is often shortened by the use of the vacuum extractor or obstetric forceps. This reduces or eliminates the need for bearing down and decreases the swings in hemodynamic performance associated with the Valsalva maneuver. The proper choice of anesthetic can do much to stabilize the patient. With proper hemodynamic monitoring and anesthetic selection, the overall risk and stress for both mother and infant may well be reduced by an elective cesarean section performed under controlled conditions.[27]

THE FOURTH RISK PERIOD

The final major risk period occurs during the first few hours postpartum. The hemodynamic changes are rapid and unpredictable. Cardiac output may rise as much as 60% as a result of the alterations discussed above. The patient may experience substantial blood loss at delivery or surgery and oxytoxic drugs may be given rapidly to control hemorrhage. The effects of anesthetics will be dissipating. This is a time when the cardiac patient should be in an intensive care unit or similar setting.

The potential risks to the patient who has heart disease and is pregnant can certainly be minimized by a team approach to her care. However, during gestation, the patient may decompensate and require hospitalization with potent pharmacological therapy or even cardiac surgery. While the effects of the commonly used drugs are well known for the primary patient, i.e., the mother, their influence on the fetus needs to be considered also. Similarly, the effects of car-

diopulmonary bypass on the fetus need to be assessed. These issues will now be explored.

PHARMACOLOGICAL CONSIDERATIONS

The proper management of the obstetric cardiac patient not only involves monitoring and observation, but frequently requires the use of potent specific agents to adjust cardiac performance. These drugs, in addition to their beneficial effect on maternal hemodynamics may exert a negative effect on the developing fetus or the newborn infant. This may occur directly as the result of placental transfer of the agent, or indirectly due to impairment of uteroplacental blood flow. Many of these responses are transient, but a proper perspective must be maintained. Maternal well-being is, of course, the first priority. The following review of the more commonly utilized cardiovascular drugs will highlight some of the potential fetal and neonatal effects.

Propranolol

Propranolol has found wide application in the management of many diseases affecting the cardiovascular system. Its use for the pregnant patient has, however, been quite controversial. The concerns have been focused on fetal development and on immediate neonatal responses after acute administration to the mother prior to delivery. There have been several case reports of intrauterine fetal growth retardation in babies of patients who have received propranolol throughout pregnancy.[28,29] The proposed mechanism by which the beta-blockade would induce this phenomenon includes reduction in uteroplacental blood flow by the unopposed alpha-adrenergic system,[29] and the possibility of reduced umbilical blood in the fetus, which deprives it of adequate intrauterine nutrition.[28] While there is laboratory evidence to support both of these concepts, a prospective study in humans suggests that propranolol does not cause intrauterine fetal growth retardation.[30]

The immediate effects in the newborn

period are predictable and the infant warrants close observation by the pediatrician. Bradycardia and hypoglycemia are both likely to occur if the mother receives a large parenteral dose of propranolol before delivery. The resting heart rate in the newborn is under minimum beta-adrenergic control; therefore, with proper management no untoward effects should occur.[30] The drug is secreted in the breast milk and in some cases has been reported to reach therapeutic levels,[31] although this is probably a rarity. The overall conclusion is that the use of propranolol during pregnancy is appropriate for patients such as those with idiopathic hypertrophic subaortic stenosis who require beta-adrenergic blockade. The effect on the fetus and newborn should be minimum.

Lidocaine

This very popular local anesthetic is one of the most widely used antiarrhythmic agents. When administered in the normal therapeutic range, the blood level is maintained at 2 to 5 μgm/ml and no fetal effects of significance should occur. Levels higher than this may induce central nervous system toxicity in the mother, and have been associated with a decrease in the normal variability of the fetal heart rate and bradycardia. This is a direct effect of the drug on both the central nervous and cardiovascular systems and reflects placental transfer of the drug in sufficient quantities to induce these effects. Very high doses of lidocaine result in a reduction in uteroplacental blood flow. This occurs because the local anesthetics cause constriction, rather than the usual vasodilitation, of the uterine vessels. In addition, they have been shown to elevate the resting tone of the myometrium.[32] This could lead to hypoxia and acidosis in the fetus. These types of stress would be manifested by an alteration in the normal fetal heart rate pattern, e.g., bradycardia, as observed on the fetal heart rate monitor. This can easily be applied to the mother's abdomen. Fortunately, those levels of lidocaine which are deleterious to the fetus are also deleterious to the mother, so the usual therapeutic approaches need not be modified.

Vasoactive Substances

The vasopressor substances are occasionally required to support the blood pressure after some cardiovascular incidents. This might be the result of the disease, anesthesia for labor, delivery, or cesarean section, or to support the patient during or following cardiopulmonary bypass for corrective surgery. The specific actions of these drugs on the uterine arteries must be considered as they may compromise the fetus by reducing uteroplacental perfusion even in the face of restoring maternal perfusion pressure. The uteroplacental bed has very limited capacity for autoregulation, therefore, it is a pressure-dependent circulation. Anything which reduces mean arterial pressure may reduce uteroplacental perfusion. It is believed that under normal circumstances the blood flow is normal if mean arterial pressure is maintained between 70 and 115 torr. A normal fetus can tolerate as much as 40% reduction in uteroplacental flow for a short period of time without substantial ill effect. The compromised fetus, however, may not tolerate even a few minutes of reduced flow. Since the fetus of a cardiac patient is often at increased risk, we must assume it falls into the latter category. Therefore, when the vasoactive amines are necessary, they should be used but the fetus should be carefully monitored and therapy altered if possible if fetal distress should occur. The specific drugs to be reviewed have their actions summarized in Table 2.1.

ALPHA-ADRENERGIC AGONISTS

The alpha-adrenergic agonists cause the greatest reduction of uterine blood flow. The representative examples of this group are phenylephrine, norepinephrine, and methoxamine. These drugs cause arteriolar constriction and a rise in systemic vascular resistance. This results in an increase in maternal arterial pressure. The uterine vessels also constrict and this causes a reduction in uterine blood flow.[33] The reduction in uterine blood flow has been shown to parallel the percentage increase in maternal mean arterial pressure in the normovolemic

Table 2.1
Effects of Vasoactive Drugs in the Pregnant Patient*

Agent	Cardiac Output	Systemic Vascular Resistance	Systolic/Diastolic Pressure	Uterine Blood Flow
Alpha-adrenergic				
Norepinephrine	0/↓	↑	↑/↑	↓
Phenylephrine	↓	↑	↑/↑	↓
Methoxamine	↓	↑	↑/↑	↓
Beta-adrenergic				
Isoproterenol	↑	↓	0↑/↓	↓
Mixed action				
Epinephrine	↑	↓ or ↑	↑/↓	↑ or ↓
Ephedrine	↑	↑	↑/↑	↑ or 0
Dopamine	↑	0 or ↑	↑0/0↓	0 or ↓
Metaraminol	0/↑	↑	↑/↑	↑/0/↓

* Symbols used are: ↑ = increase; 0 = no change; ↓ = decrease.

pregnant ewe. In the hypotensive ewe treated with these agents, maternal arterial pressure is restored with no increase in uterine blood flow and occasionally a further decrease occurs. The net result could be significant fetal bradycardia induced by hypoxemia and acidosis. These agents should be used only when specifically indicated for maternal well-being as demonstrated by invasive monitoring and a calculated low systemic vascular resistance.

BETA-ADRENERGIC AGONISTS

The classical representative of this group is isoproterenol which is a pure beta-agonist. This drug produces both an inotropic and chronotropic response in the myocardium. Its peripheral effects result in venoconstriction, thus an increased cardiac return, and arteriolar dilation. Thus, peripheral vascular resistance is reduced and mean arterial pressure should be decreased. This was studied in the nonpregnant ewe and a 20% decrease in arterial pressure was observed as well as a 15% reduction in uterine blood flow.[34] The pregnant animal, however, showed only a 10% reduction in arterial pressure with essentially no alteration in uteroplacental flow when isoproterenol was infused. This was thought to be due to the fact that the uteroplacental bed is already maximally dilated during pregnancy and that the peripheral vascular resistance is already reduced during pregnancy. The difference in the nonpregnant animal is ex-

plained as a redistribution of blood flow to newly dilated vascular beds rather than to specific vascular response by the uterine vessels. However, beta-adrenergic agents must be administered to the pregnant patient who requires them with caution; if the blood volume is reduced for any reason a serious decrease in uteroplacental perfusion may occur.

The uterus itself responds to beta-adrenergic substances by relaxing myometrial tone.[35] This had led to their widespread use to suppress premature labor by obstetricians.[36] They have also been used to reduce excessive uterine tone which has compromised a fetus via the mechanism of decreased uteroplacental flow.[37]

COMBINATION AGENTS

Drugs with a combination of both alpha- and beta-adrenergic activity find wide utility as resuscitative agents for many threatening cardiovascular events. The predominating effect depends on the cause of the problem and the condition of the patient, the dosage and rate of administration, and the route by which the drug is given. The following drugs have been used and studied a great deal.

Ephedrine

This vasopressor is one of the most popular drugs used to treat hypotension, especially that associated with regional block during pregnancy. The beta-adrenergic effect of ephedrine is mediated by a direct stimulation of the beta$_1$-receptors in the heart. Its alpha-adrenergic effect is the result of stimulation of the norepinephrine release from the sympathetic nerve endings, thus leading to peripheral vasoconstriction and a decrease in venous capacitance. Thus, cardiac return is improved, heart rate and contractility are increased, and peripheral vascular resistance is slightly increased. Uterine blood flow is not negatively affected by ephedrine.[33] A proposed explanation for this is that there are alpha-adrenergic receptors in the uteroplacental bed but no sympathetic nerve terminals present. Therefore, drugs with direct alpha-adrenergic action will affect uteroplacental flow, but indirect acting agents like ephedrine will not.[38] Ephedrine does cross the placenta and may increase fetal heart rate and its variability but no adverse effect has been demonstrated. While this is the preferred drug during pregnancy by anesthesiologists, it may not be the best choice for some cardiac patients who might not tolerate the heart rate increase and another drug should then be selected.

Epinephrine

Epinephrine is a drug which has a multiplicity of effects on the uteroplacental circulation dictated by the dosage which is administered. In very low doses the beta-adrenergic action is predominant and cardiac output increases. The dilating effects on the peripheral vasculature may reduce mean arterial pressure under some circumstances and lead to a decrease in uterine blood flow. High doses of epinephrine manifest a substantial alpha-effect and uterine blood flow decreases.[34] Therefore, this mixed-function catecholamine has a range of effects on uteroplacental flow depending on the dose and rate of administration. It can be safely used when indicated by controlled infusion coupled with fetal heart rate monitoring. It does cross the placenta to a limited degree.

Metaraminol

This vasopressor, while mixed in function, is predominantly alpha-adrenergic

throughout its useful dosage range. It has been found to reduce uterine blood flow when administered to pregnant animals in quantities sufficient to elevate the maternal arterial blood pressure.[33] However, when given to animals made hypotensive with spinal anesthesia, the uterine blood flow was increased to within 70 to 80% of the control value.[39] A pressor response has also been observed in the fetus, thus suggesting placental transfer.[33] This drug is the vasopressor often selected for restoration of maternal blood pressure when ephedrine is contraindicated.

Dopamine

Dopamine is often used to maintain cardiac output in critically ill patients. It has been evaluated for use as a vasopressor in obstetrics using the pregnant ewe model. It appears that in doses which are adequate to support the cardiac output but do not raise blood pressure there is little effect on uteroplacental flow. When an amount sufficient to correct hypotension from spinal anesthesia is given, an alpha-adrenergic effect is demonstrated, i.e., the uterine blood flow is not increased toward normal as the maternal arterial pressure is raised or it is decreased even further.[40]

Digitalis

The digitalis preparations have specific medical indications and these are not changed by pregnancy. They do not appear to have a negative impact on uteroplacental blood flow. Digoxin appears to be quite safe, and digitoxin, while safe in the usual clinical range, has been associated with fetal death from digitalis intoxication when a maternal overdose was consumed.[26] These preparations do cross the placenta and equilibration in fetal tissues does take place. This has lead some investigators to believe that if a diagnosis of fetal congestive heart failure is made then maternal digitalis administration might be therapeutic.

An interesting aspect of digitalis use in the cardiac patient who becomes pregnant is the required dose. The blood level achieved with a fixed dose of oral digoxin was nearly 50% lower during pregnancy.[42]

This is presumed to be a function of the increased maternal blood volume and increased glomerular filtration. It has also been suggested that the decreased gastric emptying time in pregnancy may contribute to this.

ANTICOAGULANTS

Patients who have undergone prior cardiac surgery and have a prosthetic valve often need anticoagulation. This form of therapy does carry significant hazards for the fetus. The coumarin group of oral anticoagulants are of small molecular size and cross the placenta. They appear to be teratogenic during the first trimester when organogenesis is taking place. They may also anticoagulate the developing fetus during the remainder of pregnancy and can cause bleeding and anomaly formation.[43] The results of one study showed a combined neonatal morbidity and mortality of 41.8% for patients taking coumadin throughout pregnancy.[44] This has caused many obstetricians and cardiologists to stop coumadin therapy as soon as pregnancy is diagnosed and to place the patient on heparin therapy for at least the first trimester, although several continue it now throughout pregnancy. Heparin has a large molecular weight and does not cross the placenta. There has been an increase in spontaneous abortion rate noted in patients on chronic heparin treatment. Heparin is the drug of choice in the peripartal periods as it can be temporarily reversed for the vaginal delivery or cesarean section. Infants born of mothers taking coumarin have a high incidence of intracranial hemorrhage. This drug is also actively secreted in breast milk in quantities which will anticoagulate the newborn.

ANTIHYPERTENSIVE AGENTS

The antihypertensive drugs may be used to treat pre-existing hypertension or to decrease the peripheral vascular resistance both acutely and chronically for patients with valvular insufficiency. Those agents in common use today will be considered, although some of the newer drugs such as clonidine have yet to be assessed in the pregnant patient.

Thiazide Diuretics

The thiazides have been commonly used forms of antihypertensive therapy for years. They appear to have a relaxing effect on the peripheral vasculature and they decrease intravascular volume. This latter effect is not beneficial to the mother and the concurrent electrolyte disturbances of hyponatremia, hypokalemia, and hyperglycemia are also undesirable. Neonatal thrombocytopenia and, rarely, agranulocytosis have been reported. These side-effects have lead to diminishing use of diuretics during pregnancy and they are now reserved for cases of acute decompensation or refractile pathological edema.[1,6,34]

Methyldopa

This well known antihypertensive agent acts by inhibiting the synthesis of norepinephrine as well as by causing the formation of alpha-methylnorepinephrine, a false transmitter, at the nerve endings of the sympathetic nervous system. It also crosses the blood-brain barrier and depletes the brain of biogenic amines.[45] This ability to cross the blood-brain barrier indicates that the drug can cross the placenta also. It exerts a reserpine-like action on the fetus due to the depletion of catecholamines. Therefore, the infant whose mother has been on chronic methyldopa therapy may demonstrate lethargy, bradycardia, hypothermia, and nasal congestion at birth. The latter is more significant than it first appears because newborn infants are obligate nose breathers.

Hydralazine

This direct-acting vasodilator is frequently used in pregnancy because it maintains both renal and uterine blood flows. It is most often used to treat the hypertension associated with severe pre-eclampsia. It may be given orally, intravenously, or intramuscularly and is being used for some cardiac patients who require a decrease in systemic vascular resistance. Long-term therapy with this drug may result in a lupus erythematosis-like syndrome in the mother. While uteroplacental blood flow is preserved with judicious therapy,[46] excessive doses given parenterally will cause precipitous decreases in blood pressure and fetal distress, particularly in the parturient with the decreased blood volume of severe pre-eclampsia. It does cross the placenta and the neonate may demonstrate tachycardia and/or hypotension.

Sodium Nitroprusside

This very potent direct-acting vasodilator is extremely popular for the treatment of hypertensive emergencies and for the reduction of peripheral vascular resistance in congestive heart failure from a variety of lesions including mitral and aortic insufficiency. It is extremely rapid in response and evanescent in action. In spite of these very definite advantages its use for the obstetric patient has not been widely recommended for two reasons. The first is based on an animal model which shows that uteroplacental blood flow is not restored when sodium nitroprusside is administered to a pregnant ewe made hypertensive by the infusion of phenylephrine.[46] The second concern is that of potential cyanide toxicity in the fetus which has again been demonstrated in the pregnant ewe.[47] The data obtained from these models may not apply directly to the human situation. Indeed, the drug has been used on a short-term basis with excellent results in human pregnant patients for the management of severe hypertension and acute congestive heart failure without fetal compromise and with no evidence of cyanide formation in the umbilical cord blood.[48] Therefore, it seems appropriate to use this agent for the pregnant cardiac patient when indicated, providing that the proper maternal and fetal monitoring modalities are utilized.

Nitroglycerine

Nitroglycerine has potent vasodilating properties on both the systemic and pulmonary vasculature. It is broken down in the body to various nitrates and nitrites which are then excreted. There have not been any toxic effects of these breakdown products demonstrated in the fetus to date. The uteroplacental circulation does not appear to be adversely affected by the administration of this drug when given properly.[49]

As with the other potent vasodilators, precipitous hypotension could result in a reduction in uterine blood flow. Therefore, careful monitoring of both the maternal cardiovascular system and the fetal heart rate is indicated.

CARDIAC SURGERY DURING PREGNANCY

Surgery of any type is avoided during pregnancy because of potential compromise to the unborn infant. The developing fetus may experience teratogenic effects from drugs administered in the course of anesthesia. This has been demonstrated in animals with a multitude of anesthetic adjuvants but has never been clearly documented in humans.[50-52] Teratogenic changes may also be induced by hypoxia during the procedure as the result of maternal hypoxia or by decreased uteroplacental perfusion. Premature labor is often associated with surgery during pregnancy, particularly abdominal procedures.[53] Thus, if surgery is indicated during the course of pregnancy, it is usually performed during the second trimester whenever possible. This avoids the period of organogenesis and premature labor is said to be less likely. Many centers utilize tocolytic therapy as part of their routine for the surgical patient who is pregnant. While this may be useful for patients without cardiovascular disease, most of these drugs have potent side-effects, particularly for the cardiovascular system, and would prove less desirable for the patient with heart disease.[54]

The pregnant patient with heart disease is usually managed with medical therapy including long periods of bedrest if necessary. If a surgical lesion is present, every attempt to delay the definitive procedure until after delivery is made. However, there are patients who decompensate so severely from the cardiovascular stresses imposed by pregnancy that their chance of survival is very small unless surgical correction is accomplished. These patients are usually those with rheumatic valvular disease, particularly mitral stenosis.

The first cardiac operations undertaken

during pregnancy were closed mitral commissurotomy for severe congestive failure from mitral stenosis in 1952. A review of 514 cases undergoing mitral valvotomy during pregnancy revealed a maternal mortality of 1.75% and a fetal loss of 8.6%.[4] This was quite favorable when compared to a maternal mortality rate of from 4.2 to 18.7% in pregnant patients with Class III and IV cardiac disease managed with medical therapy. The fetal loss in these patients is approximately 50%. The extremely good surgical survival figures are attributed to the fact that the patients are young and have relatively healthy hearts which have been overburdened by the circulatory overload imposed by pregnancy.

The use of cardiopulmonary bypass for open heart procedures in the pregnant patient soon followed. The risk for both mother and fetus increases with this more complex situation. A multi-institutional survey has revealed a maternal mortality rate of about 5% and a fetal loss of approximately 33%.[55] The high fetal loss has been attributed to several factors which might affect fetal oxygenation. These are nonpulsatile perfusion, inadequate perfusion pressure, inadequate blood flow, embolic phenomena to the uteroplacental bed, alterations in uteroplacental flow patterns due to the insertion of the cannulae, and the release of catecholamines and renin as the result of nonpulsatile flow.[56] Many of these potential hazards could be minimized or completely eliminated by proper monitoring of the fetus. The use of the external fetal heart rate monitor as well as the tocodynamometer can alert the surgical team to alterations in fetal heart rate and heart rate variability, which signify hypoxia and acidosis, and to the presence of premature labor. When a fetus becomes hypoxic and acidotic, the heart rate initially increases and beat-to-beat variability may be decreased. As the situation continues, the fetal heart decreases below the usual baseline rate of 120 to 160 beats per minute. When contractions are present in the presence of hypoxia, the fetal heart rate decreases from baseline beginning near the peak of the contraction and persisting through the remainder of the

contraction. It slowly returns to baseline after the contraction is over. This is called a late deceleration and is the result of cessation of blood flow across the myometrium as the pressure generated from the contraction exceeds the pressure in the arterioles supplying the uteroplacental bed (Fig. 2.4). Decreases in heart rate variability may also be caused by anything which would decrease central nervous system activity in the fetus, such as sedative drugs and by anticholinergic drugs like atropine.

Several reports of fetal monitoring for patients requiring cardiopulmonary bypass have appeared in the literature.[2,56–59] They all attest to its usefulness in assessing the condition of the fetus. In addition, all have observed a persistent bradycardia throughout the period of cardiopulmonary bypass even with adequate maternal oxygenation and acid-base balance. This resolves quickly with the resumption of normal maternal circulation. This may be due to the moderate hypothermia which is utilized. The heart rate is usually between 80 and 100 beats per minute. If the fetal heart rate falls to 60 or less, the fetal cardiac output is significantly reduced as the fetus has little or no capacity for increasing stroke volume. One author found that increasing his pump flow from 3100 ml/minute to 3600 ml/minute resulted in the correction of a bradycardia of 60 back to a rate of over 100.[58]

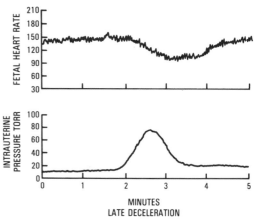

Figure 2.4. The diagram represents a late, uniform deceleration of fetal heart rate which indicates fetal hypoxia and acidosis.

Based on the available knowledge about the physiological changes of pregnancy, the pharmacology of the drugs used, the physiology of extracorporeal circulation, and the experiences reported, the following recommendations for the use of open-heart surgery with cardiopulmonary bypass during pregnancy can be made. Although it would be preferable to avoid such surgery during pregnancy, no pregnant patient should be denied a definitive operation because of her gestation. The procedure should be performed after the first trimester to avoid the period of organogenesis and before the third trimester when cardiac demands and blood volume are reaching their peaks whenever possible.

Every effort must be made to ensure adequate fetal oxygenation. This is a direct function of maternal oxygenation, acid-base status, and uteroplacental blood flow. The maternal inspired oxygen concentration should be maintained as high as possible and arterial blood gases checked frequently. Once on bypass this becomes critical. Maternal ventilation before and after bypass should be carefully adjusted to avoid respiratory alkalosis. This causes a shift in the oxyhemoglobin dissociation curve to the left, thus decreasing available oxygen for transfer to the fetus and may lead to a reduction in umbilical blood flow. Acidosis should also be avoided because this leads to a fetal acidosis as well. Aortocaval compression by the uterus must be avoided by placing a wedge of foam or rolled blankets or an inflatable device under the right hip until the patient is tilted to the left between 15 and 30 degrees. This should displace the uterus away from the inferior vena cava, thus allowing for adequate venous return, and away from the aorta, thus allowing for adequate perfusion of the kidneys, the uteroplacental circulation, and the lower extremities. The efficacy of this maneuver may be assessed by palpating the right femoral pulse and observing its quality before and after the maneuver.

Calculation of flows to be used during cardiopulmonary bypass should include compensation for the 30 to 50% increase in cardiac output during pregnancy. This means that flows will have to remain high. Perfusion pressure should also be maintained at high enough levels to maintain perfusion of the uteroplacental bed. The current experience suggests that this is 60 torr. Perfusion times should be kept to a minimum. Electrolyte balance should be maintained and glucose provided for both maternal and fetal nutrition. If vasopressors or vasodilators are required both during and after cardiopulmonary bypass, select them carefully with thought to possible fetal effects.

Electronic fetal heart rate monitoring with a strip chart record should be utilized with a member of the health care team who is experienced at interpretation available. Monitoring for uterine contractions is also desirable. The heart rate pattern has alerted surgical teams to problems with perfusion or maternal hypoxia and acidosis before any significant changes in vital signs took place in the mothers.[59,60] If uterine suppressants are needed, this agent should be carefully selected due to the wide range of potential side-effects. The beta-sympathomimetics, while the most popular, are associated with maternal pulmonary edema and myocardial ischemia. Ethanol or magnesium sulfate infusion may prove more appropriate. Volatile anesthetics suppress uterine activity, and halothane has been used at the termination of an open heart case to suppress labor successfully.[59]

The care of a pregnant patient who is quite ill from cardiac disease is indeed a challenging problem. The maternal physiology and fetal concerns add significantly to the complexity of the situation. There is, unfortunately, no single approach that is successful with all patients as the lesions, their severity, and the obstetric situation vary widely. We must make use of the available knowledge and our consultants in order to assure the optimum management for each individual patient.

References

1. Szekely P, Snaith L: *Heart Disease and Pregnancy.* Edinburgh and London, Churchill Livingstone, 1974.
2. Eilen B, Kaiser IH, Becker RM, et al: Aortic valve replacement in the third trimester of pregnancy:

Case report and review of the literature. *Obstet Gynecol* 57:119, 1981.

3. Oakley GDG, McGarry K, Limb DG, et al: Management of pregnancy in patients with hypertrophic cardiomyopathy. *Br Med J* 1:1749, 1979.

4. Ueland K: Cardiac surgery and pregnancy. *Am J Obstet Gynecol* 92:148, 1975.

5. Kahler RL: Cardiac disease. In (eds): Burrow GN, Ferris TF *Medical Complications during Pregnancy*, Philadelphia, W.B. Saunders Co., 1975.

6. Ueland K: Cardiovascular diseases complicating pregnancy. *Clin Obstet Gynecol* 21:429, 1978.

7. Burch GE: Heart disease and pregnancy. *Am Heart J* 93:104, 1977.

8. Peck TM, Arias F: Hematologic changes associated with pregnancy. *Clin Obstet Gynecol* 22:785, 1979.

9. Ueland K: Maternal cardiovascular dynamics. VII. Intrapartum blood volume changes. *Am J Obstet Gynecol* 126:671, 1976.

10. Rubler S, Prabodkumar M, Dumani M, et al: Cardiac size and performance during pregnancy estimated with echocardiography. *Am J Cardiol* 40:534, 1977.

11. Ueland K, Metcalfe J: Circulatory changes in pregnancy. *Clin Obstet Gynecol* 18:41, 1975.

12. Burwell CS, Metcalfe J: *Heart Disease and Pregnancy: Physiology and Management*. Boston, Little, Brown and Co., 1958.

13. Resnick R, Battaglia FC, Makowski EL, et al: The effect of actinomycin-D on estrogen-induced uterine blood flow. *Gynecol Invest* 5:24, 1974.

14. Roy SB, Malkain PK, Virik R: Circulatory effects of pregnancy. *Am J Obstet Gynecol* 95:221, 1966.

15. Rovinsky JJ, Jaffin H: Cardiovascular hemodynamics in pregnancy. *Am J Obstet Gynecol* 95:781, 1966.

16. Cutforth R, MacDonald CB: Heart sounds and murmurs in pregnancy. *Am Heart J* 71:741, 1966.

17. Turner AF: The chest radiograph in pregnancy. *Clin Obstet Gynecol* 18:65, 1975.

18. Milne JA: The respiratory response to pregnancy. *Postgrad Med J* 55:318, 1979.

19. Ueland K, Novy MJ, Metcalfe J: Hemodynamic responses of patients with heart disease to pregnancy and exercise. *Am J Obstet Gynecol* 113:47, 1972.

20. Freeman RK: Intrapartum management of the pregnant patient with heart disease. *Clin Obstet Gynecol* 18:75, 1975.

21. Weis FR, Markello R, Mo B, et al: Cardiovascular effects of oxytocin. *Obstet Gynecol* 46:211, 1975.

22. Hendriks CH, Brenner WE: Cardiovascular effects of oxytoxic drugs used post partum. *Am J Obstet Gynecol* 108:751, 1970.

23. Johnstone M: The cardiovascular effects of oxytoxic drugs. *Br J Anaesth* 44:826, 1972.

24. Young BK, Weinstein HM: Effects of magnesium sulfate on toxemic patients in labor. *Obstet Gynecol* 49:681, 1977.

25. Ostheimer GW, Alper MH: Intrapartum anesthetic management of the pregnant patient with heart disease. *Clin Obstet Gynecol* 18:81, 1975.

26. Jacobi AGM: Obstetric anesthesia and the cardiac patient. *Perinat Neonatol* 6:51, 1982.

27. Mendelson CL: *Cardiac Disease in Pregnancy*. Philadelphia, F.A. Davis, 1960.

28. Pruyn SC, Phelan JP, Buchanan GD: Long-term propranolol therapy in pegnancy: Maternal and fetal outcome. *Am J Obstet Gynecol* 135:485, 1979.

29. Reed RL, Cheney CB, Fearon RE, et al: Propranolol therapy throughout pregnancy: A case report. *Anesth Analg* 53:214, 1974.

30. Rubin PC: Beta-blockers in pregnancy. *N Engl J Med* 305:1323, 1981.

31. Levitan AA, Manion JC: Propranolol therapy during pregnancy and lactation. *Am J Cardiol* 32:247, 1973.

32. James FM: Anesthesia for vaginal delivery. *Seminars in Anesthia* 1:112, 1982.

33. Ralston DH, Shnider SM, deLorimer AA: Effects of equipotent ephedrine, metaraminol, mephentermine, and methoxamine on uterine blood flow in the pregnant ewe. *Anesthesiology* 40:354, 1974.

34. Brinkman CR, Woods JR: Effects of cardiovascular drugs during pregnancy. *Cardiovasc Med* 1:231, 1976.

35. Mahon WA, Reid DWJ, Day RA: The *in vivo* effects of beta-adrenergic stimulation and blockade on the human uterus at term. *J Pharmacol Exp Ther* 156:178, 1967.

36. Caritis SN, Edelstone DI, Mueller-Heubach E: Pharmacologic inhibition of pre-term labor. *Am J Obstet Gynecol* 133:557, 1979.

37. Arias F: Intrauterine resuscitation with terbutaline: A method for the management of acute intrapartum fetal distress. *Am J Obstet Gynecol* 131:39, 1978.

38. Conklin KA, Murad SHN: Pharmacology of drugs in obstetric anesthesia. *Seminars in Anesthia* 1:83, 1982.

39. James FM, Greiss FC, Kemp RA: An evaluation of vasopressor therapy for maternal hypotension during spinal anesthesia. *Anesthesiology* 33:25, 1970.

40. Rolbin SH, Levinson G, Shnider SM, et al: Dopamine treatment of spinal hypotension decreases uterine blood flow in the pregnant ewe. *Anesthesiology* 51:36, 1979.

41. Hernandez A, Burton RM, Goldring D, et al: The effects of maternally administered digoxin upon the cardiovascular hemodynamics of the fetal lamb. *Am Heart J* 85:511, 1973.

42. Rogers MC, Willerson JT, Goldblatt A, et al: Serum digoxin concentrations in the human fetus, neonate, and infant. *N Engl J Med* 287:1010, 1972.

43. Stevenson RE, Burton M, Feriauto GJ, et al: Hazards of oral anticoagulants during pregnancy. *JAMA* 243:1549, 1980.

44. Harrison EC, Roschke EJ: Pregnancy in patients with cardiac valve prostheses. *Clin Obstet Gynecol* 18:107, 1975.

45. Ferris TF: Toxemia and hypertension. In Burrow GN, Ferris TF (eds). *Medical Complications During Pregnancy*. Philadelphia,W. B. Saunders Co. 1975.

46. Ring G, Krames E, Shnider SM, et al: Comparison of nitroprusside and hydralazine in hypertensive pregnant ewes. *Obstet Gynecol* 50:598, 1977.

47. Naulty JS, Cefalo RC, Lewis P: Fetal toxicity of

nitroprusside in the pregnant ewe. *Am J Obstet Gynecol* 139:708, 1980.

48. Stempel JE, O'Grady JP, Morton MJ, et al: Use of sodium nitroprusside in complications of gestational hypertension. *Obstet Gynecol* 60:533, 1982.

49. Wheeler AS, James FM, Meis PJ, et al: Effects of nitroglycerine and nitroprusside on the uterine vasculature of pregnant ewes. *Anesthesiology* 52:390, 1980.

50. Pedersen H, Finster M: Anesthetic risk in the pregnant surgical patient. *Anesthesiology* 51:439, 1979.

51. Levinson G, Shnider SM: Anesthesia for operations during pregnancy. In: Shnider SM, Levinson G (eds). *Anesthesia for Obstetrics*. Baltimore, Williams & Wilkins, 1979.

52. Reisner LS: The pregnant patient and the disorders of pregnancy. In Katz J, Benumof J, Kadis LB (eds). *Anesthesia and Uncommon Diseases*. Philadelphia, W. B. Saunders Co., 1981.

53. Levine W, Diamond B: Surgical procedures during pregnancy. *Am J Obstet Gynecol* 81:1046, 1961.

54. Ravindran R, Viegas OJ, Padilla LM, et al: Anesthetic considerations in pregnant patients receiving terbutaline therapy. *Anesth Analg* 59:391, 1980.

55. Zitnik RS, Brandenberg RO, Sheldon R, et al: Pregnancy and open-heart surgery. *Circulation* 39 (Suppl I):I257, 1969.

56. Levy DL, Warriner RA, Burgess GE: Fetal response to cardiopulmonary bypass. *Obstet Gynecol* 56:112, 1980.

57. Trimakas AP, Maxwell KD, Berkay, et al: Fetal monitoring during cardiopulmonary bypass for removal of a left atrial myxoma during pregnancy. *Johns Hopkins Medical Journal* 144:156, 1979.

58. Koh KS, Friesen RM, Livingstone RA, et al: Fetal monitoring during maternal cardiac surgery with cardiopulmonary bypass. *Can Med Assoc J* 112:1102, 1975.

59. Werch A, Lambert HM, Cooley D, et al: Fetal monitoring and maternal open heart surgery. *South Med J* 70:1024, 1977.

60. Katz JD, Hook R, Barash PG: Fetal heart rate monitoring in pregnant patients undergoing surgery. *Am J Obstet Gynecol* 125:267, 1976.

61. Bonica JJ: *Obstetric Analgesia and Anesthesia*. World Federation of Societies of Anesthesiologists, 1980.

62. Bromage PR: *Epidural Analgesia*. Philadelphia, W. B. Saunders Co., 1978.

CHAPTER 3

ARTERIAL BARORECEPTORS AND CARDIAC RECEPTORS, THEIR PHYSIOLOGY AND PATHOPHYSIOLOGY

JOHN C. LONGHURST, M.D., PH.D.

Regulation of blood pressure is of major importance in maintaining adequate blood supply to the body's vital organs. To accomplish this task compensatory adjustments in cardiac output and systemic vascular resistance occur whenever blood pressure is altered. Short-term adjustments in blood pressure occurring in response to normal physiological or pathophysiological events frequently are mediated through neural reflexes. These reflexes consist of strategically placed receptor regions which respond to changes in blood pressure by altering the frequency of discharge of afferent nerves. These afferents relay information to the central nervous system. The information is processed by the central nervous system and the discharge of efferent or autonomic nerves which impinge the heart and blood vessels is altered. This chapter reviews the function of arterial or high-pressure as well as cardiopulmonary or low-pressure baroreceptors and cardiac chemosensitive receptors in physiological as well as pathophysiological conditions.

ANATOMY OF ARTERIAL AND CARDIAC RECEPTORS

Anatomists have identified two areas which are considered to be the predominant high-pressure barosensitive regions. One region is the carotid sinus, which has been identified as a segmental enlargement of the internal carotid artery at its origin from the common carotid. In humans, the carotid sinus likely comprises both the region of the bifurcation and the proximal portion of the external carotid branch.[1] The other region is the aortic arch. The aortic arch baroreceptors are located between two parallel lines that extend downward from the brachiocephalic trunk and upward from the ligamentum arteriosum, with the bulk of the endings found in the area directly facing the ligamentum arteriosum.[2] Receptors in both the carotid sinus and the aortic arch are located in the adventitia immediately adjacent to the media.[3, 4]

Afferent impulses are generated by stretch of the arterial walls and transmitted by both myelinated fibers and nonmyelinated sensory or afferent fibers of the carotid sinus nerve.[5, 6] Fibers from the carotid sinus nerve travel mainly with the glossopharyngeal nerve in humans, although some fibers also may travel with the cervical sympathetics and the pharyngeal and superior laryngeal branches of the vagus nerve.[7] The afferent innervation of the aortic arch is similar to that of the carotid sinus in terms of fiber size. In both systems, the

C fibers predominate.[8] In humans, there is no distinct afferent pathway for the aortic arch stretch receptors such as exists for the carotid sinus, and it seems that the aortic fibers are distributed in various morphological nerves, including the vagus and the sympathetics.[2] After projecting to various centers in the brain, the final efferent pathway consists of the sympathetic adrenergic nerves to the heart, resistance, and capacitance vessels of the body and cardiac vagus nerve.[9, 10]

Studies of the anatomy of cardiac receptors have documented two major types of endings within the heart. These are in the form of complex unencapsulated endings of either the diffuse or compact type and the nerve net.[11–19] Both types of endings are present in humans.[20] It is not clear from the histological studies whether these endings subserve different functions according to their morphology. However, interconnections have been found between the unencapsulated endings and the nerve net suggesting that they are similar functionally.[15]

Nerve receptors in the arterial baroreceptor regions act as deformation, or stretch, receptors rather than as the pressure receptors.[21] Stimulation or stretch of the arterial baroreceptors greatly affects arterial pressure, heart rate, myocardial performance, cardiac output, arterial resistance, and venous capacitance.[22–26] The resultant change in arterial pressure opposes the original change in transmural pressure.[27]

In humans, carotid sinus nerve stimulation causes a 23% decrease in arterial pressure, which is a result of a 14% decrease in peripheral vascular resistance and an 8% decrease in cardiac output.[28] Contractility in animals is increased as carotid sinus pressure is decreased. The increased contractility results from increased sympathetic discharge as well as from parasympathetic withdrawal. The effect from parasympathetic nerves becomes significant when sufficient sympathetic background activity is present.[23, 29, 30] Lowering carotid sinus pressure in animals increases the mean systemic (venous) pressure by decreasing the unstressed vascular volume through the mechanism of venoconstriction. An increase in venous pressure of 1 to 2 mm Hg, which occurs during carotid sinus hypotension, increases cardiac output by as much as 30%. Thus, a small degree of venoconstriction in response to carotid sinus hypotension substantially enhances cardiac output.[31] The heart rate response to tilt or to lower body negative pressure in humans is thought by some investigators to be a sympathetic response when blood pressure is lowered and to be a parasympathetic response when blood pressure is raised.[32] Other investigators, however, believe that the heart rate response is parasympathetic in origin, regardless of the direction of change.[33] Several studies have concluded that the reflex response of heart rate generally is less than the blood pressure response to changes in carotid sinus pressure in humans.[28, 34] Therefore, studying heart rate alone does not accurately assess all aspects of reflex control by the baroreceptors. Work from several groups of investigators indicates that the reflex control of heart rate in humans lies chiefly in baroreceptor areas other than the carotid sinus.[35–37]

ORTHOSTATIC FUNCTION OF ARTERIAL BARORECEPTORS

Since the primary function of the baroreceptors is to oppose changes in blood pressure, a decrease in arterial blood pressure causes reflex increases in heart rate and myocardial performance and a decrease in venous capacitance that, together with the tachycardia effect, increases cardiac output. Increased cardiac output combined with an increase in vascular resistance drives arterial blood pressure back toward the original level. The sum of these effects, therefore, is to increase blood pressure when receptor stretch is decreased. Humans have an upright posture, and in this position large amounts of blood are pooled in the extremities. When a person stands up, particularly when standing still, there is a decreased venous blood return to the heart. In this situation, the importance of the baroreflexes is their capacity to return decreased arterial pressure back toward normal. Homeostasis of pressure and perfusion of vital organs, such as the heart and brain, are thus maintained.

ATRIAL RECEPTORS

Based on the relation of discharge patterns of afferent nerves to atrial pressure waves, two types of atrial receptors, Types A and B, have been described.[16,38] Type B and Type A receptor endings are located largely in pulmonary venous and caval-atrial junctions and to a lesser extent in the bodies and appendages of the atria.[15,17,39–42] Both types are innervated by myelinated afferent fibers located in the vagus nerve.

Atrial Type B endings are stretch receptors which respond to pulsatile changes in atrial pressure.[43] Their discharge activity is related closely to the volume of the atrium.[15,39,44–46] Thus, the atrial v wave, to which these endings respond, appears to be a fairly accurate reflection of atrial volume.[47–50] Type B endings also respond to the amplitude of the v wave and to the rate of rise of the v wave.[51]

Arrhythmias which raise atrial volume can increase the discharge of Type B receptors.[16] Several other maneuvers also stimulate Type B receptors. These include distention of the atria by infusion of saline, by inflation of a balloon, or by negative pressure breathing.[44,52] Conversely, hemorrhage decreases the activity of these receptors.

Type A receptors discharge in time with the atrial a wave. Because they actually begin to discharge before the start of the atrial a wave, the natural stimulus to atrial Type A receptors may be atrial contraction which increases wall tension.[53,54] However, absolute atrial pressure also may be an important stimulus since the terminal burst of impulses of the Type A receptor is related closely to the a wave of the atrial pressure pulse.[16]

Ectopic atrial contractions produce a burst of firing of type A receptors but do not cause a sustained increase in firing such as occurs with Type B receptors. Unlike Type B receptors, Type A receptors do not change their firing rate with either volume infusion or hemorrhage.[54] However, they do respond positively to interventions which increase systolic function such as infusion of isoproterenol or stimulation of the stellate ganglion and negatively to interventions that decrease systolic function such as infusion of propranolol or removal of the stellate

ganglion.[54] Differences between Type A and B receptors, as described, are controversial since one study has demonstrated that under certain circumstances one receptor type can be converted to the other.[55] However, it has yet to be proven that such changes in discharge patterns occur in normal physiological situations.[56]

ATRIAL REFLEXES

In 1915 Bainbridge[57] noted that venous filling caused the heart rate to increase. He postulated that this effect might be caused by a neural reflex. In fact, there are two possible mechanisms which could increase heart rate during volume loading. One possibility is local stretch of the pacemaker region which enhances automaticity and increases heart rate. A second possibility is a reflex response originating in the heart that causes a cardiocardiac reflex to augment heart rate. The Bainbridge reflex also occurs in humans who have been volume loaded.[58,59]

The anatomy and physiology of this reflex has been investigated by distending the atriocaval or pulmonary vein junctions with small balloons. Stimulation of either right or left atrial receptors in this manner increases heart rate in 1 to 2 minutes.[17,42,52,60] With regard to other cardiovascular manifestations of this reflex, distention of such well-localized regions of the atria does not consistently change arterial pressure, systemic vascular resistance, or myocardial contractility, even if there are large increases in heart rate.[61–66]

Some of the reflex tachycardia caused by venoatrial distention may come from activation of sympathetic afferent fibers,[67] but the major afferent pathway consists of myelinated afferent fibers in the vagus nerves.[52,68–70] The efferent limb of this reflex is mediated by increased sympathetic activity.[52,71,72] The physiological importance of the Bainbridge reflex may be to increase cardiac output during situations of increased venous return.[15,72]

Atrial receptor stimulation associated with expanded intravascular volume causes a diuresis.[73] Although the diuresis may be mediated by a reduction in circulating antidiuretic hormone (ADH),[74] there is some evidence that a reduction in ADH is not necessary since diuresis will occur after ablation of the posterior pituitary.[72,75,76] Distention of the entire left atrium with large balloons causes bradycardia, hypotension, and a decrease in systemic vascular resistance.[60,63,77,78]

VENTRICULAR RECEPTORS

Ventricular receptors innervated by myelinated fibers frequently discharge in isovolumic systole.[79] They are tension- or pressure-sensitive receptors since they begin to discharge at the onset of left ventricular contraction which is at or just before the increase in ventricular pressure. However, the frequency of discharge of some myelinated ventricular afferent fibers also is related to the rate of rise of pressure.[80]

The functional importance of these fibers is uncertain.[81] However, premature atrial contractions decrease firing of these receptors, probably because ventricular pressure is reduced. Also, their discharge is enhanced when aortic blood pressure is increased and the ventricle is distended.[40,79,82]

There are two types of unmyelinated ventricular afferent fibers. One type innervates mechanoreceptors since they frequently respond to constriction of the aorta or epinephrine injection. Fewer of these fibers innervate the right than the left ventricle.[13,40,83,84]

Unmyelinated mechanoreceptors innervated by vagal afferent fibers can be stimulated by myocardial ischemia, hypoxia, severe hemorrhage, or hyperkinetic ventricular contractions.[85-87] The response of these receptors to hypoxia probably is related to altered wall motion rather than to an altered oxygen tension.[88] They respond to gradual occlusion of the aorta with their discharge activity increasing in parallel to changes in the left ventricular end-diastolic pressure.[89] They also respond to digitalis glycosides.[84]

The response characteristics of ventricular mechanoreceptors are altered markedly by changes in ventricular contractility.[88] Presently, there is evidence that these respond to changes in diastolic pressure as well as to changes in systolic pressure.[88]

A second type of receptor innervated by unmyelinated vagal afferent fibers generally displays an irregular discharge which has no obvious relationship to the cardiac cycle.[40] These fibers are believed to innervate chemosensitive receptors (to be distinguished from aortic and carotid body chemoreceptors) since they can be stimulated by chemicals such as veratradine, capsaicin, and phenyldiguanide. They also respond to constriction of the coronary arteries and to hypoxia possibly because these conditions cause the formation of bradykinin and/or prostaglandins (see below).[90-92]

VENTRICULAR REFLEXES

Distention of the left ventricle causes reflex vasodepression.[93] The afferent pathway for this reflex lies in the vagus nerve. Peripheral vasodilation is caused by withdrawal of sympathetic vasoconstrictor activity and bradycardia by increased parasympathetic discharge to the heart.[62,86,89,94-97] The reflex vasodepression is less pronounced from the right than from the left ventricle.[89,98,99] The bradycardia and the reflex renal vasodilation elicited by stimulation of ventricular receptors during constriction of the aorta is greater than the bradycardia and the reflex vasodilation caused by stimulation of carotid baroreceptors.[86] Because the direct effect of stimulating the myelinated fibers is weak and excitatory rather than inhibitory, it is more likely that unmyelinated vagal afferent fibers transmit this response.[85]

This is tonic inhibitory input from unmyelinated cardiac afferent nerve fibers.[85,86,100-103] This inhibition comes equally from atria and ventricles. It is greatest when there is increased pressure or volume in the ventricles or during myocardial ischemia.[85,86,100] The tonic reflex effect is to cause a reduction of blood flow to skeletal muscle, kidney, intestine, and a depression of myocardial contractility.[104] However, the tonic reflex inhibition of myocardial contractility from the cardiopulmonary region is less than the tonic inhibitiory activity from the carotid sinus afferents.[104]

In addition to the vagus, cardiac sympathetic nerves form an important afferent pathway.[11,12] Receptor endings of these fibers consist of free, unmyelinated terminals scattered diffusely in the extracellular spaces of the heart. Both thinly myelinated and unmyelinated sympathetic afferents innervate the heart.[105,106] Cell bodies of these sensory nerves are located in the upper five thoracic dorsal root ganglia.[107] Sympathetic afferents particularly seem to innervate epicardial receptors located on the surface of the left ventricle.[108-110]

Myelinated sympathetic afferents from the heart discharge spontaneously in phase with the cardiac cycle at normal blood pressures. They respond to changes in blood pressure and coronary flow, but ony when the latter is reduced sufficiently to cause cardiac failure.[111]

Unmyelinated sympathetic afferent fibers from the heart have been studied by several groups of investigators.[19,109,112,113] They can be subdivided into fibers which innervate mechanosensitive and chemosensitive receptors.[87,108,114,115] Mechanosensitive endings are scattered widely over the atria, ventricles, vena cavae, pulmonary arteries, and veins and pericardium.[87,108,114] This wide distribution of receptive endings for single unmyelinated fibers results from branching of these fibers.[87,114] The endogenous peptide, bradykinin, sensitizes these unmyelinated afferent fibers and causes them to discharge rhythmically with the cardiac cycle.[116-118]

In addition to the mechanosensitive receptors in the ventricle, there is a smaller group of chemosensitive receptors which are innervated by unmyelinated sympathetic afferent fibers. Both bradykinin and prostaglandins stimulate these receptors.[90,91] Coronary chemosensitive receptors, as described by the Coleridges,[91] may be the mechanically insensitive receptors described by others[119] that respond to acetylcholine, sodium cyanide, and asphyxia.

Stimulation of sympathetic afferent fibers causes mainly excitatory or pressor reflexes.[109,113,120,121] The excitation response includes increases in heart rate and myocardial contractility, effects which are mediated by an increased discharge of sympathetic efferent nerves.[109,113,121,122] Thus, volume infusion into cats with a high spinal transection causes a reflex tachycardia and pressor response due to stimulation of sympathetic afferents.[67] Occlusion of a coronary artery or coronary sinus increases in coronary pressure mechanically stimulate these fibers,[120,121] while lactic acid and potassium chemically stimulate them.[123,124] Tugging or occluding the left main coronary artery in lightly anesthetized cats or intracoronary injection of lactic acid in lightly anesthetized dogs cause pain-like responses.[125-127] Thus, sympathetic afferent fibers signal pain, particularly during myocardial ischemia.[108,120,125]

ARTERIAL BARORECEPTOR FUNCTION IN HYPERTENSION

The relation of the arterial baroreceptors to systemic hypertension has interested physiologists and clinicians for many years. Arterial baroreceptors have not been implicated as causal factors in hypertension in humans or in animals.[128] The high-pressure baroreceptors do, however, adapt to a chronically hypertensive state. The baroreceptor system maintains its capacity to buffer acute changes in arterial pressure but it does so at a higher set point.[33,129-132] In this respect, therefore, baroreceptors contribute to sustained elevation of blood pressure and are not able to return the system back toward normal blood pressure levels.[133]

Possible explanations for the altered baroreceptor function in chronic systemic hypertension are: (a) morphological changes in the baroreceptor filaments that are thought to be degenerative in nature and that have been described in humans, as well as in other species[134]; (b) a selective loss of baroreceptor units, particularly the low-threshold type[135]; (c) reduced sensitivity of individual receptor units[136]; (d) alterations in central integration and efferent limb function[137]; and (e) reduced compliance of the aorta and carotid sinus so that receptors are stretched less for any increase in pressure.[131,132,138-140]

ARTERIAL BARORECEPTOR FUNCTION IN CONGESTIVE HEART FAILURE

The sensitivity of the baroreflex system is significantly decreased in experimental chronic heart failure in dogs.[141] This reduced sensitivity impairs the ability of baroreceptors to respond to changes in arterial pressure. The cause of this reduced sensitivity is not known yet. However, there are certain experimental observations suggesting that reduced sensitivity may result from alterations in several components of the baroreceptor reflex. For instance, animals in congestive heart failure retain salt and water. This retention decreases compliance or increases stiffness of the vessel walls.[142] Furthermore, histological studies have demonstrated a degeneration of nerve endings in the baroreceptor areas in patients with a history of heart failure.[134] Altered central integration of the baroreflex has also been suggested.[133]

There is abundant evidence indicating that the efferent limb of the reflex arc, including both the sympathetic and parasympathetic divisions of autonomic nervous system, is altered in chronic congestive heart failure. For instance, norepinephrine stores in the myocardium are significantly depleted.[143, 144] Reduced catecholamine stores are probably both functionally significant and causally related to the reduced chronotropic and inotropic responses to cardiac sympathetic nerve stimulation in animals in chronic congestive heart failure.[145] This mechanism, however, does not explain decreased peripheral vascular responsiveness, because norepinephrine stores in resistance vessels are not reduced in congestive heart failure and neurotransmitter activity actually may be enhanced.[146, 147] The other branch of the autonomic nervous system, that of parasympathetic innervation, also is altered in patients with heart disease. Atropine administration increases heart rate by approximately 55% in normal persons but by only 23% in patients with heart disease. It is possible that, along with the impaired contractile state that limits stroke volume, a

defective control of heart rate may contribute to the inability for these individuals to raise their cardiac outputs in response to hypotension.[148]

There are important interactions of the digitalis glycosides with the baroreceptors. Pressor and inotropic responses to ouabain are attenuated by baroreflexes[149-151] partly because intravenous administration of these agents directly stimulates the baroreceptors. However, in contrast to the reduction of the pressor effect, it is unlikely that the direct inotropic action of these preparations is significantly modified because the baroreceptors normally exert only a small effect on myocardial performance.[151, 152]

BARORECEPTOR FUNCTION IN SHOCK

Prominent manifestations of the shock syndrome are hypotension and a narrowing of the pulse pressure due to a reduction of cardiac output. Baroreceptors significantly compensate for a 20% loss of blood by increasing total peripheral resistance by 55 to 70%, a tachycardia, and by increasing in cardiac output 20 to 25%.[153] Thus, the blood pressure reduction is lessened substantially by arterial baroreceptors. In the range between 60 and 150 mm Hg, it is probable that mean arterial pressure and pulse pressure are important contributory factors to baroreceptor stimulation.[154-157] However, changes in pulse pressure are of little importance when mean arterial pressures are less than 60 mm Hg.[153] Carotid baroreceptors may be qualitatively more important than are aortic arch baroreceptors, because the stimulation threshold in the latter regions is higher (probably in the range of 100 mm Hg) and because changes in pulse pressure normally have little influence on the aortic arch receptors.[29, 158-160] However, the low pressure baroreceptor in the heart and lungs as well as chemoreceptors in the aorta and carotid arteries, and central nervous system reflexes probably contribute to the reflex adjustments during cardiovascular shock. When a substantial hemorrhage occurs and the duration of arterial hypotension is prolonged, reflex compensatory mechanisms fail.[151] Which portion of the reflex fails is not known, although in some situations it may result from a decrease in norepinephrine concentration at the tissue level.[161] Downing[133] has suggested that the tissue hypoxia and metabolic acidosis that accompany hemorrhagic shock may be the most important factors in blunting the response to efferent sympathetic stimulation during hemorrhagic shock. In contrast with sympathetic function, parasympathetic function remains intact and actually may be enhanced by acidosis. This enhancement would contribute to the terminal bradycardia and circulatory collapse present in end-stage shock.[162–165]

In contrast with the evidence demonstrating an abnormality in the response to efferent limb stimulation, there is little or no evidence that implicates pathophysiological abnormalities occurring in either the receptor units or the afferent limb of the baroreflexes.

BARORECEPTOR FUNCTION IN CORONARY ARTERY DISEASE

Wasserman[166] has noted that externally applied carotid sinus pressure frequently decreases or abolished angina. Several other investigators have subsequently confirmed this finding.[167–169] Lown and Levine[169] have found that this maneuver was helpful in the diagnosis of rest angina rather than effort-induced angina. They have recommended that first right then left carotid sinus pressure (CSP) be applied and then the patient be asked whether the pain has become worse. If the patient is not misled but states that there is improvement, the test is considered positive. If the pain worsens or is unrelieved with slowing of the heart, however, the pain is likely not angina. Lastly, if the heart does not slow, the test is inconclusive. These and other investigators have noted that rarely is there improvement of the angina without slowing of the heart. This situation could be due to coronary vasodilatation.[170]

Lown and Levine[169] as well as several other groups of investigators[171–175] have noted that patients with coronary disease are more sensitive to carotid sinus pressure and respond with a greater bradycardia or even with asystole than do patients with normal hearts.

Many clinicians believe that CSP is useful in the differential diagnosis of arrhythmias. Heart rates of 120 to 180 beats/min are usually interpreted as sinus tachycardia or paroxysmal atrial tachycardia (PAT). However, sharp triangular P waves in limb lead II suggest atrial flutter, an arrhythmia that can be confirmed when CSP increases the AV block and reveals a typical sawtooth baseline undulation of atrial flutter. In addition, it has been demonstrated that atrial flutter and paroxysmal atrial tachycardia can be abolished by the vagontonia induced by CSP.

Lown and Levine[169] recognized the fact that digitalis enhances the sensitivity of the carotid sinus reflex. They and other clinicians have thought that CSP could help diagnose digitalis intoxication. For instance, prolonged cardiac standstill, ventricular premature beats, and excessive AV block may all indicate digitalis intoxication. Lown and Levine popularized the fact that PAT with block also signifies digitalis toxicity. This arrhythmia is often difficult to diagnose since the P waves that are blocked may be hidden in the T waves. However, CSP increases the block and thus separates the P and T waves and allows the arrhythmia to be diagnosed.

The presence of heart block often is difficult to diagnose when there is a rapid junctional or ventricular rate. However, if the atrial rate is slowed during CSP but the ventricular rate is unchanged, a diagnosis of complete heart block with ventricular tachycardia or a diagnosis of junctional tachycardia with aberrancy is established.

It is well known that left bundle branch block may mask the electrocardiographic evidence of a myocardial infarction.[169,176] Since bundle branch block can be rate-related in some instances, it is occasionally possible to slow the heart by CSP to view complexes of normal duration and to look for evidence of a myocardial infarction.

THE TECHNIQUE OF APPLYING CAROTID SINUS PRESSURE

Carotid sinus stimulation is an important procedure that must be performed with strict clinical indications under appropriate monitoring conditions. Most patients, particularly those with a history of syncope, should be tested in the recumbent position. The one exception is the patient with suspected angina, in whom the test is better performed in the sitting position.[169] The head should be tilted back and to one side until the bifurcation of the carotid can be palpitated. The sinus is known to be situated just below the angle of the jaw and above the edge of the sternocleidomastoid muscle at the upper level of the thyroid cartilage. Prior to massage, each patient should be attached to an electrocardiograph since this permits accurate assessment of the effect of CSP on the cardiac rhythm. In addition to gently palpating the arteries to locate the bulb of the carotid sinus, the observer should note the intensity of the pulsations of both carotid arteries. Lastly, the observer should carefully auscultate over both carotid vessels to determine the presence of any bruits that might signify carotid atherosclerotic disease. If there is a significantly reduced pulsation on one side or if there is any other evidence of intrinsic carotid disease, CSP should not be performed. In the absence of these excluding criteria, CSP should be performed by compressing the bulb against the vertebral spine with a rapid on-off rhythm and with pressure directed both posteriorly and medially. Massage is applied for no more than 5 seconds at a time, and the pressure is always applied unilaterally, never bilaterally. After several seconds of rest, the procedure may be repeated on the ipsilateral or contralateral side. Generally, both sides should be massaged separately, since it has been recognized that one side may cause larger reflex cardiovascular alterations than the other. Carotid sinus massage should not be performed without the immediate availability of adequate resuscitation equipment.

The dangers of CSP include cerebrovascular accidents[177,178] and death.[179,180] These situations occur when the carotid arteries are not carefully examined prior to compression, when CSP is carried on for more than 5 seconds, when CSP is not stopped with the appearance of arrhythmias, and lastly, when proper resuscitation equipment is unavailable.

HYPERSENSITIVE CAROTID SINUS SYNDROME

It is important to differentiate between the hypersensitive reflex and the hypersensitive syndrome. Nathanson[174] studied the reflex in 115 patients. He noted that all patients developed cardiac standstill of at least 5 seconds, whereas only 23 had evidence of dizziness or syncope. Thus, the majority of his patients had the hypersensitive carotid sinus reflex but not the syndrome. He reported one example of asystole that occurred for 7.6 sec without symptoms. Thus, the hypersensitive carotid sinus reflex is without symptoms, whereas the hypersensitive syndrome is associated with dizziness, syncope, and often convulsions. The importance of differentiating between these two reactions is that the reflex requires no treatment, and the syndrome frequently requires therapy.[175]

In the early 1930s, Weiss and coworkers[171,172] described their extensive experience with three groups of patients who had developed the carotid sinus syndrome. The patients were broadly classified as: (a) the vagal or cardioinhibitory type; (b) the vasodepressor type; or (c) the cerebral type. All types produced unconsciousness and convulsions or at least severe dizziness. More recent studies, however, have concluded that the cerebral form of carotid sinus hypersensitivity is nonexistent.[169,175,181-183] Although the relative incidences of the other two types of carotid sinus hypersensitivity are not well known, most investigators believe that the cardioinhibitory form is most common, occurring in 34 to 78% of cases, whereas the pure vasodepressor type is somewhat less common, occurring in 5 to 10% of cases. Although the symptoms rarely occur in a pure form, generally there is either predominant brady-cardia or vasodepression.[184–186]

Diagnosis of the hypersensitive carotid sinus syndrome rests on a careful observation of the cardiovascular response to CSP. If this syndrome is strongly suspected as being the cause of the patient's syncope, it is perhaps the one indication for which CSP should be performed longer than 5 seconds. Thomas[175] suggests that light brief stimulation of each carotid sinus be carried out (up to 10 sec). If no unusual cardiac response occurs, the stimulus intensity should be increased and the sinus massaged for a maximum of 20 seconds. As the sinus is massaged, constant electrocardiographic monitoring is required along with cuff blood pressure recording done during the peak bradycardia response or, in the absence of a bradycardia response, approximately 15 seconds after the start of massage. The test should be terminated immediately if bradycardia occurs or if there is vasodepression.

Patients with a hypersensitive carotid sinus syndrome present with a variety of symptoms. In a summary of several of their previous studies, Weiss and colleagues[187] noted all patients presented with fainting, dizziness, weakness and convulsions, and, less commonly, with other symptoms.

Attacks of syncope or dizziness generally occur when the patient is in the upright position and can be relieved by lying down.[171,172] Such attacks can be related to factors such as neck movement, pressure on or blows to the neck, and sudden changes in position.[188] Several types of drugs, including methyldopa,[189] digitalis,[172] and propranolol,[190] have been incriminated as agents that predispose patients to the development of the hypersensitive carotid sinus syndrome. With discontinuation of each of these agents, the syndrome disappears.

In general, the hypersensitive carotid sinus syndrome occurs in patients 55 years of age or older. A number of cases studied have demonstrated pathological abnormalities localized to the region of the carotid sinus. These include a dilated sinus, cervical adenitis, and local atherosclerotic changes. Several other groups of investigators have confirmed the finding that older men with atherosclerotic heart disease or hypertension or both most commonly develop this syndrome.[173–175,191]

Both medical and surgical therapies have been advocated for this syndrome. Medical therapy consists of withdrawing digoxin or other drugs that may be causing sensitization. Patients are warned not to put pressure on their neck, turn their head, or put themselves into other similar situations that might directly stimulate the carotid sinus.[171,172,186] Atropine appears to prevent bradycardia in 70 to 90% of patients with the vagal form of this syndrome.[171,172,188,191,192] The vasodepressor form of the syndrome does not respond to atropine but can be prevented effectively in some situations with sympathomimetic agents or amphetamines.[171,172]

Permanent demand pacemaker implantation has proved useful, particularly with the vagal type of this syndrome.[192–195] Other forms of surgical therapy have included transection of the glossopharyngeal nerve[196,197] and surgical stripping of the adventitia of the carotid artery.[187,198] It is recommended that: (a) a preoperative carotid angiogram be performed to exclude the presence of atherosclerotic carotid artery disease, (b) endocardial pacing be available during surgery, and (c) both electrical and mechanical stimulation of the carotid sinus be performed with electrocardiographic monitoring to determine the areas of sensitivity during surgery.[199]

CARDIAC RECEPTOR FUNCTION IN ISCHEMIC HEART DISEASE

Occlusion of a coronary artery stimulates receptive endings of vagal afferent fibers from the heart.[85,86,100,200–204] The increased discharge of unmyelinated vagal afferents occurs with a rhythmicity that is directly related to the cardiac cycle and is in parallel with the ischemic bulging of the myocardium. This suggests that mechanical rather than chemical factors activate these receptors.[203,204] Also, the discharge rate of mechanoreceptors with myelinated sympathetic afferent fibers is increased during occlusion of a coronary artery.[205]

Myocardial ischemia either could increase or decrease blood pressure because stimulation of sympathetic afferents reflexly increases and stimulation of vagal afferent fibers reflexly decreases the discharge of sympathetic efferent nerves.[206] However, to be able to demonstrate a pressor response to occlusion of a coronary artery it is usually necessary to cut the vagal afferent fibers.[120,207,208] It has been suggested that depressor responses mediated by vagal afferent fibers are manifested as excess vasodilation and could contribute to cardiogenic shock associated with a myocardial infarction.[209]

A greater reflex bradycardia, systemic vasodepression, decrease in renal nerve activity, and gastric relaxation can be elicited by occlusion of the circumflex than by left anterior descending coronary artery. This differential reflex effect most likely is caused by differences in numbers of receptors present in these two locations rather than differences in drug concentration or muscle mass perfused. The observation that posterior ischemia causes gastric relaxation is interesting since another symptom that frequently bothers patients, particularly those with posterior-inferior myocardial infarctions, is nausea and vomiting.[210–212]

It has been speculated that the reflex vasodilation in the kidney may be beneficial in protecting patients with cardiogenic shock. For instance, in one series of patients with acute renal failure, the cause of the failure could be related to coronary ischemia (i.e., postmyocardial infarction shock) in only 2% of cases.[213] Also, comparison of hypotension caused by hemorrhage to that caused by coronary artery embolization demonstrates that in the latter situation, renal blood flow and urine-concentrating capability are better maintained.[214] The difference between these two forms of shock may be that myocardial ischemia causes a cardiac reflex which reduces renal sympathetic efferent discharge.[215] Decreased efferent nerve discharge to the kidney can be reversed by vagus nerve transection suggesting that stimulation of cardiac receptors by coronary occlusion buffers the increased sympathetic discharge resulting from the hypotension-

induced stimulation of high-pressure arterial baroreceptors.[216]

Consistent with the hypothesis of cardiovascular depression originating from stimulation of receptors located on the inferior-posterior myocardium and cardiovascular excitation from receptors located on the anterior myocardium is the finding that patients with Prinzmetal's angina can manifest reflex bradycardia in association with spasm of vessels supplying the inferior wall and tachycardia in association with spasm of vessels supplying the anterior wall.[217]

Sympathetic afferent fibers may transmit the sensation of pain which is associated with coronary artery occlusion.[108,120,125] Thus, occlusion of a coronary artery in lightly anesthetized dogs or cats causes a pain-like response which is associated with increased sympathetic efferent nerve activity.[107] The afferent pathways for these responses are, in part, located in the stellate and upper four thoracic ganglia. Distal to these ganglia, the afferents pass through the upper three or four thoracic and the lower two cervical dorsal spinal cord roots.[218] Removal of the stellate ganglia and the entire length of the cervical chains does not relieve angina as long as the upper three thoracic ganglia are left intact.[218] However, removal of both stellate ganglia and excision of the first to the fifth thoracic sympathetic ganglia relieves cardiac pain in man.[219] Other operations which were used to control angina pectoris in humans in the late 1940s and 1950s were a paravertebral anesthetic block and posterior rhizotomy of appropriate dorsal roots of the spinal cord.

Clinical Studies of Cardiac Receptors in Ischemic Heart Disease

Successful reperfusion of the right coronary artery following intracoronary thrombolytic therapy frequently causes bradycardia and hypotension.[220] In contrast, successful left coronary artery reperfusion only infrequently causes this hemodynamic pattern. In fact, left coronary artery reperfusion is more frequently associated with hypertension, tachycardia, or an increase in ventricular ectopy. Thus, reperfusion of the acutely ischemic posterior-inferior myocardium causes a Bezold-Jarish-like reflex while reperfusion of the anterior myocardium more commonly causes an excitatory reflex.

As many as 77% of patients with acute posterior myocardial infarctions develop bradyarrhythmias and/or hypotension.[221-223] Conversely, only 30% of patients with acute anterior infarctions experience these problems. Bradyarrhythmias occur even when hypotension would be expected to cause a reflex tachycardia through stimulation of high-pressure arterial baroreceptors. One potential cause of the bradyarrhythmias could be a cardiac depressor reflex.

Other patients may develop hypertension spontaneously during angina pectoris.[224] The angina cannot be reproduced simply by elevating the blood pressure to the same level as the patient experienced during the spontaneous episode of chest pain. Also, the onset of chest pain and increase in blood pressure frequently occur simultaneously, suggesting that the increase in blood pressure is unlikely to be the cause of the chest pain.[225-227] It appears, therefore, that some patients, particularly those with variant angina, develop an increase in blood pressure as a consequence of a cardiac reflex and not as a cause of angina. Hypertension also may be associated with a myocardial infarction.[228] In some patients, blood pressure increases before the onset of chest pain, again suggesting that pain is not the etiology of the hypertensive response in these patients.

In the immediate postoperative period after cardiopulmonary bypass, especially after coronary artery bypass surgery, a significant number of patients develop hypertension.[229-232] This clinical situation is quite serious since it can be associated with hemorrhage, myocardial decompensation, and/or arrhythmias.[229,233,234] These patients have an unchanged cardiac output and an increased total peripheral vascular resistance.[230] The hypertension usually is not related to overtransfusion.[230] Anesthetic blockade of either the right or left stellate ganglion causes a rapid return of the blood pressure to normotensive levels and returns vascular resistance to normal in two-thirds of patients. Return of systemic vascular resistance to normal is not caused by a reduction of cardiac output although heart rate significantly decreases. These data suggest that the phenomenon of postbypass hypertension is a cardiogenic reflex which is conducted by sympathetic afferent fibers traveling through the stellate ganglion.

Potential Chemical Mediators of Cardiac Reflexes in Ischemic Heart Disease

There are several potentially important factors produced by the ischemic myocardium that could cause cardiovascular reflexes. The candidates include bradykinin, prostaglandins (PG), potassium, hydrogen ions, lactate, and carbon dioxide.

Increased concentrations of bradykinin efflux from the coronary sinus following coronary occlusion.[235,236] This peptide stimulates chemosensitive sensory endings in the heart which are innervated by unmyelinated afferents in the vagus nerve.[118] Reflex bradycardia (and occasionally tachycardia) and hypotension are caused when it is injected into the coronary circulation.[237-239]

Although there is some controversy, bradykinin probably is one of the mediators of the sensation of pain in the skin[240,241] and possibly in the heart.[126,242] In this context, bradykinin is produced in the condition of inflammation.[243]

Prostaglandins are produced in the myocardium, smooth muscle of the coronary arteries, and platelets in the blood. These compounds are released in response to hypoxia, myocardial ischemia, increased preload, and collagen-induced aggregation of platelets.[238,239,244,245] PGE_2, PGA, $PGF_{2\alpha}$, PGI_2, and TxB_2 are released in experimental animals following coronary artery occlusion.[244,246-249] In addition, atrial pacing causes release of $PGF_{2\alpha}$ in patients with coronary artery disease who have stable angina pectoris.[245] Thus, prostaglandins are produced in the heart of patients with ischemic heart disease when there is an imbalance between myocardial oxygen supply and demand.

Prostaglandins stimulate atrial, ventricular, pulmonary arterial, and aortic chemosensitive receptors innervated by vagal afferent fibers.[87,90,91] The receptor's discharge frequently remains elevated for several minutes after stimulation even though the prostaglandins are rapidly destroyed. The most consistent stimulation comes from PGE_2 and less frequently from $PGF_{2\alpha}$. In cats, but not in dogs, $PGF_{2\alpha}$ injected into the coronary circulation causes a reflex bradycardia and hypotension which is mediated by vagal afferent fibers.[250] More recently, it has been suggested that prostacyclin (PGI_2), perhaps a more potent coronary vasodilator than the other prostaglandins, stimulates unmyelinated vagal afferent fibers.[251] PGI_2 causes a vagally mediated reflex bradycardia and hypotension when it is injected into the left atrium of dogs.[252-254]

The excitatory reflex elicited by application of bradykinin to the epicardial surface of the heart can be reduced by the pretreatment with indomethacin. This suggests that formation of prostaglandins may be necessary for this reflex. Consistent with this hypothesis is the demonstration that PGE_1 and PGE_2 (but not $PGF_{2\alpha}$) potentiate the discharge of sympathetic afferent nerves and the excitatory response caused by application of bradykinin to the epicardium.[239,255] Prostaglandins applied topically generally do not cause a reflex response.[239]

It is possible that the ischemic myocardium releases bradykinin and prostaglandins which, in concert, stimulate sympathetic afferent nerves and thus signal pain during myocardial ischemia.[239,246,256,257] This hypothesis is consistent with the observation by Uchida and Murao[124] that aspirin inhibits prostaglandin synthesis and reduces stimulation of sympathetic afferents during coronary artery occlusion. Thus, in the setting of coronary stenosis a heavy workload placed on the heart may decrease oxygen tension and thereby stimulate bradykinin production. Bradykinin, in turn, may induce local release of prostaglandins. These two factors acting separately or together may cause local coronary vasodilation. They also may stimulate sympathetic afferent fibers within the myocardium and elicit pain. Lastly, these two factors may cause a reflex bradycardia and depressor response which would lessen the myocardium's demand for oxygen.[238]

Mechanosensitive and, less commonly, chemosensitive vagal afferents can be stimulated by hypoxia.[87] The response of the mechanosensitive afferent vagal fibers probably results from a wall motion abnormality. The chemosensitive fibers which are stimulated by hypoxia, may be aberrantly located aortic body glomus tissue and perhaps should be called chemoreceptors rather than receptors with chemosensitive endings.[87] Local myocardial hypoxia and hypercapnia in animals with and without vagotomy ($Po_2 = 43$ mm Hg, $Pco_2 > 100$ mm Hg, pH = 6.96) does not cause any reflex hemodynamic effects.[258] Although a similar gas mixture profoundly stimulates aortic chemoreceptors, more severe degrees of hypoxia are necessary to cause cardiovascular reflexes by other regions of the body such as skeletal muscle.[259] The reflex effect of severe myocardial hypoxia is not known.

Aggregation of human platelets causes release of serotonin.[260] Serotonin can induce a hypertensive cardiogenic chemoreflex when it is infused into the proximal left coronary artery of dogs.[261-265] The afferent pathway for this reflex lies in the vagus nerve. The actual receptive area for this response very likely is the aortic body which is supplied by a small branch of the proximal left coronary artery.[266] The reflex is diminished in the conscious dog which shows an initial depressor and a later small pressor response.[267] It has been postulated that a reflex increase in blood pressure is caused by release of serotonin by aggregated platelets. A hypertensive response could help to preserve coronary flow by dislodging the platelet aggregation. Similar types of responses have been noted with $PGF_{2\alpha}$ which, along with serotonin, is released by platelets in animals.[260,268] A coronary hypertensive reflex caused by local release of $PGF_{2\alpha}$ or serotonin within the coronary vascular bed also may be responsible for the early hypertension which occurs in some patients soon after a myocardial infarction.

ROLE OF CARDIAC RECEPTORS IN PRODUCTION OF ARRHYTHMIAS

Atrial fibrillation increases left atrial pressure and thereby stimulates Type B receptors causing them to discharge in an asynchronous pattern.[269] This situation could cause erroneous information to be sent to the central nervous system and result in an inappropriate diuresis.[270] In fact, polyuria occurs with many forms of paroxysmal tachycardia lasting over 20 minutes, particularly if the associated heart rate is greater than 110/min.[270]

The possibility of cardio-cardiac reflexes may be important in the genesis of ventricular arrhythmias. Studies have demonstrated that cardiac sympathetic nerves and the left stellate ganglion, in particular, are important for the development of arrhythmias.[271-275] In this regard, occlusion of a coronary artery in vagotomized animals substantially decreases the absolute number of ectopic beats after transection of dorsal roots C_8-T_5.[276] Thus, it is very likely that ischemia of the myocardium leads to an excitatory reflex which is transmitted by sensory fibers traveling with sympathetic nerves. Excitation of these fibers leads to increased efferent sympathetic tone and production of arrhythmias.

CARDIAC RECEPTOR FUNCTION IN CONGESTIVE HEART FAILURE

Patients with heart failure have high left atrial pressures and high ADH levels.[277,278] Inappropriately high ADH levels may contribute to the peripheral edema, ascites, and hyponatremia which often occurs in patients with heart failure.[279] Although ADH levels would be expected to decrease as a result of increased stretch of the left atrium, left atrial receptors may adapt or may be reset when they are subjected to chronic stretch.[279-283]

In addition to altered compliance of the left atrium, the axons which terminate in the atria are diffuse and fragmented in chronic heart failure.[284] It is not known if these histological findings are truly abnormal since normally there are a variety of types of endings and the diffuse fragmented endings observed in the condition of heart failure may be simply one end of this spectrum.

Approximately 50% of unmyelinated vagal afferent fibers demonstrate an increased discharge rate following application of acetylstrophathidin to the epicardial surface of the heart.[285] The reflex hypotension, brady-cardia, and decreased renal sympathetic nerve activity caused by this glycoside is mediated by vagal afferent fibers.[286,287] These ventricular receptors not only are stimulated by digitalis glycosides but are sensitized by these drugs so that they respond more vigorously to other stimuli such as constriction of the aorta.[84]

The discharge of myelinated atrial Type B receptors also is enhanced by cardiac glycosides.[267] The augmented discharge of atrial receptors occurs over a broad range of atrial pressures and occurs without accompanying changes in heart rate or mean atrial pressure. This digitalis-induced heightened sensitivity of left atrial receptors may reduce plasma ADH and partially restore renal function in patients with congestive heart failure.

There may be increased activity of cardiac afferent nerves during the early hypervolumic phase of heart failure.[288] This could result in a decreased neurohumoral drive to the circulation. In more chronic heart failure there likely is decreased cardiac afferent nerve activity which causes increased neurohumoral drive with associated vasoconstriction, sodium retention, and augmentation of certain excitatory reflexes.[212,289,290] In humans this would be manifest by increased circulating norepinephrine, plasma renin activity, and angiotensin.[291-294] Treatment with digitalis, diuretics, and sodium restriction may restore cardiac afferent nerve stimulation, thereby inhibiting the prevailing neurohumoral excitatory state of heart failure. The result would be peripheral vasodilation, naturesis, diuresis, and decreased afterload presented to the heart.

CARDIAC RECEPTOR FUNCTION IN AORTIC STENOSIS

Patients with severe aortic stenosis commonly experience syncope. The syncope could be caused by sudden failure of the myocardium which leads to decreased cardiac output, decreased cerebral blood flow, and loss of consciousness. However, during exercise, patients with aortic stenosis and syncope develop a significantly decreased forearm vascular resistance whereas normal subjects develop an increased forearm vascular resistance.[295] Apparently, patients with aortic stenosis who experience syncope are unable to vasoconstrict these inactive regional circulations during exertion. In this regard, stimulation of cardiac receptors in dogs causes reflex withdrawal of alpha-adrenergic vasoconstrictor tone in muscles and to a lesser extent in skin.[296] It is likely, therefore, that the observed vasodilation is caused by excessive increases in left ventricular systolic and end-diastolic pressures which stimulate cardiac receptors to reflexly decrease vascular resistance and blood pressure. Thus, paradoxical vasodilation caused by cardiac receptor stimulation may explain some cases of syncope in patients with aortic stenosis, particularly those associated with exercise.

Acknowledgment. The author wishes to thank Ms. Lynne Keith for her secretarial assistance.

References

1. Binswanger O: Anatomische Untersuchungen uber die Ursprungsstelle und den Anfangstheil der Carotis Interna. *Arch Psychiatr Nervenkr* 9:351, 1979.
2. Abraham A: *Microscopic Innervation of the Heart and Blood Vessels in Vertebrates Including Man.* Oxford, Pergamon Press, 1969, pp. 260–304.
3. Abraham A: Blood pressure and peripheral nervous system. *Acta Biol Acad Sci Hung* 4:307, 1953.
4. Abraham A: Die Innervation der Blutgetabl. *Acta Biol Acad Sci Hung* 4:69, 1953.
5. Sato A, Fidone S, Eyzaguirre C: Presence of chemoreceptor C-fibers in the carotid nerve of the cat. *Brain Res* 11:459, 1968.
6. Fidone SJ, Sato A: A study of chemoreceptor and baroreceptor A- and C- fibers in the cat carotid nerve. *J Physiol* (London) 205:527, 1969.
7. Sheehan D, Mulholland JH, Safiroff B: Surgical anatomy of the carotid sinus nerve. *Anat Rec* 80:431, 1941.
8. Gerard MW, Billingsley PR: The innervation of the carotid body. *Anat Rec* 25:391, 1923.
9. Heymans C, Neil E: *Reflexogenic Areas of the Cardiovascular System.* Boston, Little, Brown and Co., 1958.
10. Gunn CG, Sevelius G, Puiggari MJ: Vagal cardiomotor mechanisms in the hind brain of the dog and cat. *Am J Physiol* 214:258, 1968.
11. Nettleship WA: Experimental studies on the afferent innervation of the cat's heart. *J Comp Neurol* 64:115, 1936.
12. Nonidez JF: Studies on the innervation of the heart. II. Afferent nerve endings in the large arteries and veins. *Am J Anat* 68:151, 1941.
13. Sleight P, Widdicombe JG: Action potentials in fibers from receptors in the epicardium and myocardium of the dog's left ventricle. *J Physiol* (London) 181:235, 1965.
14. Whitteridge D: Afferent nerve fibers from the heart and lungs in the cervical vagus. *J Physiol* (London) 107:496, 1948.
15. Coleridge JCG, Hemingway A, Holmes RL, et al: The location of arterial receptors in the dog: A physiological and histological study. *J Physiol* (London) 136:174, 1957.
16. Paintal AS: Vagal afferent fibers. *Ergebn Physiol* 52:74, 1963.
17. Linden RJ: Function of cardiac receptors. *Circulation* 48:463, 1973.
18. Floyd K, Linden RJ, Saunders DA: The morphological variation of nervous structures in the atrial endocardium of the dog. *J Physiol* (London) 238:19, 1974.
19. Tranum-Jensen J: The ultrastructure of the sensory (baroreceptors) in the atrial endocardium of young. *J Anat* 119:255, 1975.
20. Johnston BD: Nerve endings in the human endocardium. *Am J Anat* 122:621, 1968.
21. Hauss WH, Kreuziger H, Asteroth H: Uber die Reizung per Pressorezeptoren im Sinus Caroticus beim Hund. *Z Kreislaufforsch* 38:28, 1949.
22. Sarnoff SJ, Gilmore JP, Brockman SK, et al: Regulation ventricular contraction by the carotid sinus: Its effects on atrial and ventricular dynamics. *Circ Res* 8:1123, 1960.
23. DeGeest H, Levy MN, Zieske Jr H: Carotid sinus baroreceptor reflex effects upon myocardial contractility. *Circ Res* 15:327, 1964.
24. Kumada M, Iriuchijima J: Cardiac output in carotid sinus reflex. *Jpn J Physiol* 15:397, 1965.
25. Schmidt RM, Kumada M, Sagawa K: Cardiac output and total peripheral resistance in the carotid sinus reflex. *Am J Physiol* 221:480, 1967.
26. Shoukas AA, Sagawa K: Control of total systemic vascular capacity by the carotid sinus baroreceptor reflex. *Circ Res* 33:22, 1973.
27. Sagawa K, Kumada M, Schramm LP: Nervous control of the circulation. In Guyton AC, Jones CE (eds): *Cardiovascular Physiology.* Vol. 1, Baltimore, University Park Press, 1975, pp. 197–232.
28. Bohm E, Strang RR: Glossopharyngeal neuralgia. *Brain* 85:371, 1962.
29. Levy MN, Ng ML, Zieske H: Cardiac and respiratory effects of aortic arch baroreceptor stimulation. *Circ Res* 19:930, 1966.
30. Randall WC, Armour JA, Geis WP, et al: Regional cardiac distribution of the sympathetic nerves. *Fed Am Soc Exp Biol* 31:1199, 1972.
31. Kumada M, Okai O, Gunji A: Mean circulatory pressure in carotid sinus reflex. *Jpn J Physiol* 21:591, 1971.
32. Scher AM, Ohm WW, Bumgarner K, et al: Sympathetic and parasympathetic control of the heart rate in the dog, baboon and man. *Fed Proc* 31:1912, 1972.
33. Pickering TG, Gribbin B, Oliver DO: Baroreflex sensitivity in patients on long-term hemodialysis. *Clin Sci* 43:645, 1972.
34. Bevegard BS, Shepherd JT: Circulatory effects of stimulating the carotid arterial stretch receptors

in man at rest and during exercise. *J Clin Invest* 45:132, 1966.

35. Glick G, Covell JW: Relative importance of the carotid and aortic baroreceptors in the reflex control of heart rate. *Am J Physiol* 214:955, 1968.

36. Mancia G: Riflessi barocettivi seno-aortici nell'uomo,. In Bartorelli C, Motolese M, Zanchetti A (eds): *Meccanismi Adrenergici e Terapia Cardiovascolare*. Florence, Ciba-Geigy, 1977, pp. 61–76.

37. Mancia G, Iannos J, Jamieson CG, et al: Effect of isometric hand-grip exercise on the carotid sinus baroreceptor reflex in man. *Clin Sci Mol Med* 54:33, 1978.

38. Arndt JO: Neurophysiological properties of atrial mechanoreceptors. In Hainsworth R, Kidd C, Linden RJ (eds): *Cardiac Receptors*. Cambridge, Cambridge University Press, 1979, pp. 89–115.

39. Paintal AS: A study of right and left arterial receptors. *J Physiol* (London) 120:596, 1953.

40. Coleridge HM, Coleridge JCG, Kidd C: Cardiac receptors in the dog with particular reference to two types of afferent ending in the ventricular wall. *J Physiol* (London) 174:323, 1964.

41. Langrehr D: Entladungsmuster und allgemeine Reizbedingunen von Vorhofsreceptoren bei Hund und Katze. *Pflugers Arch ges Physiol* 271:257, 1960.

42. Kappagoda CT, Linden RJ, Saunders DA: The effect on heart rate of distending the atrial appendages in the dog. *J Physiol* (London) 225:705, 1972.

43. Arndt JO, Brambring P, Hindorf K, et al: The afferent impulse traffic from atrial A-type receptors in cats. Does the A-type receptor signal heart rate? *Pflugers Arch, Europ J Physiol* 326:300, 1971.

44. Henry JP, Pearce JW: The possible role of cardiac atrial stretch receptors in the induction of changes in urine flow. *J Physiol* (London) 131:572, 1956.

45. Muhl N, Scholderer I, Kramer K: Uber die aktivitat der intrathorakalen gefa β-rezeptoren und ihrc beziehung zur herzfrequenz bei anderung des blut volumens. *Verh Dtsch Ges Kreisl-Forsch* 22:S122, 1956.

46. Kramer K: Die afferente innervation und die reflex von herz und venosem system. *Verh Dtsch Ges Kreisl-forsch* 25 Tagg:S142, 1959.

47. Opdyke DF, Duomarco J, Dillon WH, et al: Study of simultaneous right and left arterial pressure pulses under normal and experimentally altered conditions. *Am J Physiol* 154:258, 1948.

48. Little RC: Volume elastic properties of the right and left atrium. *Am J Physiol* 158:237, 1949.

49. Little RC: Volume pressure relationships of the pulmonary-left heart vascular segment. *Circ Res* 8:594, 1960.

50. Irisawa H, Greer AP, Rushmer RF: Changes in the dimensions of the vena cavae. *Am J Physiol* 196:741, 1959.

51. Paintal AS: Natural and paranatural stimulation of sensory receptors. In Zotterman Y (ed): *Sensory Functions of the Skin*. London, Pergamon Press, 1976, pp 3–12.

52. Ledsome JR, Linden RJ: A reflex increase in heart rate from distension of the pulmonary vein-atrial junction. *J Physiol* (London) 170:456, 1964.

53. Paintal AS: Natural stimulation of type B arterial receptors. *J Physiol* (London) 169:116, 1963.

54. Recordati G, Bishop VS, Lombardi F, et al: Mechanical stimuli exciting type A atrial vagal receptors in the cat. *Circ Res* 38:397, 1976.

55. Kappagoda CT, Linden RJ, Mary DASG: Atrial receptors in the cat. *J Physiol* (London) 262:431, 1976.

56. Paintal AS: Electrophysiology of atrial receptors. In Linden RJ (ed): *Cardiac Receptors*. Cambridge, Cambridge Univ Press, 1979, pp. 73–87.

57. Bainbridge FA: The influence of venous filling upon the rate of the heart. *J Physiol* (London) 50:65–84, 1915.

58. Giuntini C, Maseri A, Bianchi R: Pulmonary vascular distensibility and lung compliance as modified by dextran infusion and subsequent atropine injection in normal subjects. *J Clin Invest* 45:1770, 1966.

59. Koubenec HJ, Riseh WD, Crauer O: Effective compliance of the circulation in the upright sitting posture. *Pflugers Arch Ges* 374:121, 1978.

60. Pelletier CL, Shepherd JT: Circulatory reflexes from mechanoreceptors in the cardio-aortic area. *Circ Res* 33:131, 1973.

61. Daly IDB, Ludany G, Todd A, et al: Sensory receptors in the pulmonary vascular bed. *J Exp Physiol* 27:123, 1937.

62. Doutheil U, Kraver K: Uber die Differenzierung Kreislaufregulie render reflexe aus dem linken Herzen. *Pflugers Arch ges Physiol* 269:114, 1959.

63. Edis AJ, Donald DE, Shepherd JT: Cardiovascular reflexes from stretch of pulmonary vein-atrial junctions in the dog. *Circ Res* 27:1091, 1970.

64. Ledsome JR, Hainsworth R: The effects upon respiration of distension of the pulmonary vein-atrial junctions. *Respir Physiol* 9:86, 1970.

65. Furnival CM, Linden RJ, Snow HM: Reflex effects on the heart of stimulating left atrial receptors. *J Physiol* (London) 218:447, 1971.

66. Carswell F, Hainsworth R, Ledsome JR: The effects of distension of the pulmonary vein-atrial junctions upon peripheral vascular resistance. *J Physiol* (London) 207:1, 1970.

67. Bishop VS, Lombardi F, Malliani A, et al: Reflex sympathetic tachycardia during intravenous infusions in chronic spinal cats. *Am J Physiol* 230:25, 1976.

68. Kappagoda CT, Linden RJ, Sivananthan N: Atrial receptors and the urine response. *J Physiol* (London) 282:49P, 1978.

69. Kappagoda CT, Linden RJ, Sivananthan N: The nature of the atrial receptors responsible for a reflex increase in heart rate in the dog. *J Physiol* (London) 291:393, 1979.

70. Linden RJ, Mary ASG, Weatherill D: The nature of the atrial receptors responsible for a reflex decrease in activity in the renal nerves in the dog. *J Physiol* (London) 300:31, 1980.

71. Karim F, Kidd C, Malpus CM, et al: The effects of stimulation of the left atrial receptors on sympathetic efferent nerve activity. *J Physiol* (London) 227:243, 1972.

72. Linden RJ: Reflexes from the heart. *Prog Cardiovasc Dis* 18:201, 1975.

73. Gauer OH, Henry JP: Circulatory basis of fluid volume control. *Physiol Rev* 63:423, 1963.

74. DeTorrente A, Robertson GL, McDonald KM, et al: Mechanism of diuretic response to increased left atrial pressure in anesthetized dog. *Kidney Int* 8:355, 1975.

75. Goetz KL, Bond GC, Bloxham DD: Atrial receptors and renal function. *Physiol Rev* 55:157, 1975.

76. Kappagoda CT, Linden RJ, Snow HM, et al: Effect of destruction of the posterior pituitary on the diuresis from left atrial receptors. *J Physiol* (London) 244:757, 1975.

77. Lloyd TC Jr: Control of systemic vascular resistance by pulmonary and left heart baroreflexes. *Am J Physiol* 225:1511, 1972.

78. Thoren P, Ricksten S: Cardiac C-fiber ending's in cardiovascular control under normal and pathophysiological conditions. In Abboud FM, Fozzard HA, Gilmore JP, Reis DJ (eds): *Disturbances in Neurogenic Control of the Circulation*. Bethesda, American Physiological Society, 1981, pp. 17–31.

79. Paintal AS: The study of ventricular pressure receptors and their role in the Bezold reflex. *Quart J Exp Physiol* 40:348, 1955.

80. Kolatat TK, Kramer K, Muhl N: Uber die aktivitat sensibler herznerven des Frosches und ihre Beziehungen zur Herzdynamik. *Pflugers Arch ges Physiol* 264:127, 1957.

81. Coleridge HM, Coleridge JCG: Cardiovascular receptors. In Downman CBB (ed): *Modern Trends in Physiology*. London, Butterworths, 1972, pp. 245–257.

82. Gupta BN, Thames MD: Behavior of left ventricular mechanoreceptors with myelinated and non myelinated afferent vagal fibers in cats. *Circ Res* 52:291, 1983.

83. Muers MF, Sleight P: Action potentials from ventricular mechanoreceptors stimulated by occlusion of the coronary sinus in the dog. *J Physiol* (London) 221:283, 1972.

84. Oberg B, Thoren P: Studies on left ventricular receptors, signalling in non-medullated vagal afferents. *Acta Physiol Scand* 85:145, 1972.

85. Oberg B, Thoren P: Circulatory responses to stimulation of medullated and non-medullated afferents in the cardiac nerve in the cat. *Acta Physiol Scand* 87:121, 1973.

86. Oberg B, Thoren P: Circulatory responses to stimulation of left ventricular receptors in the cat. *Acta Physiol Scand* 88:8, 1973.

87. Baker DG, Coleridge HM, Coleridge JCG: Vagal afferent C fibers from the ventricle. In Hainsworth R, Kidd C, Linden RJ (eds): *Cardiac Receptors*. Cambridge, Cambridge University Press, 1979, pp. 117–137.

88. Thoren PN: Characteristics of left ventricular receptors with nonmedullated vagal afferents in cats. *Circ Res* 40:415–421, 1977.

89. Thoren PN: Role of cardiac vagal C-fibers in cardiovascular control. *Rev Physiol Biochem Pharmacol* 86:1, 1979.

90. Baker DG, Kaufman MP, Coleridge HM, et al: Prostaglandin E₂ stimulates vagal chemical-sensitive C-fiber in the heart and great vessels. (Abstr). *Fed Proc* 38:1322, 1979.

91. Coleridge HM, Coleridge JCG: Cardiovascular afferents involved in regulation of peripheral vessels. *Ann Rev Physiol* 42:413, 1980.

92. Kaufman MP, Baker DG, Coleridge HM, et al: Stimulation by bradykinin of afferent vagal C-fibers with chemosensitive endings in the heart and aorta of the dog. *Circ Res* 46:476, 1980.

93. Daly IDB, Verney EB: The localization of receptors involved in the reflex regulation of the heart rate. *J Physiol* (London) 62:330, 1926, 1927.

94. Aviado Dm, Schmidt CF: Cardiovascular and respiratory reflexes from the left side of the heart. *Am J Physiol* 196:726, 1959.

95. Salisbury PF, Cross EC, Rieben PA: Reflex effects of left ventricular distention. *Circ Res* 8:530, 1960.

96. Ross J Jr, Frahm CJ, Braunwald E: The influence of intracardiac baroreceptors on venous return, systemic vascular volume and peripheral resistance. *J Clin Invest* 40:563, 1961.

97. Bergel DH, Makin GS: Central and peripheral cardiovascular changes following chemical stimulation of the surface of the dog's heart. *Cardiovasc Res* 1:80, 1967.

98. Aviado DMJ, Schmidt CF: Reflexes from stretch receptors in blood vessels, heart and lungs. *Physiol Rev* 35:247, 1955.

99. Abramhamsson H, Thoren P: Reflex relaxation of the stomach elicited from receptors located in the heart. An analysis of the receptors and afferents involved. *Acta Physiol Scand* 84:197, 1972.

100. Oberg B, Thoren P: Increased activity in left ventricular receptors during hemorrhage or occlusion of caval veins in the cat—a possible cause for the vaso-vagal reaction. *Acta Physiol Scand* 85:164, 1972.

101. Mancia G, Donald DE: Demonstration that the atria, ventricles, and lungs each are responsible for a tonic inhibition of the vasomotor center in the dog. *Circ Res* 36:310, 1975.

102. Thoren PN, Mancia G, Shepherd JT: Vasomotor inhibition in rabbits by vagal nonmedullated fibers from cardiopulmonary area. *Am J Physiol* 229:1410, 1975.

103. Thoren PN, Shepherd JT, Donald DE: Anodal block of medullated cardiopulmonary vagal afferents in cats. *J Appl Physiol* 42:461, 1977.

104. Shimizu T, Bishop VS: Role of carotid sinus and cardiopulmonary reflexes on left ventricular dP/dt in cats. *Am J Physiol* 238:H93, 1980.

105. Emery DG, Foreman RD, Coggeshall RE: Fiber analysis of the feline inferior cardiac sympathetic nerve. *J Comp Neurol* 166:457, 1976.

106. Emery DG, Foreman RD, Coggeshall RE: Categories of axons in the inferior cardiac nerve of the cat. *J Comp Neurol* 117:301, 1976.

107. White JC, Garny WE, Atkins JA: Cardiac innervation. *Arch Surg* 26:765, 1933.

108. Ueda H, Uchida Y, Kamisaka K: Distribution and responses of the cardiac sympathetic receptors to mechanically induced circulatory changes. *Jpn Heart J* 10:70, 1969.

109. Malliani A, Recordati G, Schwartz PJ: Nervous activity of afferent cardiac sympathetic fibers with atrial and ventricular endings. *J Physiol* (London) 229:457, 1973.

110. Hess GL, Zuperku EJ, Coon RL, et al: Sympathetic afferent nerve activity of left ventricular origin. *Am J Physiol* 227:543, 1974.
111. Malliani A, Parks M, Tuckett RP, et al: Reflex increases in heart rate elicited by stimulation of afferent cardiac sympathetic nerve fibers in the cat. *Circ Res* 32:9, 1973.
112. Hirsch EF, Borghard-Erdle AM: The innervation of the human heart. *Arch Pathol* 71:384, 1961.
113. Peterson DF, Brown AM: Pressor reflexes produced by stimulation of afferent fibers in the cardiac sympathetic nerves of the cat. *Circ Res* 28:605, 1971.
114. Nishi K, Sakanashi M, Takenaka F: Afferent fibers from pulmonary arterial baroreceptors in the left cardiac sympathetic nerve of the cat. *J Physiol* (London) 240:53, 1974.
115. Casati R, Lomardi F, Malliani A: Afferent sympathetic unmyelinated fibers with left ventricular endings in cats. *J Physiol* (London) 292:135, 1979.
116. Uchida Y, Murao S: Bradykinin-induced excitation of afferent cardiac sympathetic nerve fibers. *Jpn Heart J* 15:84, 1974.
117. Nishi K, Sakanashi M, Takenaka F: Activation of afferent cardiac sympathetic nerve fibers of the cat by pain producing substances and by noxious heat. *Pflugers Arch ges Physiol* 372:53, 1977.
118. Baker DG, Coleridge HM, Coleridge JCG, et al: Search for a cardiac nociceptor: Stimulation by bradykinin of sympathetic afferent nerve endings in the heart of the cat. *J Physiol* (London) 306:519, 1980.
119. Nishi K, Takenaka F: Chemosensitive afferent fibers in the cardiac sympathetic nerve of the cat. *Brain Res* 55:214, 1973.
120. Brown AM, Malliani A: Spinal sympathetic reflexes initiated by coronary receptors. *J Physiol* (London) 212:685, 1971.
121. Malliani A, Peterson DF, Bishop VS, Brown AM: Spinal sympathetic cardiocardiac reflexes. *Circ Res* 30:158, 1972.
122. Pagani M, Schwartz PJ, Banks R, et al: Reflex responses of sympathetic preganglionic neurones initiated by different cardiovascular receptors in spinal animals. *Brain Res* 68:215, 1974.
123. Uchida Y, Murao S: Excitation of afferent cardiac sympathetic nerve fibers during coronary occlusion. *Am J Physiol* 226:1094, 1974.
124. Uchida Y, Murao S: Acid-induced excitation of afferent cardiac sympathetic nerve fibers. *Am J Physiol* 228:27, 1975.
125. Brown AM: Excitation of afferent cardiac sympathetic nerve fibers during myocardial ischemia. *J Physiol* (London) 190:35, 1968.
126. Guzman F, Lim RKS: Visceral pain and the pseudoaffective response to intra-arterial injection of bradykinin and other algesic agents. *Arch Intern Pharmacodyn* 136:353, 1962.
127. Guzman F, Braun C, Lim RKS, et al: Narcotic and non-narcotic analgesic which block visceral pain evoked by intra-arterial injection of bradykinin and other algesic agents. *Arch Intern Pharmacodyn* 149:571, 1964.
128. Cowley AW, Liard JF, Guyton AC: Role of the baroreceptor reflex in daily control of arterial blood pressure and other variables in dogs. *Circ Res* 32:564, 1973.
129. Kezdi P: Sinoaortic regulatory mechanisms: Role in pathogenesis of essential and malignant hypertension. *Circ Res* 91:26, 1953.
130. McCubbin MW, Green JH, Page IH: Baroreceptor function in chronic renal hypertension. *Circ Res* 4:205, 1956.
131. Bristow JD, Honour J, Pickering GW, et al: Diminished baroreflex sensitivity in high blood pressure. *Circulation* 39:48, 1969.
132. Gribbon B, Pickering TG, Sleight P, et al: Effect of age and high blood pressure on baroreflex sensitivity in man. *Circ Res* 29:424, 1971.
133. Downing SE: Baroreceptor regulation of the heart. In Berne RM, Sperelakes N, Geiger SR (eds): *Handbook of Physiology, Section 2: The Cardiovascular System*, Vol. 1, *The Heart*. Bethesda, American Physiological Society, 1979, pp. 621–652.
134. Abraham A: The structure of baroreceptors in pathological conditions in man. In Kezdi P (ed): *Baroreceptors and Hypertension*. Oxford, Pergamon, 1967, pp. 273–291.
135. Kezdi P: Resetting of the carotid sinus in experimental renal hypertension. In Kezdi P (ed): *Baroreceptors and Hypertension*. Oxford, Pergamon Press, 1967, p. 305.
136. Nosaka S, Wang SC: Carotid sinus baroreceptor functions in the spontaneously hypertensive rat. *Am J Physiol* 222:1079, 1972.
137. Lazarus JM, Hampers CL, Lowrie EG, et al: Baroreceptor activity in normotensive and hypertensive uremic patients. *Circulation* 47:1015, 1973.
138. Wolinsky H: Response of the rat aortic media to hypertension: Morphological and chemical studies. *Circ Res* 26:507, 1970.
139. Aars H: Relationship between blood pressure and diameter and ascending aorta in normal and hypertensive rabbits. *Acta Physiol Scand* 75:397, 1969.
140. Angell-James JE: Characteristics of single aortic and right subclavian baroreceptor fiber activity in rabbits with chronic renal hypertension. *Circ Res* 32:149, 1973.
141. Higgins CB, Vatner SF, Eckberg DL, et al: Alterations in the baroreceptor reflex in conscious dogs with heart failure. *J Clin Invest* 51:715, 1972.
142. Zelis R, Delea CS, Coleman HN: Arterial sodium content in experimental congestive heart failure. *Circulation* 41:213, 1970.
143. Chidsey CA, Kaiser GA, Sonnenblick EH, et al: Cardiac norepinephrine stores in experimental heart failure in the dog. *J Clin Invest* 43:2386, 1964.
144. Vogel JHK, Jacobowitz D, Chidsey CA: Distribution of norepinephrine in the failing bovine heart: Correlation of chemical analysis and fluorescene microscopy. *Circ Res* 24:71, 1964.
145. Covell JW, Chidsey CA, Braunwald E: Reduction of the cardiac response to postganglionic sympathetic nerve stimulation in experimental heart failure. *Circ Res* 19:51, 1966.
146. Chidsey CA, Braunwald E: Sympathetic activity and neurotransmitter depletion in congestive heart failure. *Pharmacol Rev* 18:685, 1966.

147. Kramer RS, Mason DT, Braunwald E: Augmented sympathetic neurotransmitter activity in the peripheral vascular bed of patients with congestive heart failure and cardiac norepinephrine depletion. *Circulation* 38:629, 1968.

148. Eckberg DL, Brabinsky M, Braunwald E: Defective cardiac parasympathetic control in patients with heart disease. *N Engl J Med* 285:877, 1971.

149. Gillis RA, Quest JA, Standaert FG: Depression by reflexes of the pressor and cardiotoxic responses to ouabain. *J Pharmacol Exp Ther* 170:294, 1969.

150. Quest JA, Gillis RA: Carotid sinus reflex changes produced by digitalis. *J Pharmacol Exp Ther* 177:650, 1971.

151. Quest JA, Gillis RA: Effect of digitalis on carotid sinus baroreceptor activity. *Circ Res* 35:247, 1974.

152. Vatner SF, Higgins CB, Franklin D, et al: Extent of carotid sinus regulation of the myocardial contractile state in conscious dogs. *J Clin Invest* 51:995, 1972.

153. Kumada M, Schmidt RM, Sagawa K, et al: Carotid sinus reflex in response to hemorrhage. *Am J Physiol* 219:1373, 1970.

154. McCrea FD, Wiggers CJ: Rhythmic atrial expansion as a factor in the control of heart rate. *Am J Physiol* 103:417, 1933.

155. Ead HW, Green JH, Neil E: A comparison of the effects of pulsatile and nonpulsatile blood flow through the carotid sinus on the reflexogenic activity of the sinus baroreceptors in the cat. *J Physiol* (London) 118:509, 1952.

156. Schmidt RM, Kumada M, Sagawa K: Cardiovascular responses to various pulsatile pressures in the carotid sinus. *Am J Physiol* 223:1, 1972.

157. Kenner T, Baertschi AJ, Allison JL, et al: Amplitude dependence of the carotid sinus reflex. *Pfluegers Arch* 346:49, 1974.

158. Angell-James JE, Daly M deB: Comparison of the reflex vasomotor responses to separate and combined stimulation of the carotid sinus and aortic arch baroreceptors by pulsatile and non-pulsatile pressure in the dog. *J Physiol* (London) 209:257, 1970.

159. Donald DE, Edis AJ: Comparison of aortic and carotid baroreflexes in the dog. *J Physiol* (London) 215:521, 1971.

160. Pelletier CL, Clement DL, Shepherd JT: Comparison of afferent activity of canine aortic and sinus nerves. *Circ Res* 31:557, 1972.

161. Glaviano VV, Coleman B: Myocardial depletion of norepinephrine in hemorrhagic hypotension. *Proc Soc Exp Biol Med* 107:761, 1961.

162. Campbell GS: Cardiac arrest: Further studies on the effect of pH changes on vagal inhibition of the heart. *Surgery* 38:615, 1955.

163. Ng ML, Levy MN, Zieske HA: Effects of changes of pH and of carbon dioxide tension of left ventricular performance. *Am J Physiol* 213:115, 1967.

164. Linden RJ, Norman J: The effect of acidaemia on the response to stimulation of the autonomic nerves to the heart. *J Physiol* (London) 200:51, 1969.

165. Downing SE, Milgram EA, Halloran KH: Cardiac responses to autonomic nerve stimulation during acidosis and hypoxia in the lamb. *Am J Physiol*

166. Wasserman S: Die Angina Pectoris ihre Pathogenese und Path-Physiologie. *Wien Klin Wochenschr* 41:1514, 1928.

167. Wayne EJ, Laplace LB: Observations on angina of effort. *Clin Sci* 1:103, 1933.

168. Wasserman S, Weber H: Angina pectoris und Pressorreceptoren-regulation. *Acta Med Scand* 100:589, 1939.

169. Lown B, Levine SA: The carotid sinus: Clinical value of its stimulation. *Circulation* 23:766, 1961.

170. Freedberg AS, Riseman JEF: Observations on the carotid sinus reflex and angina pectoris. *Circulation* 7:58, 1953.

171. Weiss S, Baker JP: The carotid sinus reflex in health and disease: Its role in the causation of fainting and convulsions. *Medicine* (Baltimore) 12:297, 1933.

172. Ferris EB Jr., Capps RB, Weiss S: Carotid sinus syncope and its bearing on the mechanism of the unconscious state and convulsions: A study of 32 additional cases. *Medicine* (Baltimore) 14:377, 1935.

173. Sigler LH: The cardioinhibitory carotid sinus reflex: Its importance as a vagocardiosensitivity test. *Am J Cardiol* 12:175, 1963.

174. Nathanson MH: Hyperactive cardioinhibitory carotid sinus reflex. *Arch Intern Med* 77:491, 1946.

175. Thomas JE: Hyperactive carotid sinus reflex and carotid sinus syncope. *Mayo Clin Proc* 44:127, 1969.

176. Harrington JF: Reversion of left-bundle-branch block to normal conduction by carotid-sinus pressure. *N Engl J Med* 277:37, 1977.

177. Asky JM: Hemiplegia following carotid sinus stimulation. *Am Heart J* 31:131, 1946.

178. Brannon ES: Hemiplegia following carotid sinus stimulation: Case report. *Am Heart J* 36:299, 1948.

179. Greenwood RJ, Dupler DA: Death following carotid sinus pressure. *JAMA* 181:605, 1962.

180. Hilal M, Massumi R: Fatal ventricular fibrillation after carotid-sinus stimulation. *N Engl J Med* 275:157, 1966.

181. Ask-Upmark E: Carotid sinus and the cerebral circulation: Anatomical, experimental and clinical investigation, including observations on rete mirabile caroticum. *Acta Psychiatr Scand* (Suppl) 6:1, 1935.

182. Gurdjian ES, Webster JE, Hardy WG, et al: Nonexistence of the so-called cerebral form of the carotid sinus syncope. *Neurology* (Minneap) 8:818, 1958.

183. Toole JF: Stimulation of the carotid sinus in man: I. The cerebral response; II. The significance of head positioning. *Am J Med* 27:952, 1959.

184. Greeley HP, Smedal MI, Most W: The treatment of the carotid-sinus syndrome by irradiation. *N Engl J Med* 252:91, 1955.

185. Salomon S: The carotid sinus syndrome. *Am J Cardiol* 2:342, 1958.

186. Cohen FL, Fruehan CT, Kind BB: Carotid sinus syndrome: Report of five cases and review of the literature. *J Neurosurg* 45:78, 1976.

187. Weiss S, Capps RB, Ferris EB Jr: Syncope and convulsions due to a hyperactive carotid sinus

220:1956, 1971.

reflex. *Arch Intern Med* 58:407, 1936.

188. Draper AJ: The cardioinhibitory carotid sinus syndrome. *Ann Intern Med* 32:700, 1950.

189. Bauernfeind R, Hall C, Denes P, et al: Carotid sinus hypersensitivity with alpha methyldopa. *Ann Intern Med* 88:214, 1978.

190. Reyes Al: Propranolol and the hyperactive carotid sinus reflex syndrome. *Br Med J* 2:662, 1973.

191. Walter PF, Crawley IS, Dorney ER: Carotid sinus hypersensitivity and syncope. *Am J Cardiol* 42:396, 1978.

192. Hartzler GO, Maloney JD: Cardioinhibitory carotid sinus hypersensitivity: Intracardiac recordings and clinical assessment. *Arch Intern Med* 137:727, 1977.

193. Bahl OP, Ferguson JB, Oliver GC, et al: Treatment of carotid sinus syncope with demand pacemaker. *Chest* 59:262, 1971.

194. VonMauer K, Nelson EW, Holsinger JW, et al: Hypersensitive carotid sinus syncope treated by implantable demand cardiac pacemaker. *Am J Cardiol* 29:109, 1972.

195. Thormann J, Schwarz F: Vagal role and pacemaker indication in hypersensitive carotid sinus reflex. *Eur J Cardiol* 3:47, 1975.

196. Herbert C, Zahn D, Ryan J, et al: Treatment of carotid sinus sensitivity by intracranial section of the glossopharyngeal nerve. *Trans Am Neurol Assoc* 68:29, 1942.

197. Ray BS, Stewart JH: Observations and surgical aspects of the carotid sinus reflex in man. *Surgery* 11:915, 1942.

198. Turner R, Learmonth JR: Carotid sinus syndrome: Case treated by bilateral denervation. *Lancet* 2:644, 1948.

199. Gardner RS, Magovern GJ, Park SB, et al: Carotid sinus syndrome: New surgical considerations. *Vasc Surg* 9:204, 1975.

200. Brown AM: Mechanoreceptors in or near the coronary arteries. *J Physiol* (London) 177:203, 1965.

201. Brown AM: The depressor reflex arising from the left coronary artery of the cat. *J Physiol* (London) 184:825, 1966.

202. Recordati G, Schwartz PJ, Pagani M, et al: Activation of cardiac vagal receptors during myocardial ischemia. *Experientia* 27:1423, 1971.

203. Thoren P: Left ventricular receptors activated by severe asphyxia and by coronary artery occlusion. *Acta Physiol Scand* 85:455, 1972.

204. Thoren P: Activation of left ventricular receptors with non-medullated vagal afferents during occlusion of a coronary artery in the cat. *Am J Cardiol* 37:1046, 1976.

205. Bosnjak ZJ, Zuperku EJ, Coon RL, et al: Acute coronary artery occlusion and cardiac sympathetic afferent nerve activity. *Proc Soc Exp Biol Med* 161:142, 1979.

206. Malliani A, Schwartz PJ, Zanchetti A: A sympathetic reflex elicited by experimental coronary occlusion. *Am J Physiol* (London) 217:703, 1969.

207. Weaver LC, Danos LM, Oehl RS, et al: Contrasting reflex influences of cardiac afferent nerves during coronary occlusion. *Am J Physiol* 240:H620, 1981.

208. Pelletier C: Vagal inhibitory effects on peripheral circulation in acute coronary occlusion. *Can J Pharmacol* 57:547 1979.

209. Constantin L: Extra cardiac factors contributing to hypotension during coronary occlusion. *Am J Cardiol* 11:205, 1963.

210. Chadda KD, Lichstein E, Gupta PK, et al: Bradycardia-hypotension syndrome in acute myocardial infarction. *Am J Med* 59:158, 1975.

211. Thames MD, Klopfenstein HS, Abboud FM, et al: Preferential disruption of inhibitory cardiac receptors with vagal afferents to the inferoposterior wall of the left ventricle activated during coronary occlusion in the dog. *Circ Res* 43:512, 1978.

212. Thames MD, Abboud FM: Reflex inhibition of renal sympathetic nerve activity during myocardial ischemia mediated by left ventricular receptors with vagal afferents in dogs. *J Clin Invest* 63:395, 1979.

213. Hanley HG, Raizner AE, Inglesby TV, et al: Response of the renal vascular bed to acute experimental coronary arterial occlusion. *Am J Physiol* 29:803, 1972.

214. Gorfinkel HJ, Szidon JP, Hirsch LJ, et al: Renal performance in experimental cardiogenic shock. *Am J Physiol* 222:1260, 1972.

215. Kezdi P, Kordenat RK, Mismara SN: Reflex inhibitory effects of vagal afferents in experimental myocardial infarction. *Am J Cardiol* 33:853, 1974.

216. Donald DF, Shepard JT: Cardiac receptors: normal and disturbed function. *Am J Cardiol* 44:873, 1979.

217. Perez-Gomez F, Garcia-Aquado A, Deios R, et al: Prinzmetal's angina: Reflex cardiovascular response during episode of pain. *Br Heart J* 42:81, 1979.

218. White JC: Cardiac pain: Anatomic pathways and physiologic mechanisms. *Circulation* 16:644, 1957.

219. Lindgren I, Olivecrona H: Surgical treatment of angina pectoris. *J Neurosurg* 4:19, 1947.

220. Wei JY, Markis JE, Malagold M, et al: Cardiovascular reflexes stimulated by perfusion of ischemic myocardium in acute myocardial infarction. *Circulation* 67:796, 1983.

221. George M, Greenwood TW: Relation between bradycardia and the site of myocardial infarction. *Lancet* 2:739, 1967.

222. Adgey AAJ, Geddes JS, Webb SW, et al: Acute phase of myocardial infarction. *Lancet* 2:501, 1971.

223. Webb SW, Adgey AA, Pantridge JF: Autonomic disturbance at onset of acute myocardial infarction. *Br Med J* 3:89, 1972.

224. Figueras J, Cinca J: Acute arterial hypertension during spontaneous angina in patients with fixed coronary stenosis and exertional angina: An associated rather than a triggering phenomenon. *Circulation* 64:60, 1981.

225. Guazzi M, Polese A, Fiorentini C, et al: Comparison between angina with ST-segment depression and angina with ST-segment elevation. *Br Heart J* 37:401, 1975.

226. Scheidt S, Wolk M, Killip T: Unstable angina pectoris natural history, hemodynamics, uncertainties of treatment and the ethics of clinical

study. *Am J Med* 60:409, 1976.

227. Figueras J, Singh BN, Ganz W, et al: Mechanisms of rest and nocturnal angina: observations during continuous hemodynamic and electrocardiographic monitoring. *Circulation* 59:955, 197ᵒ.

228. Dye LE, Urthaler F, MacLean WAH, et al: New arterial hypertension during myocardial infarction. *South Med J* 71:289, 1978.

229. Estafanous FG, Tarazi RC, Vilijoen JF, et al: Systemic hypertension following myocardial revascularization. *Am Heart J* 85:732, 1973.

230. Fouad FM, Estafanous FG, Tarazi RC: Hemodynamics of postmyocardial revascularization hypertension. *Am J Cardiol* 41:564, 1978.

231. Fouad FM, Estafanous FG, Gravo EL, et al: Possible role of cardioaortic reflexes in postcoronary bypass hypertension. *Am J Cardiol* 44:866, 1979.

232. Tarazi RC, Estafanous GF, Fouad FM: Unilateral stellate block in the treatment of hypertension after coronary bypass surgery. *Am J Cardiol* 42:1013, 1978.

233. Chaptal PA, Grolleau-Raoux D, Millet F: Les crises hypertensives dans la chirurgie de linsuffisance coronarienne. Prevention par le diazepam. *Ann Chir Thorac Cardiovasc* 14:255, 1975.

234. Viljoen JF, Estafanous FG, Tarazi RC: Acute hypertension immediately after coronary artery surgery. *J Thorac Cardiovasc Surg* 71:548, 1976.

235. Furukawa S, Hashimoto K, Hayakawa H, et al: Changes in bradykinogen bradykinin and bradykinase after experimental coronary artery ligation. (Abstr). *Jpn Circ J* 33:866, 1969.

236. Kimura E, Hashimoto K, Furukawa S, et al: Changes in bradykinin level in coronary sinus blood after the experimental occlusion of a coronary artery. *Am Heart J* 85:635, 1973.

237. Neto FR, Brasil JCF, Antonio A: Bradykinin induced coronary chemoreflex in the dog. *Naunyn-Schmiedeberg's Arch Pharmacol* 283:135, 1974.

238. Needleman P: The synthesis and function of prostaglandins in the heart. *Fed Proc* 35:2376, 1976.

239. Staszewska-Barezak J, Ferreira SH, Vane JR: An excitatory nociceptive cardiac reflex elicited by bradykinin and potentiated by prostaglandins and myocardial ischemia. *Cardiovasc Res* 10:314, 1976.

240. Beck PW, Handwerker HO: Bradykinin and serotonin effects on various types of cutaneous nerve fibers. *Pflugers Arch ges Physiol* 347:209, 1974.

241. Guilbaud G, LeBars D, Besson JM: Bradykinin as a tool in neurophysiological studies of pain mechanisms. In Bonica JJ, Albe-fessard D (eds): *Advances in Pain Research and Therapy.* New York, Raven Press, 1976, pp. 67–73.

242. Vogt A, Vetterlein F, et al: Excitation of afferent fibers in the cardiac sympathetic nerves induced by coronary occlusion and injection of bradykinin. The influence of acetylsalicylic acid and dipron. *Arch Int Pharmcodyn* 239:86, 1979.

243. Lewis GP: Kinins in inflammation and tissue injury. In *Handbook of Experimental Pharmacology.* New York, Springer-Verlag, 1970, pp. 516–530.

244. Berger HJ, Zaret BL, Speroff L, et al: Regional cardiac prostaglandin release during myocardial ischemia in anesthetized dogs. *Circ Res* 38:566,

1976.

245. Berger HJ, Zaret BL, Speroff L, et al: Cardiac prostaglandin release during myocardial ischemia induced by atrial pacing in patients with coronary artery disease. *Am J Cardiol* 39:481, 1977.

246. Alexander RW, Kent KM, Pisano JJ, et al: Regulation of canine coronary blood flow by endogenously synthesized prostaglandins. (Abstr). *Circulation* (Suppl). IV:107, 1973.

247. Kraemer RJ, Phernelton TM, Folts JD: Prostaglandin-like substances in coronary venous blood following myocardial ischemia. *J Pharm Exp Ther* 199:611, 1976.

248. Ogawa K, Ito T, Enomoto I, et al: Increase of coronary flow and levels of PGE, and PGF_2 from the ischemic area of experimental myocardial infarction. *Adv Prostaglandin Thromboxane* 7:665, 1980.

249. Chierchia S, Decaterina R, Brunelli C, et al: Low dose aspirin prevents thromboxane A_2 synthesis by platelets but not attacks of Prinzmetal's angina. (Abstr). *Circulation* 62:III, 1980.

250. Koss MC, Nakamo J: Reflex bradycardia and hypotension produced by prostaglandin F_2 in the cat. *Br J Pharmacol* 56:245, 1976.

251. Roberts AM, Coleridge JCG, Coleridge HM, et al: Prostacyclin stimulates vagal C-fibers with chemosensitive endings in the heart. (Abstr). *Fed Proc* 39:839, 1980.

252. Hintze TH, Martin EG, Messina EJ, et al: Prostacyclin (PGI_2) elicits reflex bradycardia in dogs: evidence for vagal mediation. *Proc Soc Exp Biol Med* 162:96, 1979.

253. Hintze TH, Panzenbeck MJ, Messina EJ, et al: Prostacyclin (PGI_2) lowers heart rate in the conscious dog. *Cardiovasc Res* 15:538, 1981.

254. Chapple DJ, Dusting GJ, Hughes R, et al: Some direct and reflex cardiovasc actions of prostacyclin (PGI_2) and prostaglandin E_2 in anaesthetized dogs. *Br J Pharmacol* 68:437, 1980.

255. Baker DG, Nerdrum T, Coleridge HM, et al: Potentiating role of prostaglandin E, in the action of bradykinin on sympathetic afferent endings in the heart. (Abstr). *Fed Proc* 37:701, 1978.

256. Block AJ, Poole S, Vane JR: Modification of basal release of prostaglandins from rabbit isolated hearts. *Prostaglandins* 7:473, 1974.

257. Wennmalon A, Chanh PH, Justad M: Hypoxia causes prostaglandin release from perfused rabbit hearts. *Acta Physiol Scand* 91:133, 1974.

258. Mark AL, Abboud FM, Heistad DD, et al: Evidence against the presence of ventricular chemoreceptors activated by hypoxia and hypercapnia. *Am J Physiol* 227:178, 1974.

259. Longhurst JC, Zelis R: Cardiovascular responses to local hindlimb hypoxemia, relation to the exercise reflex. *Am J Physiol* 237:H359, 1979.

260. Smith JB, Ingerman C, Koesis JJ, et al: Formation of prostaglandins during the aggregation of human blood platelets. *J Clin Invest* 52:965, 1973.

261. Eckstein RW, Shintani F, Rowen HE Jr., et al: Identification of left coronary blood supply of aortic bodies in anesthetized dogs. *J Appl Physiol* 30:488, 1971.

262. James TN, Isobe JH, Urthaler F: Analysis of com-

ponents in cardiogenic hypertensive chemoreflex. *Circulation* 52:179, 1975.

263. Hageman GR, Urthaler F, James TN: Neural pathways of a cardiogenic hypertensive chemoreflex. *Am J Physiol* 235:H345, 1978.

264. Urthaler F, Hageman GR, James TN: Hemodynamic components of a cardiogenic hypertensive chemoreflex in dogs. *Circ Res* 42:135, 1978.

265. Parker RE, Strandhoy JW: A vasoconstrictor cardiogenic chemoreflex induced by prostaglandin F$_{2\alpha}$. *Am J Physiol* 240:H528, 1981.

266. Coleridge HM, Coleridge JCG, Howe A: A search for pulmonary arterial chemoreceptors in the cat, with a comparison of the blood supply of the aortic bodies with newborn and adult animal. *J Physiol* (London) 191:353, 1967.

267. Zucker IH, Peterson TV, Gilmore JP: Ouabain increases left atrial stretch receptor discharge in the dog. *J Pharmacol Exp Ther* 212:320, 1980.

268. Hamberg M, Samuelsson B: Prostaglandin endoperoxides VII. Novel transformations of arachidonic acid in guinea pig lung. *Biochem Biophys Res Commun* 61:942, 1974.

269. Zucker IH, Gilmore JP: Left atrial receptor discharge during atrial arrhythmias in the dog. *Circ Res* 33:672, 1973.

270. Wood P: Polyuria in paroxysmal tachycardia and paroxysmal atrial flutter and fibrillation. *Br Heart J* 25:273, 1963.

271. Schwartz PJ, Snebold NG, Brown AM: Effects of unilateral cardiac sympathetic denervation on the ventricular fibrillation threshold. *Am J Cardiol* 37:1034, 1976.

272. Kliks BR, Burgess MJ, Abildskov JA: Influence of sympathetic tone on ventricular fibrillation threshold during experimental coronary occlusion. *Am J Cardiol* 36:45, 1975.

273. Armour JA, Hageman GR, Randall WC: Arrhythmias induced by local cardiac nerve stimulation. *Am J Physiol* 223:1068, 1972.

274. Hageman GR, Goldberg JM, Armour JA: Cardiac dysrhythmias induced by autonomic nerve stimulation. *Am J Cardiol* 32:823, 1973.

275. Schwartz PJ, Malliani A: Electrical alternation of the T-wave: clinical and experimental evidence of its relationship with the sympathetic nervous system and with the long Q-T syndrome. *Am Heart J* 89:378, 1975.

276. Schwartz PJ, Foreman RD, Stone HL, Brown AM: Effect of dorsal root section on the arrhythmias associated with coronary occlusion. *Am J Physiol* 231:923, 1976.

277. Stein M, Schwartz R, Mirsky IA: The antidiuretic activity of plasma of patients with hepatic cirrhosis, congestive heart failure, hypertension, and other clinical disorders. *J Clin Invest* 33:77, 1954.

278. Yamane Y: Plasma ADH level in patients with chronic congestive heart failure. *Jpn Circ J* 32:745, 1968.

279. Zucker IH, Earle AM, Gilmore JP: The mechanism of adaptation of left atrial stretch receptors in dogs with chronic congestive heart failure. *J Clin Invest* 60:323, 1977.

280. Greenberg TT, Richmond WH, Stocking RA, et

al: Impaired atrial receptor responses in dogs with heart failure due to tricuspid insufficiency and pulmonary artery stenosis. *Circ Res* 32:424, 1973.

281. Aujuchovskij EP, Beloshepico GG, Yasinovskuya FP: Characteristics of atrial mechanoreceptor and elastic feature following heart failure. *Sechenov Physiol J USSR* 62:1210, 1976.

282. Zehr JE, Hawe A, Isakiris AG, et al: ADH levels following nonhypotensive hemorrhage in dogs with chronic mitral stenosis. *Am J Physiol* 221:312, 1971.

283. Zucker IH, Earle AM, Gilmore JP: Changes in sensitivity of left atrial receptors following reversal of heart failure. *Am J Physiol* 237:H555, 1979.

284. Zucker IH, Gilmore JP: Atrial receptor modulation of renal function in heart failure. In Abboud FM, Fozzard HA, Gilmore JP, Reis DJ (eds): *Disturbances in Neurogenic Control of the Circulation.* Bethesda, American Physiological Society, 1981, pp. 1–16.

285. Sleight P, Lall A, Muers M: Reflex cardiovascular effects of epicardial stimulation by acetylstrophanthidin in dogs. *Circ Res* 25:705, 1969.

286. Thames MD: Acetylstrophanthidin-induced reflex inhibition of canine renal sympathetic nerve activity mediated by cardiac receptors with vagal afferents. *Circ Res* 44:8, 1979.

287. Thames MD, Waickman LA, Abboud FM: Sensitization of cardiac receptors (vagal afferents) by intracoronary acetylstrophanthidin. *Am J Physiol* 239:H628, 1980.

288. Watkins L Jr., Burton JP, Haber E, et al: The renin angiotensin-aldosterone system in congestive failure in conscious dogs. *J Clin Invest* 57:1606, 1976.

289. Thames MD, Schmid PG: Cardiopulmonary receptors with vagal afferents tonically inhibit ADH release in the dog. *Am J Physiol* 237:H299, 1979.

290. Abboud FM, Thames MD, Mark AL: Role of cardiac afferent nerves in regulation of circulation during coronary occlusion and heart failure. In Abboud FM, Fozzard HA, Gilmore JP, Rees DJ (eds): *Disturbances in Neurological Control of the Circulation.* Bethesda, American Physiological Society, 1981, pp. 65–86.

291. Chidsey CA, Harrison DC, Braunwald E: Augmentation of the plasma norepinephrine response to exercise in patients with congestive heart failure. *N Engl J Med* 267:650, 1962.

292. DeChamplain J, Boucher R, Genest J: Arterial angiotensin levels in edematous patients. *Proc Soc Exp Biol Med* 113:932, 1963.

293. Genest JP, Granger P, Champlain JD, et al: Endocrine factors in congestive heart failure. *Am J Cardiol* 22:35, 1968.

294. Levine TB, Gross KA, Cohn JN: Sympathetic and renin response to orthostasis in congestive heart failure. (Abstr.) *Am J Cardiol* 45:433, 1980.

295. Mark AL, Kioschos MJ, Abbound MF, et al: Abnormal vascular responses to exercise in patients with aortic stenosis. *J Clin Invest* 52:1138, 1973.

296. Mark AL, Abboud FM, Schmid PG, et al: Cardiovascular responses to left ventricular outflow obstruction and activation of ventricular baroreceptors in dogs. *J Clin Invest* 52:1147, 1973.

CHAPTER 4

RECENT ADVANCES IN BALLOON COUNTERPULSATION

DAVID BREGMAN, M.D.

In 1981 it was estimated that 1.5 million Americans sustained an acute myocardial infarction.[1] In the same year more than 100,000 cardiac surgical procedures were performed.[1] The development of direct techniques for coronary revascularization has resulted in a multitude of critically ill patients requiring open heart surgery. In an effort to deal with the increasing numbers of patients who present with the many complicated patterns of coronary artery or valvular heart disease, or both, and require urgent open heart surgery, a spectrum of cardiac support measures, ranging from simple pharmacological maneuvers to a variety of mechanical assist devices, have been devised.

Temporary mechanical assist devices that employ the principle of arterial counterpulsation have met with the most consistent clinical success.[2] Early cardiogenic shock has been reversed, coronary catheterization and anesthetic induction have been carried out in acutely ill patients with coronary insufficiency syndromes, and patients undergoing cardiotomy have been successfully freed from the extracorporeal pump with the help of these devices.

The concept of counterpulsation, which forms the basis for intra-aortic balloon pumping (IABP), was first described by Harken in 1958.[3] As originally proposed, blood removed from the body via the femoral artery during ventricular systole was rapidly reinfused during diastole to augment coronary perfusion pressure. By this method, in the normotensive preparation, one could decrease left ventricular work while increasing coronary blood flow. However, the prolonged use of this form of circulatory support was limited because of excessive hemolysis. Furthermore, bilateral femoral arteriotomies were required and in the hypotensive state counterpulsation via the femoral route was shown to produce no increase in coronary blood flow.[4]

In 1962, Moulopoulos et al.[5] suggested the use of an intra-aortic balloon (IAB) positioned in the descending thoracic aorta to accomplish the same purpose as external counterpulsation but without the drawbacks. The balloon was inflated in diastole at the closure of the aortic valve, augmenting coronary perfusion. With the onset of systole the balloon collapsed, creating a "vacuum" effect, which decreased left ventricular afterload. After a hiatus of 7 years, Kantrowitz et al.[6] reported the first successful clinical application of the IAB in a patient with cardiogenic shock.

The findings that counterpulsation decreased the extent and severity of ischemic injury[7-10] and opened dormant coronary collateral vessels[11] were intriguing. These facts suggested to others that perhaps counterpulsation should be considered not only in patients with cardiogenic shock, but also early in the course of patients sustaining uncomplicated infarcts, to minimize the quantity of myocardium that ultimately becomes necrotic.[12]

However, in spite of its acceptance, indications for IABP remain unclear and continue to evolve as experience accumulates. Although initially employed in patients with cardiogenic shock, careful follow-up of such patients showed that mortality was largely unaltered.[2] Nevertheless, application of the IAB has expanded to prophylactic management of patients with mild-to-moderate hemodynamic decompensation. At the present time, IABP is widely used for circulatory support in patients with postoperative left ventricular failure, unstable angina refractory to medical treatment, and recurrent myocardial ischemia following acute myocardial infarction.

Conventional insertion of the IAB devices requires surgical exposure of the common femoral artery and end-to-side anastomosis of a prosthetic graft to the artery with vascular surgical techniques. Subsequent removal of the balloon necessitates a second surgical procedure that requires either oversewing or removal of the graft. Most clinical series estimated that complications occurred in 20% of patients undergoing conventional IABP.[13-24] However, necropsy evaluation suggests that the actual complication rate is much higher and most mishaps occurred as a result of device insertion.[25]

A single-chambered 40-cc percutaneous IAB has been constructed around a central guidewire.[26] The balloon can be furled around the guidewire enabling percutaneous insertion into the femoral artery through a 12 F (French) sheath by the Seldinger technique. Volume displacement and hemodynamic augmentation are similar to that produced by the standard IAB. Percutaneous balloon insertion requires approximately 5 to 10 minutes and has been successfully performed in the cardiac catheterization laboratory, coronary care unit, operating suite, and recovery room. From early clinical experience it appears that complications related to balloon insertion are reduced by the percutaneous approach.

Thus, circulatory support can now be safely and rapidly instituted by any physician familiar with the Seldinger technique.

TECHNIQUE OF PERCUTANEOUS INTRA-AORTIC BALLOON INSERTION AND REMOVAL

Employing the Seldinger method,[27] the percutaneous intra-aortic balloon is inserted utilizing the following technique: After the inguinal region is prepared and draped, the common femoral artery is punctured with a standard 18-gauge arterial needle, and a 0.038-inch (0.097 cm), J-tip guidewire is introduced through the needle. After removal of the needle, an 8 F dilator is passed over the guidewire to predilate the subcutaneous tissues and the arterial puncture site. The dilator is then exchanged for a 12 F dilator-sheath combination, which is advanced over the guidewire into the artery. To control hemorrhage, 1 inch of the sheath is left exposed.

The percutaneous balloon is then prepared in the following manner: The balloon is moistened in saline solution and furled while an assistant holds the distal tip of the balloon catheter immobile. The deflated balloon is furled by wrapping it around the balloon catheter, starting at the distal end and proceeding proximally (Fig. 4.1). Any air remaining in the balloon is completely evacuated with a syringe and stopcock. The guidewire and 12 F dilator are then removed, leaving the 12 F sheath in place. Bleeding is controlled by firmly compressing the exposed sheath. The furled balloon is then inserted through the sheath (Fig. 4.2) and positioned under fluoroscopy in the descending thoracic aorta. After removal of the stopcock, the balloon catheter is attached to the pumping console and intra-aortic pumping is initiated. If resistance is encountered in passage through the aorto-iliac bifuraction, the catheter can be rotated, but no force is imparted lest dissection occur. The appropriate length of catheter to be inserted may be estimated by placing the catheter on the patient's abdomen and chest with the tip 1 cm below the angle of Louis marking the catheter at the end of the 12 F

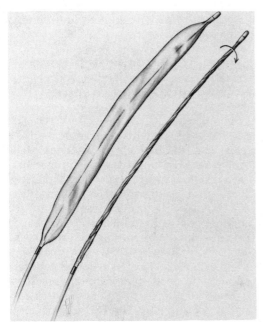

Figure 4.1. IAB furled for percutaneous insertion.

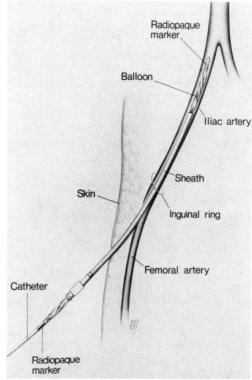

Figure 4.2. The Safety guidewire and 12 F dilator have been removed leaving 12 F sheath *in situ* through which furled percutaneous IAB is passed into descending thoracic aorta.

intravascular sheath. Sometimes the tip of the catheter may be felt against the aortic arch and the catheter is withdrawn about 1 inch outward so that the tip will lie just below the left subclavian artery. Correct inflation and deflation of the balloon may be confirmed with fluoroscopic visualization. The 12 F sheath and balloon catheter are ligated with umbilical tape to prevent bleeding around the catheter, and a sterile dressing is applied to the sheath and balloon catheter assembly. Management of patients on the IABP has been described elsewhere.[28]

Before removal of the balloon catheter, the balloon is completely collapsed by aspiration with a syringe. The balloon is pulled down to (but not into) the sheath. The femoral artery immediately distal to the balloon is tightly compressed and the balloon and sheath are then removed as a unit. Blood is allowed to spurt from the artery for a few seconds and the compression is shifted over the puncture site for 30 minutes. Distal pulses are monitored with a Doppler apparatus and manual compression is adjusted so that an audible pulse is registered. A compression dressing is affixed

to the puncture site for 24 hours. Weaning from percutaneous IABP is accomplished in the same manner as previously described for the standard IAB pump.[29]

The other balloon designs have become available and are currently being used. One is a 10.5 F percutaneous balloon with automatic wrapping. The others are the Percor-DL and DL II, both with an inner lumen to facilitate balloon insertion and which gives the operator the ability to monitor central aortic pressure through the balloon catheter. Our initial experience with these balloons has been satisfactory.[30, 31]

A long (45-cm) 12 F sheath-dilator combination (Fig. 4.3) which extends up to the descending aorta and protects the iliac artery and aorta from injury during insertion of the balloon catheter may also be em-

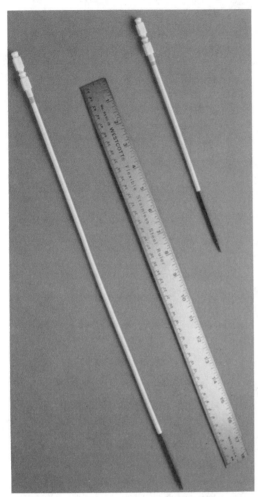

Figure 4.3. Two 12 F dilator-sheath combinations are shown which are used for percutaneous IAB catheter insertion. The long (45-cm) sheath is compared to the standard (15-cm) sheath.

ployed.[32] In patients with severe acute myocardial ischemia in whom insertion of IAB catheters is not possible by the conventional percutaneous technique, use of the long sheath approach permits rapid institution of circulatory support. Placement of the IAB using the long sheath technique is performed in a manner similar to conventional percutaneous balloon insertion. However, following proper positioning of the balloon and catheter in the descending thoracic aorta, the long sheath is withdrawn into the iliac artery to allow complete unfurling of the balloon membrane.

CLINICAL EXPERIENCE WITH PERCUTANEOUS INTRA-AORTIC BALLOON INSERTION

Percutaneous IAB insertion was attempted in 133 patients from February 1979 to July 1982 at Columbia Presbyterian Medical Center (Table 4.1). Successful insertion was accomplished in 120 of 133 patients (90%). In 10 patients the initial insertion attempt failed. However, four of the 10 patients eventually underwent successful IAB implantation by the long insertion technique.

Ten of the 120 patients required counterpulsation for end-stage cardiomyopathies. Of these 10 patients, three underwent cardiac transplantation. The IAB was percutaneously inserted for preoperative pump failure in one and acute rejection in the other two. All three succumbed and the overall mortality of the 10 patients was 100% despite circulatory assist.

If patients with cardiomyopathies are excluded, then 123 patients required IAB counterpulsation for ischemic myocardial dysfunction. Insertion was successful in 110 of 123 patients. Indications in these patients were broadly divided among medical and surgical groups. Of the 110 patients, 47 received the IAB for a surgical indication. Surgical indications were intraoperative low cardiac output in 45, and cardiac arrest in two. Medical indications for counterpulsation included unstable angina in 20, postinfarction angina in 17, cardiogenic shock in nine, acute ventricular septal defect complicating myocardial infarction in four, recurrent ventricular tachycardia in one, and three unsuccessful Gruntzig procedures. When hemodynamic decompensation occurred in the three patients undergoing transluminal angioplasty, the IAB was inserted and emergency coronary revascularization was carried out. The patients subsequently were discharged from the hospital. Only one patient received the IAB prophylactically for unstable angina prior to a general surgical procedure. This patient sur-

Table 4.1

Successful Percutaneous IAB Pump Insertion at Columbia Presbyterian Medical Center (Excluding Patients with Cardiomyopathies)

PERCUTANEOUS IABP
Columbia Presbyterian – St. Josephs Medical Center
1979–1982

	SUCCESSFUL INSERTIONS	CCU	Cath Lab
PREOP	Unstable angina with general surgery	1	—
	Unstable angina with cardiac surgery	9	7
	Unstable angina — treated with medication	2(1)	1
	Postinfarction angina — treated with medication	1	4(1)
	Postinfarction angina with surgery	10(1)	2
	Cardiogenic shock — treated with medication	2	3(2)
	Cardiogenic shock with surgery	1	3(1)
	Recurrent ventricular tachycardia — medication	1	—
	Failed Gruntzig Procedure with emergency surgery	—	3
	Acute VSD with surgery	1	2(1)
	Acute VSD without surgery	—	1(1)
	Anesthesia support for open heart surgery	1	8
PERIOP	Low output — OR	36(21)	
POSTOP	Low output	9(4)	
	Cardiac arrest	2(1)	

Total Number Assisted — **110**

Total Number Discharged — **76(69%)**

(parentheses indicate number of deaths)

vived and the balloon was removed in the immediate postoperative period.

The location of the balloon insertion varied. Thirty-six patients had the balloon implanted in the operating room, 11 in the open heart recovery room, 34 in the cardiac catheterization laboratory, and 29 in the cardiac care unit.

Of the 63 patients in whom the IAB was successfully inserted for a medical indication, 48 (76%) eventually underwent a cardiac surgical procedure whereas 15 were treated medically. Only three of the 48 patients undergoing preoperative IAB support combined with definitive surgical procedures died. In contrast, 26 of 47 patients (55%) requiring intraoperative or postoperative IAB died.

Complications of percutaneous IAB insertion occurred in 15 of the 120 patients (12.5%). However, only one guidewire perforation of the aorta occurred as a result of insertion of the device. Complications related to balloon use and removal included femoral thrombi in five patients, asymptomatic iliac occlusion in one, and one weak dorsalis pedis pulses.

There were no false aneurysms, aortic dissections, or septic complications in this series. However, extensive necropsy examination was not performed.

Four patients in whom percutaneous IAB insertion by conventional approach was unsuccessful underwent successful balloon implantion by the long insertion technique. There were no insertion-related complications in these patients. One patient had an improperly positioned IAB which intermittently occluded the origin of the superior mesenteric artery. The resulting abdominal pain was relieved upon advancing the balloon to its correct position.[33]

PERIOPERATIVE INTRA-AORTIC BALLOON PUMPING

Only recently has it been realized that death from acute cardiac failure soon after cardiac operations is related to new and often extensive perioperative myocardial necrosis.[34] Thus, despite the low mortality associated with open heart surgery, a substantial number of patients are unable to be weaned from cardiopulmonary bypass or develop low cardiac output syndrome in the early postoperative period. Myocardial failure was found to occur in 4% of all bypass operations performed at the Massachusetts General Hospital since 1971.[13] McEnany et al.,[13] reported in their review of 728 cases of IABP that the most common indication for balloon insertion was cardiac failure following open heart surgery. Of those patients assisted with the IAB, 54.2% survived. Seventy-three percent of the cases of perioperative IABP were for coronary artery disease, while 24.4% were for patients who had undergone valve replacement. Of note is the fact that of the fatalities, 79% occurred in the operating room, while only 21% took place during the duration for balloon counterpulsation.

The most successful clinical application of the IAB has been in helping to wean those patients from cardiopulmonary bypass in whom intraoperative myocardial ischemia or necrosis precludes autonomous perfusion. It is believed that the balloon acts as a temporizing device, supporting the patient at lower levels of myocardial work and oxygen demands, while ischemia is reversed by augmented coronary perfusion. Although perioperative IABP may reduce the occurrence of myocardial ischemia during induction of anesthesia and performance of an operation, it cannot compensate for inadequate surgical treatment. Thus, surgical re-establishment of coronary perfusion is essential. Most cardiac surgeons now believe that the availability of a balloon pump in a center performing open heart surgery should be mandatory.

In high-risk cardiac surgical patients undergoing open heart surgery in whom an IAB was not inserted before anesthetic induction, it is recommended that femoral artery access be obtained with an arterial needle and guidewire, which are maintained in the sterile operative field. If IABP is subsequently required for separation from cardiopulmonary bypass, arterial access is then already established for IABP insertion.

CARDIOGENIC SHOCK

The outlook of patients in cardiogenic shock is largely unaltered by conventional counterpulsation techniques. There is no reason to expect an improved prognosis with conversion to the percutaneous approach, as circulatory hemodynamics are unchanged. However, some evidence is available which suggests that earlier institution of counterpulsation may enhance survival of patients with cardiac pump failure.

Ischemic damage to the myocardium may be sublethal and reversible or more intense and prolonged, resulting in cell death. It is exceedingly difficult to define the boundaries which separate reversible from irreversible injury. Thus, the injured and failing heart exists along a continuum of progressive decompensation. Presumably, there is a point of time when the stressed myocardium still has the potential for recovery. By lowering the pressure against which the ventricle must expel its volume and decreasing the pressure within the ventricle itself, the IAB reduces the workload of the ailing heart. In addition, the inadequate perfusion of the brain, heart, and kidneys is augmented by counterpulsation with further reduction in myocardial work and oxygen consumption. Consequently, available chemical energy is diverted to synthetic and reparative cellular processes and the injured heart is allowed to recuperate.

In practice, it is recommended that circulatory support be instituted in all patients afflicted with cardiogenic shock, those who are refractory to maximal medical therapy.

Subsequently, such patients are subjected to coronary angiography and cardiac catheterization. If contrast studies reveal a surgically amendable lesion, corrective operation is carried out. Survival following coronary revascularization in these patients has been reported to approach 50%.[13]

PREOPERATIVE INTRA-AORTIC BALLOON PUMPING

Preoperative IABP in high-risk patients undergoing cardiac catheterization, in patients with unstable angina, and in patients with angina following an acute myocardial infarction has been successfully employed. The rapidity of insertion makes the percutaneously inserted balloon most useful in supporting patients with an acute coronary ischemic syndrome.

In patients with refractory angina after acute myocardial infarction, the risks of coronary arteriography are increased (38%). In this group of patients, the IAB may be inserted percutaneously in the catheterization laboratory prior to coronary arteriography. This approach allows the patient to be safely guided through the angiographic study. In addition, the balloon may be left in place to provide circulatory support during induction of anesthesia and in the perioperative period. Thus, a patient who has evidence of either a significant degree of left ventricular failure, ventricular tachyarrhythmia, or one of the acute mechanical complications of myocardial infarction can be carried through cardiac catheterization without significant risk.[36-40]

Rapid percutaneous insertion of the IAB is particularly useful in patients experiencing severe myocardial ischemia or acute myocardial infarction during coronary arteriography. In these patients the coronary catheter can be rapidly exchanged for the balloon through the same puncture site in the femoral artery. In patients experiencing acute myocardial infarction during placement and pumping, the balloon can rapidly reverse cardiogenic shock and support the patient during emergency revascularization and in the postoperative period.

Some patients continue to have severe angina after infarction despite aggressive medical therapy and are candidates for coronary artery bypass surgery. Good surgical results have been achieved in such patients with reduced operative mortality.[41,42] Some authors have attributed this reduction in mortality to the liberal use of postinfarction IABP.[12,41,42] On the contrary, Brundage et al.[42] infrequently use the IAB pump in the management of postinfarction angina. Only three of their 30 patients (10%) required IABP. They advocate the use of IABP only to control hemodynamic instability, not to control angina.

In our experience and that of others, the majority of patients with unstable angina or postinfarction angina survive with intra-aortic balloon pumping.[44,45] Amsterdam et al.[43] found patients with unstable angina or postinfarction angina who underwent preoperative counterpulsation had survival rates of 78% and 100%, respectively. Of the patients in our series undergoing preoperative IABP for a medical indication, ultimately 90% were discharged from the hospital. However, no data exist which suggest that the duration of counterpulsation effects outcome. Seventy-seven percent of our patients initially assisted with the IAB for a medical indication eventually underwent a cardiac surgical procedure. Therefore, it is likely that surgery, itself, improves survival of patients receiving preoperative balloon assistance. In summary, what is truly needed is a randomized, carefully controlled, prospective trial to determine whether preoperative balloon counterpulsation in patients with either unstable angina or postinfarction angina effects ultimate survival. What is clear to us as well as to many cardiologists and cardiac surgions throughout the world is that such patients dramatically improve when IABP is commenced.

VENTRICULAR IRRITABILITY

The increase in coronary blood flow associated with IABP, as well as the decrease in myocardial wall tension secondary to acute reduction in left ventricular afterload may be beneficial in treating ventricular irritability associated with myocardial infarction. Mundth and associates[45,46] have indicated that life-threatening ventricular irritability in the early postinfarction phase resistant to a maximal medical regimen may be initially controlled with counterpulsation.

More recently, Hanson et al.[48] reported on 22 patients with medically refractory ventricular irritability after myocardial infarction who underwent IABP. Overall survival was 12 of 22 patients (55%) and survival of surgical patients was seven of 15 (47%). Survival decreased with the extent of coronary artery disease. Increased survival was seen in those patients who, after institution of IABP, had complete reversal of ischemic chest pain and in those in whom IABP could be discontinued without requiring emergency surgery. They concluded that when ventricular irritability persists in the face of maximum medical treatment, mortality is exceptionally high. In this group of high-risk patients, the ability of IABP to influence the myocardial oxygen supply/demand ratio and to reverse ischemia may improve or control ventricular irritability in the majority of such patients.

HIGH-RISK CARDIAC PATIENTS REQUIRING MAJOR NONCARDIAC SURGERY

A few reports in the literature have suggested the use of IABP in high-risk cardiac patients requiring major noncardiac surgery. Investigators have reported the use of the IABP in high-risk cardiac patients undergoing emergency gastrectomy[49] for other major abdominal surgery,[50] and in the peripartum cardiomyopathy.[51]

INTRA-AORTIC BALLOON PUMP FOR CARDIAC ARREST

Conventional balloon insertion is not feasible during resuscitation because of the time required for surgical insertion. Because percutaneous insertion can be instituted in several minutes without interfering with resuscitative efforts or closed chest massage, this approach can be used to provide mechanical circulatory support during resuscitation. In one of our patients, the IAB was inserted during closed chest cardiac massage

for treatment of cardiac arrest. The patient survived and left the hospital. Percutaneous insertion of the IAB can be performed at the bedside and may be most useful in patients for whom prolonged resuscitative efforts are anticipated. Time and further inquiry will delineate the safe and effective realm of IABP for this application.

MYOCARDIAL CONTUSION

Myocardial contusion complicates approximately 20% of cases of blunt anterior thoracic wall trauma.[52] Steering-wheel injuries are the most prevalent cause of myocardial contusion.

One of the important physiological consequences associated with severe myocardial contusion is decreased cardiac output. Proper treatment may be a major determinant of survival. While clinical IABP therapy for myocardial contusion has yet to be reported in the literature, Saunders and Doty[51] have applied this technique in dogs with experimentally induced myocardial contusion. The results of their study indicate IABP improves left ventricular performance following myocardial contusion, especially when applied early after injury.

CIRCULATORY SUPPORT IN HEART TRANSPLANT CANDIDATES

Cardiac transplantation was performed on five patients who had IABP instituted preoperatively, but could not be weaned from mechanical support and for whom no conventional operation was possible. A sixth patient while waiting for transplantation, required the insertion of an IAB when his condition suddenly deteriorated. Of these six cases, five survived the immediate postoperative period, two died within five months, and three survived into the 2nd year.[53,54]

Intra-Aortic Balloon Pumping in the Community Hospital Setting

In the medical setting, IABP has generally been a prelude to cardiac catheterization and open heart surgery. With the advent of coronary care units, many patients with acute ischemia and mechanical complications of myocardial infarction are being cared for in community hospitals. Accordingly, several community hospitals have purchased IABP equipment and have begun to insert IABs in selected patients in their coronary care units.[13,55-57] These hospitals have formed a liason with a major university center, where patients may be transferred for definitive therapy.

McEnany et al.[13] have reported that 32 of their 728 IABPs were started at peripheral community hospitals. Patients were transported to the Massachusetts General Hospital with a functioning balloon in place.

Recently, Bass et al.[52] reported on their use of IABP in a private 280-bed hospital. After thorough training of the nursing and support staff, they were able to report a survival rate of 44%, comparable to that of major centers. Hines et al.[55] inserted the IAB in 27 patients in cardiogenic shock secondary to myocardial infarction. Seventeen of these survived hospitalization and 12 were long-term survivors.

The use of IABP in noncardiac surgical centers has permitted hemodynamic support in the critically ill, safety in angiography, appropriate selection of patients for surgery, and safe transportation to a cardiac surgical center when indicated.

COMPLICATIONS OF INTRA-AORTIC BALLOON PUMPING

Initial clinical experience suggests that the vascular complications associated with conventional surgical IAB insertion may be diminished by use of the percutaneous technique.[26] Most previous reports of balloon-related complications of patients have indicated complication resulted from obstruction to the arteries supplying blood to the legs; less frequently, insertion of the device has been cited as the primary etiological factor. However, in a necropsy study of balloon-related complications, 60% resulted from conventional surgical insertion of the balloon.[25] Whether the complications result primarily from obstruction of the arteries to the legs or insertion of the device, the ultimate determinant of the balloon-related complication in most patients is the status of the native arteries.[25]

Several efforts have been directed at ameliorating complications of balloon use and insertion. Perhaps the most promising of these efforts has been the introduction of the percutaneous approach to balloon insertion, which obviated the need for surgical insertion and removal. Aorto-iliofemoral angiography, Doppler monitoring, or both have been recommended to assess more optimally the distal arteries housing the device.[58,59] The addition of a central lumen to the IAB catheter to allow pressure monitoring or guidewire placement has also helped to avoid complications related to balloon insertion.[22] To maneuver around a tortuous segment of the aortoiliac axis or negotiate passage through an eccentric arterial stenosis, the catheter tip may be bent and rotated into a modified J tip.[60]

Complication occurred in 12.5% of our patients undergoing percutaneous balloon insertion.[61] In contrast to our experience, Harvey et al.[60] evaluated complications of percutaneous balloon pumping in 71 consecutive patients and found the number and magnitude of complications were comparable to their prior experience with conventional IAB insertion. They concluded that ease of insertion alone did not justify liberalizing indications for percutaneous IABP among patients who can be managed effectively without counterpulsation.

Complications of percutaneous IABP have been classified by Subramanian et al.,[61] into major and minor types and further subdivided into immediate and delayed. Minor complications include malposition of the balloon in the ascending aorta, delay of difficulty in unfurling the balloon within the aortic lumen, transient bacteremia, and transient loss of the dorsalis pedis pulse following percutaneous removal of the device. Major complications were those associated with hemorrhage at the attempted puncture site, renal embolism, dissection of the aortoiliac axis, ischemic extremities, or balloon-related death. In their series of 71 patients undergoing percutaneous balloon insertion, limb ischemia without limb loss occurred in nine, hemorrhage at the puncture site in two, aortic dissection in two, renal embolism in one, and pseudoaneurysm at the insertion site in one. Asymptomatic loss of pedal pulses occurred in six patients. Malpositioning in the ascending aorta, which was encountered in two patients, and failure of the balloon to unwrap, which occurred in 10 patients, were successfully treated by repositioning of the device.

Bemis et al.,[44] reported a complication rate of 5% in a group of 44 patients in whom the IAB had been percutaneously implanted. Complications of percutaneous IAB implantation were found in 18.5% of 33 patients by Amsterdam et al.[43] Insertion-related complications were not separated from complications occurring with balloon use and removal. This represents a substantial reduction in insertion-related complications, however, none of our patients were subjected to an extensive necropsy analysis. Thus, percutaneous insertion of the IAB seems to diminish insertion-related complications. In contrast, complications associated with use and removal of the balloon are not decreased by percutaneous insertion.

SUMMARY

The IAB has been assigned a major role in supporting the injured myocardium. Indications for balloon placement have greatly expanded. Unfortunately, in many ways, the evolution of these indications has been sprawling and unplanned. Numerous case reports and uncontrolled, nonrandomized trials document the balloon's efficacy. Thus, despite its theoretical attractiveness, there is still no conclusive evidence that patients with mild to moderate hemodynamic decompensation require counterpulsation. Consequently, many questions remain unanswered.

Nevertheless, in many situations, balloon pumping can produce dramatic, life-saving results. In weaning patients with low cardiac output syndromes from cardiopulmonary bypass, the device is so profoundly beneficial that it is difficult to justify withholding its use in order to conduct valid prospective studies. High-risk cardiac patients can be safely guided through major general surgical procedures with prophylactic IAB. With the development of the percutaneous IAB,

physicians without surgical expertise can safely and rapidly institute circulatory support. The balloon may now be quickly inserted during resuscitation for cardiac arrest and patients with critical and unstable cardiovascular events may be transferred to tertiary centers from outlying hospitals with the IAB in place. Indications for mechanical circulatory support continue to evolve. Clarification of indications is essential to ensure rational and safe use of these devices.

References

1. Heart Facts: PR8, American Heart Association, New York, 1981.
2. Bregman D, Bailin M, Bowman FO Jr, et al: A pulsatile assist device (PAD) for improved myocardial protection during cardiopulmonary bypass. *Ann Thorac Surg* 24:547, 1977.
3. Harken DE: Presentation at the International College of Cardiology Meeting, Brussels, Belgium, 1958.
4. Dormandy JA, Goetz RH, Dripke DC: Hemodynamics and coronary blood flow with counterpulsation. *Surgery* 65:311, 1969.
5. Moulopoulos SD, Topaz S, Kolff WJ: Diastolic balloon pumping (with carbon dioxide) in the aorta— a mechanical assist to the failing circulation. *Am Heart J* 63:669, 1962.
6. Moulopoulos SD, Topaz S, Freed PS, et al: Initial clinical experience with intra-aortic balloon pumping in cardiogenic shock. *JAMA* 203:135, 1968.
7. Nachlas MM, Sieband MP: The influence of diastolic augmentation on infarct size following coronary artery ligation. *J Thorac Cardiovasc Surg* 53:698, 1967.
8. Feola M, Limet RR, Glick G: Direct and reflex vascular effects of intra-aortic balloon counterpulsation in dogs at four levels of aortic pressure. *Clin Res* 19:313, 1971.
9. Haddy FJ: Pathophysiology and therapy of the shock of myocardial infarction. *Ann Intern Med* 73:809, 1970.
10. Johnson SA, Scanlon PJ, Loeb HS, et al: Treatment of cardiogenic shock in myocardial infarction by intra-aortic counterpulsation and surgery. *Am J Med* 62:687, 1977.
11. Gold HK, Leinbach RC, Buckely MJ, et al: Refractory angina pectoris: Follow-up after intra-aortic balloon pumping and surgery. *Circulation* (Suppl III) 54:41, 1976.
12. Levine FH, Gold HK, Leinbach RC, et al: Safe early revascularization for continuing ischemia after acute myocardial infarction. *Circulation* (Suppl I), 60:I-5; 1979.
13. McEnany MT, Kay HR, Buckley MJ, et al: Clinical experience with intra-aortic balloon pump support in 728 patients. *Circulation* (Suppl I) 58:I–124, 1978.
14. Gunstensen J, Goldman BS, Scully HE, Huckell VF, Adelman AG: Evolving indications for pre-

operative intra-aortic balloon pump assistance. *Ann Thorac Surg* 22:535, 1976.

15. Cooper GN, Singh AK, Christian FC, et al: Preoperative intra-aortic balloon support in surgery for left main coronary stenosis. *Ann Surg* 185:242, 1977.

16. Scheidt S, Wilner G, Mueller H, et al: Intra-aortic balloon counterpulsation in cardiogenic shock: Report of a cooperative clinical trial. *N Engl J Med* 288:979, 1973.

17. LeFemine AA, Kosowshi B, Madoff I, et al: Results and complications of intra-aortic balloon pumping in surgical and medical patients. *Am J Cardiol* 40:416, 1977.

18. Beckman CB, Geha AS, Hammond GL, et al: Results and complications of intra-aortic balloon counterpulsation. *Ann Thorac Surg* 24:550, 1977.

19. Cleveland JC, LeFemine AA, Madoff I, et al: The role of intra-aortic balloon counterpulsation in patients undergoing cardiac operations. *Ann Thorac Surg* 20:652, 1975.

20. Dunkman WB, Seinbach RC, Buckley MJ, et al: Clinical and hemodynamic results of intra-aortic balloon pumping in surgery and cardiogenic shock. *Circulation* 46:465, 1972.

21. Leinbach RC, Gold HK, Dinsmore RE, et al: The role of angiography in cardiogenic shock. *Circulation* (Suppl III) 47, 48:III–95, 1973.

22. Wolfson S, Karsh DL, Langou RA, et al: Modifications of intra-aortic balloon catheter to permit introduction by cardiac catheterization techniques. *Am J Cardiol* 41:733, 1978.

23. Gold HK, Leinbach RC, Buckley MJ, et al: Refractory angina pectoris: Follow-up after intra-aortic balloon pumping and surgery. *Circulation* (Suppl III) 54:III–41, 1976.

24. Willerson JT, Curry GC, Watson JT, et al: Intra-aortic balloon counterpulsation in patients in cardiogenic shock, medically refractory left ventricular failure and/or recurrent ventricular tachycardia. *Am J Med* 58:183, 1975.

25. Isner JM, Cohen SR, Virmani R, et al: Complications of the intra-aortic balloon counterpulsation device: Clinical and morphologic observations in 45 necropsy patients. *Am J Cardiol* 45:260, 1980.

26. Bregman D, Casarella WJ: Percutaneous intra-aortic balloon pumping: Initial clinical experience. *Ann Thorac Surg* 29:153, 1980.

27. Seldinger SI: Catheter replacement of the needle in percutaneous arteriography: A new technique. *Acta Radiol Oncol Radiat Phys Biol* 39:368, 1953.

28. Bregman D: Management of patients undergoing intra-aortic balloon pumping. *Heart Lung* 3:916, 1974.

29. Bregman D: Mechanical support of the failing heart. In *Problems in Surgery*, Vol. 13, No. 12, Chicago, Year Book Medical Publishers, 1976.

30. Vignola PA, Swaye PS, Gosselin AJ: Guidelines for effective and safe percutaneous intra-aortic balloon pump insertion and removal. *Am J Cardiol* 48:660, 1981.

31. Merav AD, Solomon N, Montefusco CM, et al: A new guidable double lumen percutaneous intra-aortic balloon. *Trans Am Soc Artif Intern Organs* 27:593, 1981.

32. Nichols AB, Weiss MB, Bregman D, et al: Percutaneous intra-aortic balloon insertion in patients with aorto-iliac disease. *Cathet Cardiovasc Diagn* 7:443, 1981.

33. Karlson SB, Martin EC, Bregman D, et al: Superior mesenteric artery obstruction by intra-aortic balloon simulating embolism. *Cardiovasc Intervent Radiol* 4:236, 1981.

34. Kirklin JW, Conti VR, Blacksonte EH: Prevention of myocardial damage during cardiac operations. *N Engl J Med* 301:135, 1979.

35. Bregman D, Goetz RH: A new concept in circulatory assistance—the dual-chambered intra-aortic balloon. *Mt Sinai J Med* 39:123, 1972.

36. Gunstensen J, Goldman BS, Scully HS, et al: Evolving indications for preoperative intra-aortic balloon pump assistance. *Ann Thorac Surg* 22:535, 1976.

37. Lappas DG, Powell WMJ Jr, Daggett WM: Cardiac dysfunction in the perioperative period. *Anesthesiology* 47:117, 1977.

38. Webb WR, Parker FB Jr, Neville JR Jr, et al: Acute mechanical complications of coronary arterial disease. *Arch Surg* 109:251, 1974.

39. Mundth ED: Preoperative intra-aortic balloon pump assistance. *Ann Thorac Surg* 22:603, 1976.

40. Bardet J, Rigaud M, Kahn JC, et al: Treatment of post-myocardial infarction angina by intra-aortic balloon pumping in emergency revascularization. *J Thorac Cardiovasc Surg* 74:299, 1977.

41. Weintraub RM, Aroesty JR, Paulin SI, et al: Medically refractory unstable angina pectoris. Longterm follow-up of patients undergoing intra-aortic balloon counterpulsation and operation. *Am J Cardiol* 43:877, 1979.

42. Brundage BH, Ullyot DJ, Winokur S, et al: The role of aortic balloon pumping in post-infarction angina. A different perspective. *Circulation* (Suppl I) 62:I–119, 1980.

43. Amsterdam EA, Low RI, Bommer VJ, et al: Mechanical circulatory assistance by the percutaneous intra-aortic balloon pump. *Clin Res* 29:2A, 1981.

44. Bemis CE, Mindth ED, Mintz GS, et al: Comparison of techniques for intra-aortic balloon insertion. *Am J Cardiol* 47:417, 1981.

45. Mundth ED: Mechanical and surgical interventions for the reduction of myocardial ischemia. *Circulation* (Suppl 1) 53:176, 1976.

46. Mundth ED, Buckley MJ, Daggett WM, et al: Intra-aortic balloon pump assistance and early surgery in cardiogenic shock. Integrated medical-surgical care in acute coronary artery disease. *Adv Cardiol* 15:159, 1975.

47. Hanson EC, Levine FH, Kay HR, et al: Control of post-infarction ventricular irritability with the intra-aortic balloon pump. *Circulation* (Suppl 1) 62:I130, 1980.

48. Miller MG, Hall SV: Intra-aortic balloon counterpulsation in a high-risk cardiac patient undergoing emergency gastrectomy. *Anesthesiology* 42:103, 1975.

49. Baron DW, O'Rourke MF: Long term results of arterial counterpulsation in acute severe cardiac failure complicating myocardial infarction. *Br Heart*

J 38:285, 1976.

50. Brantigan CO, Grow JB Sr, Schoonmaker FW: Peripartum cardiomyopathy. *Ann Surg* 183:1, 1976.
51. Saunders CR, Doty DB: Myocardial contusion: Effect of intraaortic balloon counterpulsation on cardiac output. *J Trauma* 18:706, 1978.
52. Bass J Jr, Katzman L, Pois AJ: Experience with intra-aortic balloon counterpulsation in a community hospital. *Am Surg* 44:324, 1978.
53. Bregman D, Drusin R, Lamb J, et al: Heart transplantation in patients requiring mechanical circulatory support. *Heart Transplan* 2:154, 1982.
54. Pennock JL, Wisman CB, Pierce WS: Mechanical support of the circulation prior to cardiac transplantation. *Heart Transplan* 4:299, 1982.
55. Hines GL, Delaney TB, Goodman M, et al: Intra-aortic balloon pumping. Two year experience. *J Thorac Cardiovasc Surg* 78:140, 1979.
56. Alpert J, Ezhuthachan K, Rhaktan K, et al: Vascular complications of intra-aortic balloon pumping. *Ann Thorac Surg* 111:1190, 1976.
57. Bahn CH, Vitikainen KJ, Anderson CL, et al: Vascular evaluation for balloon pumping. *Ann Thorac Surg* 27:474, 1978.
58. Bregman D, Balooki H, Malm JR: A simple method to facilitate difficult intra-aortic balloon insertion. *Ann Thorac Surg* 15:636, 1973.
59. Bregman D, Cohen SR: Clinical experience with percutaneously inserted intra-aortic balloon. *Trans Am Soc Artif Int Organs* 26:8, 1980.
60. Harvey JC, Goldstein JC, McCabe EL, et al: Complications of percutaneous intra-aortic balloon pumping (PIABP). *Circulation* (Suppl III) 62:III–41, 1980.
61. Subramanian VA, Goldstein JE, Sos TA, et al: Preliminary clinical experience with percutaneous intra-aortic balloon pumping. *Circulation* (Suppl I) 62:I–123, 1980.

CHAPTER 5

TEMPORARY EXTRACORPOREAL POSTOPERATIVE CIRCULATORY SUPPORT USING THE ROLLER OR ROTOR IMPELLER PUMP

WALTER P. DEMBITSKY, M.D.
AIDAN A. RANEY, M.D.
PAT O. DAILY, M.D.

A recent review of 14,168 cardiac surgical patients illustrated that almost all cases were weaned from cardiopulmonary bypass without difficulty. Approximately 10% of these patients required pharmacological agents and volume loading during the weaning process. An additional 2% demonstrated inadequate response to conventional pharmacological therapy and required intra-aortic balloon (IAB) counterpulsation support during the weaning period. Approximately 1% of the patients were unresponsive to the "usual" measures of the ventricular support.[1] It has been demonstrated that a substantial fraction of this final group of patients has temporary ventricular malfunction, which is reversible enough to permit recovery.[2] A variety of mechanical support devices are available to facilitate the recovery of this small group of patients. Left ventricular (LV) balloon pumping combined with IAB pumping has been used.[3] LV copulsation technique using a pulsatile assist device has recently been described and used in animals.[4] Descending aortic pulsation was used early in the history of ventricular support.[5] The methods most widely accepted today are those employing extracorporeal pumps.

Two principles underlie the use of temporary extracorporeal circulation. First, the general support of the systemic circulation reduces the chance of multisystem failure by providing blood flow and pressure to vital organs including the heart itself, while the heart is in a recovery phase. Second, it provides a metabolic rest for the heart. This theoretically enables the myocardium to expend energy for repairing itself rather than for supporting the systemic circulation. In the normal heart, myocardial oxygen consumption (MVo_2) is equated with energy consumption. The four primary determinants of energy consumption in the heart are the ionotropic or contractile state of the heart; the heart rate; the arterial pressure or afterload; and the ventricular end-diastolic volume or preload. The relative contribution of each of these determinants is demonstrated in Figure 5.1. Note that the introduction of a high ionotropic state with the use of agents enhancing contractility such as isoproterenol (a pure beta-stimulant) markedly increases MVo_2. Similarly, introduction of an increased afterload in the form of higher blood pressure using a pure alpha-constrictor such as levarteranol also increases the MVo_2. In the ventricle with normal compliance, increased ventricular end-diastolic pressure produces an increased ventricular end-diastolic volume. As the volume increases so does the wall tension. The relationship of wall tension to MVo_2 is seen in Figure 5.2.[6]

Figure 5.3 demonstrates a reduction in oxygen consumption in the beating heart using various degrees of cardiopulmonary bypass. Left atrial (LA) to aortic bypass which assumes 85% of the total aortic flow reduces MVo_2 about 22% by eliminating the external work of the heart.[7] Since this technique does not totally drain the LV cavity, isovolemic contraction continues and wall stress remains high. LV decompression spares additional myocardial energy expenditure by reducing MVo_2 a total of 47%.[8-10] Total LV bypass using LV cannulation maximally diminishes MVo_2 by reducing the external workload of the heart by providing systemic flow and pressure and also by reducing the wall tension of the heart.

If the use of a mechanical support device reduces the oxygen consumption of the failing myocardium and allows that muscle to utilize its energy stores to repair itself, then smaller degrees of myocardial damage

RELATIVE INFLUENCE OF FACTORS AFFECTING $M\mathring{V}O_2$ IN THE NORMAL HEART

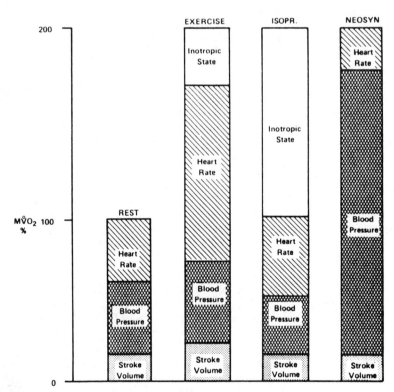

Basal and activation O_2 consumption not shown

Figure 5.1. This graph demonstrates the relative proportion of energy consumed for the four primary determinants of myocardial energy consumption ($M\mathring{V}O_2$).

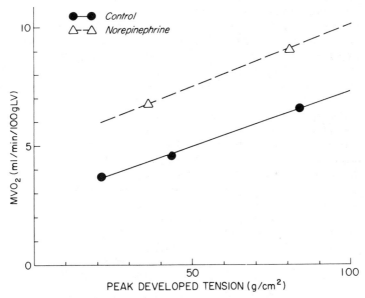

Figure 5.2. This graph demonstrates the relationship of myocardial energy consumption (MVo₂) to wall tension.

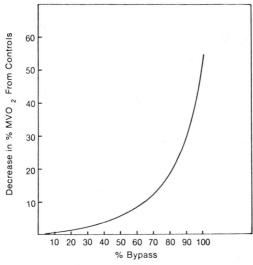

Figure 5.3. Less oxygen is consumed by the myocardium with increasing degrees of bypass.

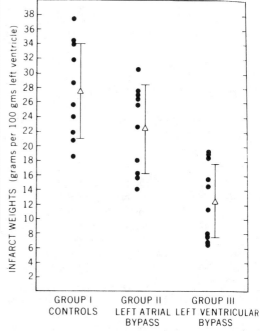

Figure 5.4. Increasing degrees of bypass reduce infarct size in animals.

should be evident in controlled injury studies comparing supported and nonsupported hearts. Figure 5.4 shows a progressive diminution in infarct size in three groups of animals. With an increase in the degree of bypass there is a progressive diminution of the infarct size.[11] In infarct models almost total bypass is necessary to benefit the injured heart significantly. The larger the infarct, the more important it becomes to increase the amount of bypass.[11,12]

Although extracorporeal ventricular support is more complex than IAB counterpulsation, it offers two advantages. Oxygen reduction by IAB counterpulsation is approximately 10%. This reduction is commensurate with the observed 19 to 25% reduction in peak LV wall tension and contractile work.[13] MVo_2 reduction is five times greater using total LV bypass. The most important advantage of extracorporeal support is that it can generate up to 6 liters of cardiac output per minute in comparison to 0.5 to 0.8 liters per minute using IAB counterpulsation.[14] It can, therefore, be utilized in instances where myocardial function is totally ineffective as in cases of sustained or recurrent ventricular fibrillation or profound power failure.

Historically, Liotta and colleagues[2] reported the first clinical use of an external left heart assist device in 1963. Spencer and associates[14] reported the first survivor in 1965 using left atrial-to-femoral artery support in a patient for 6 hours. In 1971, DeBakey[16] reported two more successes. Subsequently, numerous other reports have appeared.[13-25]

TYPES OF PUMPS

Three types of extracorporeal assist pumps are currently available for clinical use. They are the roller pump, the rotor impeller pump, and "bladder pump." The bladder is extensively discussed elsewhere in this volume. Its primary advantage for short-term use is its low thrombogenicity. This advantage is outweighed by its disadvantages. Bladder pumps are difficult to obtain because they are produced in limited quantities. All currently available models are costly because they contain expensive, nonreusable components.[9, 23, 26, 27] A nonreusable univentricular pump costs about $10,000. The reusable driver unit costs about $50,000. Even for extracorporeal univentricular assist, it is best to have two units available to minimize the risk of mechanical failure. All bladder pumps are pulsatile. Both the roller pump and the rotor impeller pump can be used in either a pulsatile or nonpulsatile mode.

Although pulsatile flow is attractive because of its similarity to the normal flow produced by the heart, its use is controversial.[28, 29] A disadvantage of pulsatile flow is that the episodic high-peak flow demands that low resistance drainage and delivery conduits be used. To provide adequate drainage at least a no. 50 French (F) caliber venous drainage tube must be used. A large caliber aortic return cannula is also necessary to prevent damping of the arterial pulses pressure. Pulsatile flow may be beneficial in vascular beds supplied by diseased vessels, especially those with collateral blood flow. Nonpulsatile flow is well tolerated by animals for periods of 30 days without adverse sequelae.[30] Because nonpulsatile flow does not seem to be a major liability to perfused tissues and because it is simple, we currently favor its use.

The roller pump has the advantage of being available and familiar to almost all cardiac surgeons. It is relatively inexpensive and much of the hardware is reusable. It does have some disadvantages when used for prolonged extracorporeal support. First the tubing used can form intraluminal balls or splinters which embolize. Although both can be filtered from the systemic circulation, this deterioration emphasizes the tenuous nature of the roller-tubing contact. If the roller pump is used for prolonged extracorporeal support, the tubing must be rotated every 6 to 8 hours to prevent rupture. Auxiliary pumps and tubing are necessary as a safety precaution. An additional disadvantage is that the roller pump is not pressure limited. It demands both unrestricted input and output. If the LA volume falls too low (usually pressure below 5 to 6 mm Hg), it is possible for the pump to aspirate air inside the heart around the cannulation site. With apical ventricular cannulation, catheter entrapment by the papillary muscles may be worse with the roller pump than with the rotor pump.

If the pump outflow is restricted in any way, severe proximal hypertension can result. Any kinking of the tubing from the pump to the patient must be corrected immediately to prevent possible rupture of tubing connections. One group experienced a fatality in a patient undergoing otherwise satisfactory prolonged support when the

IAB counterpulsation device remained distended and occluded the descending aorta. In this patient the roller pump being used to provide unlimited flow and pressure to the ascending aortic caused fatal cerebral hypertension.

The rotor impeller pump was initially manufactured by Medtronic Industries. However, a similar pump produced by Biomedicus Industries is now being used clinically. This model has the disadvantage of a slightly greater pump-blood interface area than the Medtronic pump, but does offer some distinct advantages to the clinician employing temporary extracorporeal circulation. Pressure is generated by spinning the blood approximately as a solid body vortex inside a casing. The liquid rotates at nearly the same velocity as the impeller blade resulting in minimal frictional loss and heat generation. The quantity of liquid which is tapped from the reservoir is relatively small and leaves from a relatively narrow opening in the outer wall of the scroll or casing. Kinetic energy imparted to the blood by the rotating impeller is recovered in the form of pressure in the exit diffuser. Replacement fluid enters through a central inlet.[31,32] A schematic diagram of this type of pump is seen in Figure 5.5.

The fixed expense of this pump is similar to the roller pump and the expense of nonreusable parts is relatively low. The current model has pulsatile capability if desired. It is distinctly less thrombogenic than the roller pump and has been successfully used clinically without anticoagulation for long-term support. Clot formation in the pump housing has been reported, although systemic embolization by the pump has not been recognized. Anticoagulation is currently recommended by the Biomedicus pump manufacturers. Tubing trauma with resultant embolization and fracture is nonexistent with the rotor impeller pump. Finally, the most attractive feature of the rotor impeller pump is that it is pressure limited and is tolerant of inflow fluctuations. Because high negative inflow pressure does not develop, catheter entrapment is largely prevented. If the output of the pump is occluded, flow reduces and the pressure stays the same. Conversely, if a vasodialator is given and the peripheral resistance is lowered, the flow of the pump will increase to accommodate the larger peripheral capacity. The pumped volume is dependent upon the outflow resistance and not on the revolutions per minute; therefore, a magnetic flow meter is used to measure pump output. Hemolysis is not a significant problem with either the roller or rotor impeller pump. Using the pumps in the pulsatile mode does not produce significantly more hemolysis. Table 5.1 compares the described pumps.

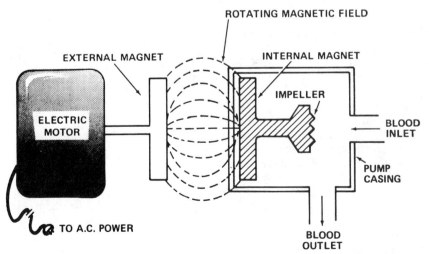

Figure 5.5. This is a schematic diagram of the rotor impeller pump.

Table 5.1
The three principle types of extracorporeal pumps available today are contrasted.

	Pulsatile	Approx. Non-Reusable Cost/Case	Approx. Reusable Cost	Thrombo-genicity	Pump Characteristics	Hemolysis	Unique Problems
Roller	Optional	$200.00	$7,500	Most of the 3.	Flow limited	Minimal	Embolization and fracture tubing
Rotor Impeller	Optional	350.00	7,500	Minimal	Pressure limited	Minimal	
Bladder	Obligatory	10,000	Pneumatic driving unit 50,000	Minimal		Minimal	Requires large drainage cannulae

INDICATIONS FOR USE

The most common indication for use is usually ventricular power failure resulting in the inability to wean a patient from cardiopulmonary bypass. Occasionally, IAB counterpulsation may be contraindicated. The presence of severe intimal aortic disease is associated with peripheral embolization to distal vascular beds if descending aortic counterpulsation is used. Friable ascending aortic intima can also be the cause of ventricular failure by embolizing to the coronary circulation. Interestingly, in animals, microembolization to the myocardium sufficient to cause myocardial failure is reversible when these animals are mechanically supported for a few days.

When ventricular power failure is present, the decision to use mechanical extracorporeal support in lieu of increased alpha- or beta-cardiac stimulation with drugs should be made early. The increased myocardial damage caused by the use of these drugs in a failing myocardium is well documented. For this reason once mechanical support has been initiated, cardiotonic drugs should be discontinued, if possible. Total circulatory support may be especially necessary to sustain a patient with recurrent or persistent ventricular tachycardia or fibrillation. Temporary lung failure as in cases of embolectomy for chronic pulmonary emboli or cases of high pulmonary resistance combined with transient right ventricular (RV) power failure might necessitate the use of an extra-corporeal pump. A clinical example is the occasional patient who acutely undergoes pulmonary embolectomy. The severe acute preoperative RV pressure load often causes transient myocardial dysfunction of the right ventricle. Since pulmonary vascular resistance remains elevated after removal of emboli in these patients, they can benefit from RV support. It is possible that some patients suffering from cardiogenic shock because of muscle failure from myocardial infarction could ultimately recover if total circulatory support is initiated early and combined with proper medical therapy.[33] Rare metabolic diseases which temporarily cause profound myocardial failure might be an indication for temporary extracorporeal ventricular support.

TYPES OF VENTRICULAR BYPASS

In a given patient the specific cause of pump failure usually dictates which techniques should be used to attach the extra-corporeal pump. Familiarity with the different assist modes will allow the surgeon to apply the pump(s) with maximum advantage for the patient.

Left Ventricular Bypass

Several methods of draining blood from the left heart have been tried. Direct drainage of the LV cavity maximally rests the myocardium and potentially allows for the greatest recovery because it compresses the ventricle. This can be accomplished in two ways. Retrograde aortic cannulation across the aortic valve has been used in animals.[31-35] Animals have been supported for 30 days without untoward effects to the aortic valve and with good drainage. It has the advantage of potentially being inserted percutaneously. The technique has not undergone clinical testing. LV apical cannulation was initially advocated by most investigators employing extracorporeal circulation.[36-38] Because of catheter entrapment by the papillary muscles as well as difficulties of insertion and removal of the apical cannula and the destruction of potentially viable myocardium in an already compromised ventricle, this method has been largely replaced by LA drainage.

LA drainage offers the distinct advantage of simplicity but the theoretical disadvantage of less than maximum support for the left ventricle.[39, 40] If no cause for aortic insufficiency is present such as the obligatory aortic insufficiency present with some prosthetic valves (like the Bjork-Shiley), the risk of damaging LV distension due to inadequate ventricular decompression is minimized and probably left atrial drainage is satisfactory. Using the nonpulsatile pump, a no. 36 F wire-wound catheter is first placed through a separate incision in the second intercostal space on the left chest. Then using a simple purse-string suture, a cannula is secured in the left atrium with a "bell tower" tip freely movable in the LA chamber. Monitoring LA pressure is necessary and much more accurate than the wedge pressure obtained from the Swan-Ganz catheter which must also be used to determine cardiac output in these patients. Measurement of the LV end-diastolic pressure is not necessary but helpful, especially during the postoperative period when weaning the patient from the pump. LV pressure development can be carefully monitored during this period if direct LV cavity pressure is obtained using either a removable micromanometer or direct pressure line introduced into the left atrium usually via the right superior pulmonary vein. Placement of the LA drainage catheter through the left atrium into the left ventricle has the potential problem of creating mitral regur-

gitation during the weaning process, especially if the drainage holes in the catheter are present in both the LA and LV sides of the mitral valve. Transmitral valvular ventricular drainage has been used with success.

With a pulsatile pump, a larger (no. 50 F) cannula must be inserted into the LA to decrease resistance during the maximal pulse drainage from the left atrium. The drainage catheter is then connected to a standard cardiopulmonary bypass venous drainage tube. Heparin-bonded tubing is a theoretical advantage. Cut sections of a Gott shunt, which is the only large-bore heparin-bonded tubing currently commercially available, can be used with the rotor impeller pump. When used with the roller pump, the tubing tends to collapse because of the high negative inflow pressure generated and is unsatisfactory for use on the drainage side of this pump. Both pumps require an arterial filter but neither requires the use of a venous reservoir. If postoperative dialysis is contemplated, an access port is placed distal to the pump but before the arterial line filter. A membrane oxygenator can also be inserted into the system at this point.

Arterial return is usually to the ascending aorta. If severe hypoxemia is not present, and a membrane lung is not being used, the arterial return need not be placed close to the aortic valve to minimize the effect of hypoxic coronary perfusion. It is preferable to direct the arterial return distal to the origin of the cerebral vessels. This can be done by passing a large return cannula such as no. 5 pediatric endotrachial tube[19] through a purse-string in the ascending aorta. Alternatively, a graft *impervious* to blood and attached to a wire-wound (no. 24 F) catheter can be sewn to the aorta using a partial occlusion clamp. Prolonged end-to-side femoral artery perfusion using such a catheter is also possible. However, even in the absence of proximal arterial obstructive disease, severe edema of the extremity perfused for many hours can occur making this route less attractive for prolonged bypass.

If the ascending aorta is used the arterial return catheter is passed through the center of the sternum by rongeuring an opening in the center of the two halves of the sternum prior to closure. The arrangement of catheters is seen in Figure 5.6.

As the patient is weaned from cardiopulmonary bypass, the LA pressure is kept between 5 and 15 mm Hg by gradually increasing the extracorporeal support pump flow as the LA pressure increases. When cardiac output and blood pressure are satisfactory, cardiopulmonary bypass is discontinued and LV bypass remains the sole systemic circulatory support. The two major problems at this point are bleeding and inflow catheter entrapment. Using the Biomedicus pump, the activated clotting time is allowed to fall transiently to near-normal

levels while hemostasis is obtained. Long-term perfusion has been reported without any anticoagulation using this pump. The roller pump requires more meticulous anticoagulation. The activated clotting time should then be kept between 160 and 180 seconds using continuous heparin infusion. Fresh frozen plasma and platelets may be necessary in large quantities as the components supplied by these blood products are initially consumed at high rates. The initial bleeding may continue at 500 to 1000 cc/hour for several hours and then subside. Blood salvage is maximized by using the cell saver and other types of reinfusion devices, such as the Sorensen device.

Catheter entrapment can be minimized by using the rotor impeller. With all pumps, the atrial pressure must be kept high to ensure the presence of an adequate pool of blood to supply the pump. A question which can arise during prolonged perfusion is whether or not a drainage problem is due to catheter entrapment or clot formation. Anticoagulation reduces the likelihood of clot formation. Reduced drainage is usually due to catheter entrapment. If entrapment is not remedied by volume expansion, temporary discontinuance of pumping may rectify it. If these measures fail, catheter repositioning may be necessary.

Although transport to the recovery room is relatively simple, two critical points deserve attention. The size of the pump must be portable; thus, the five-pump head console often used in routine cardiopulmonary bypass procedures is impractical. Smaller units such as the Cobe roller pump and the Biomedicus rotor pump heads can be placed on the patient's bed with care taken not to kink the tubing. Kinked tubing effectively discontinues the extracorporeal support with both pumps. With the roller pump, the resultant pressure buildup can be catastrophic. Both the Cobe and the Biomedicus pumps can be battery-powered during transport. Very long extension cords can be used with both pumps in lieu of a battery pack. The roller pump can easily be hand-cranked during transport, but the rotor impeller pump cannot be.

During the perfusion, blood pressure, cardiac output, LA pressure, and anticoagula-

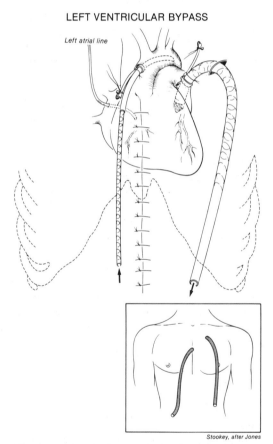

LEFT VENTRICULAR BYPASS

Left atrial line

Stookey, after Jones

Figure 5.6. Left ventricular bypass is most practical when blood is extracted from the left atrium and reinfused into the ascending aorta.

tion are all carefully monitored. Ionotropic drugs are discontinued, if possible. However, they may be occasionally necessary to support transiently a failing right ventricle so it can provide adequate flow to maintain a LA filling pressure of 5 to 15 mm Hg.

To determine the state of LV function, circulatory support can be temporarily discontinued and changes in the LA pressure, cardiac output, and blood pressure can be noted. If these parameters are satisfactory the pump is discontinued and removed in the operating room. Special cannulation techniques which allow decannulation in the recovery room have been described.[18, 22]

Right Ventricular Bypass

RV failure is manifested by low, LA pressure, high central venous pressure (CVP), with a low cardiac output and an observed RV hypocontractility. It is usually associated with a high pulmonary vascular resistance and may not be associated with hypoxemia.

When RV bypass is necessary, it may be instituted by a large-bore, venous drainage catheter passed into the right atrium through a purse-string. Return from the bypass is pumped into the pulmonary artery. A reservoir and an arterial filter is not necessary. The arrangement of catheters is seen in Figure 5.7.

Cardiopulmonary bypass is discontinued and the RV pump output is gradually increased to keep the right atrial pressure low and the LA pressure elevated to the desired level. If severe hypoxemia is present, a membrane oxygenator may be utilized.

Biventricular Bypass

Biventricular bypass is used when LV bypass with mild ionotropic support is unsuccessful. Clinically, this is manifested by a low cardiac output associated with elevated CVP and pulmonary artery pressure, the LA pressure is kept low by the output of the extracorporeal LV pump. If LV pump output is unsatisfactory because the LA volume is too low, then an additional RV pump is inserted as described.

Cardiopulmonary bypass is discontinued and the LA pressure is kept high enough to supply the LV bypass pump by gradually increasing the output of the RV pump. With

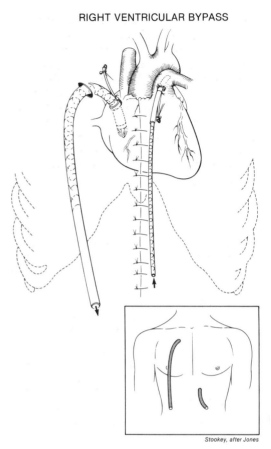

RIGHT VENTRICULAR BYPASS

Stookey, after Jones

Figure 5.7. Right ventricular bypass is shown.

the patient in regular sinus rhythm, the delay between increased RV and increased LA pressure is about 10 to 15 seconds but can vary and seems to be less when ventricular fibrillation is present. If the LA pressure begins to fall and the CVP is high, increased RV pump output will cause the LA pressure to increase to an adequate level. If the RV pump output is increased to a high level without a concomitant increase in the LV pump, the high LA pressure which results can produce severe pulmonary edema over a very brief period. If both the CVP and LA pressure are low, additional blood volume must be added.

CONCLUSION

The concept of temporary extracorporeal ventricular support should be thoroughly understood by all modern cardiac surgeons since the necessity for utilization of such a device is unpredictable and the timing urgent. The pumps and ancillary equipment described in this review are available for all concerned without significant additional cost. In the occasional patient with profound perioperative cardiac dysfunction, application of the discussed materials and principles can be life saving and the long-term result commensurate with asymptomatic survival.

References

1. Norman JC, Cooley DA, Igo SR, et al: Prognostic indices for survival during postcardiotomy intra-aortic balloon pumping. *J Thorac Cardiovasc Surg* 74:709, 1977.
2. Liotta D, Hall CW, Walter SH, et al: Prolonged assisted circulation during and after cardiac and aortic surgery. Prolonged partial left ventricular bypass by means of intracorporeal circulation. *Am J Cardiol* 12:399, 1963.
3. Bregman D, Parodi EN, Malm JR: Left ventricular and unidirectional intra-aortic balloon pumping. *J Thorac Cardiovasc Surg* 68:677, 1974.
4. Marrin CAS, Rose EA, Spotnitz HM, et al: Mechanical circulatory support via the left ventricular vent. *J Thorac Cardiovasc Surg* 84:426, 1982.
5. Kiso I, Baechler CA, Hamada O, et al: An extravascular left ventricular assist device. *Ann Thorac Surg* 21:203, 1976.
6. Braunwald E, Ross J, Sonnenblick E: *Mechanisms of the Contraction of the Normal and Failing Heart.* Little, Brown & Co., Boston, 1967.
7. Pennock JL, Pierce WS, Prophet GA, et al: Myocardial oxygen utilization during left heart bypass. Effect of varying percentages of bypass flow rate. *Arch Surg* 109:635, 1974.
8. Miller DR: Comparative effects of left atrial or left ventricular bypass on coronary sinus flow and oxygen usage in dogs. *Ann Surg* 179:830, 1974.
9. Holub DA, Hibbs DW, Sturm JT, et al: Clinical trials of the abdominal left ventricular assist device (ALVAD): Progress report. *Cardiovasc Dis Bull Texas Heart Inst* 6:359, 1979.
10. Watanabe K, Kabei N, McRea J, et al: Continuous measurement of myocardial oxygen consumption (MVO_2) and hemodynamic response during transapical left ventricular bypass (TALVB). *Trans Am Soc Artif Intern Organs* 21:566, 1975.
11. Pennock JL, Pae WE Jr, Pierce WS, et al: Reduction of myocardial infarct size: Comparison between left atrial and left ventricular bypass. *Circulation* 59:275, 1979.
12. Pennock JL, Pierce WS, Waldhausen JL: Quantitative evaluation of left ventricular bypass in reducing myocardial ischemia. *Surgery* 79:523, 1976.
13. Braunwald E, Covell JW, Maroko PR, et al: Effects of drugs and of counterpulsation on myocardial oxygen consumption. *Circulation* (Suppl IV) 39, 40:220, 1969.
14. Spencer FC, Eiseman B, Trainkle JK, et al: Assisted circulation for cardiac failure following intracardiac surgery with cardiopulmonary bypass. *J Thorac Cardiovasc Surg* 49:56, 1965.
15. Maroko PR, Bernstein EF, Libby P, et al: Effects of intraaortic balloon counterpulsation on the severity of myocardial ischemic injury following coronary occlusion. *Circulation* 45:1150, 1972.
16. DeBakey ME: Left ventricular bypass pump for cardiac assistance. Clinical experience. *Am J Cardiol* 27:3, 1971.
17. Berger RL, Merin G, Carr J, et al: Successful use of a left ventricular assist device in cardiogenic shock from massive postoperative myocardial infarction. *J Thorac Cardiovasc Surg* 78:626, 1979.
18. Litwak RS, Koffsky RM, Jurado RA, et al: Use of a left heart assist after intracardiac surgery: Technique and clinical experience. *Ann Thorac Surg* 21:191, 1976.
19. Rose DM, Colvin SB, Culliford AT, et al: Long-term survival with partial left heart bypass following perioperative myocardial infarction and shock. *J Thorac Cardiovasc Surg* 83:483, 1983.
20. Olsen EK, Pierce WS, Donachy JH, et al: A two-and-a-half year clinical experience with a mechanical left ventricular assist pump in the treatment of profound postoperative heart failure. *Int J Artif Organs* 2:197, 1979.
21. McGee MG, Zilligitt SL, Trono R, et al: Retrospective analyses of the need for mechanical circulatory support (intra-aortic balloon pump/abdominal left ventricular assist device or partial artificial heart) after cardiopulmonary bypass. *Am J Cardiol* 46:135, 1980.
22. Pierce WS, Parr GVS, Myers JL, et al: Ventricular-assist pumping in patients with cardiogenic shock after cardiac operations. *N Engl J Med* 305:1606, 1981.
23. Taguchi K, Murashita J, Maruyama T, et al: Left or biventrical bypass with local heparinization. *Trans Am Soc Artif Intern Organs* 23:498, 1977.
24. Taguchi K, Mochizuki T, Takamura K, et al: Clinical studies on the ventricular bypass with local heparinization in eight consecutive patients. *Trans Am Soc Artif Intern Organs* 23:739, 1977.
25. Pierce WS, Rosenberg G, Donachy JH, et al: Clinical experience with mechanical left ventricular assistance. International Congress Proc VIII, World Congress of Cardiology. Edited by S Hayase, S Murao.
26. Norman JC: An intracorporeal (abdominal) left ventricular assist device. *Cardiovasc Dis Bull Texas Heart Inst* 2:425, 1975.
27. Pierce WS, Brighton JA, O'Bannon W, et al: Complete left ventricular bypass with a paracorporeal pump: Design and evaluation. *Ann Surg* 180:418, 1974.
28. Edmunds LH Jr: Pulseless cardiopulmonary bypass. *J Thorac Cardiovasc Surg* 84:800, 1982.
29. Philbin DM, Hickey PR, Buckley MJ: Should we pulse? *J Thorac Cadiovasc Surg* 84:805, 1982.

30. Johnston GG, Hammill F, Marzec U, et al: Prolonged pulseless perfusion in unanesthetized calves. *Arch Surg* 111:1225, 1976.
31. Zwart JJH, Kralios AC, Eastwood N, et al: Effects of partial and complete unloading of the failing left ventricle by transarterial left heart bypass. *J Thorac Cardiovasc Surg* 68:105, 1970.
32. Bernstein EF, Dorman FD, Blackshear PL Jr, et al: An efficient, compact blood pump for assisted circulation. *Cardiovasc Surg* 63:865, 1972.
33. DeLaria GC, Johansen KH, Levine ID, et al: Reduction in myocardial ischemia by left ventricular bypass after acute coronary artery occlusion. *J Thorac Cardiovasc Surg* 67:826, 1974.
34. Schuhmann RE, Geddes LA, Hoff HE: Prolonged left ventricular bypass by transvalvular aortic catheterization. I. Physiologic effects and rationale of surgical concept. *Surgery* 67:957, 1970.
35. Bernstein EF, Cosentino LC, Reich S, et al: A compact, low hemolysis, non-thrombogenic system for non-thoiracotomy prolonged left ventricular bypass. *Trans Am Soc Artif Intern Organs* 20:643, 1974.
36. Peters JL, McRea JC, Fukumasu H, et al: Transapical left ventricular bypass (TALVB) without an auxiliary ventricle. *Trans Am Soc Artif Intern Organs* 22:357, 1976.
37. Johnston GG, Hammill FS, Johansen KH, et al: Prolonged pulsatile and nonpulsatile LV bypass with a centrifugal pump. *Trans Am Soc Artif Intern Organs* 22:323, 1976.
38. Laas J, Campbell CD, Takanashi Y, et al: Preservation of ischemic myocardium with TALVB using complete left ventricular decompression. *Trans Am Soc Artif Intern Organs* 25:220, 1979.
39. Salisbury PF, Cross CE, Rieben PA, et al: Comparison of two types of mechanical assistance in experimental heart failure. *Circ Res* 8:431, 1960.
40. Pierce WS, Aaronson AE, Prophet GA, et al: Hemodynamic and metabolic studies during two types of left ventricular bypass. *Surg Forum* 23:176, 1972.

CHAPTER 6

VENTRICULAR ASSIST DEVICES

WAYNE E. RICHENBACHER, M.D.
WILLIAM S. PIERCE, M.D.

Low cardiac output secondary to depressed myocardial function remains a major cause of death following cardiac operations. A clear example of low cardiac output is seen in the patient who cannot be weaned from cardiopulmonary bypass (CPB) upon completion of an open heart procedure. Conventional therapy for low cardiac output, including volume loading, inotropic support, and intra-aortic balloon (IAB) counterpulsation, is now available to all patients with shock following open heart operations. However, despite pharmacological support and IAB counterpulsation, 50% of these patients die.[1] The patient's demise invariably is due to inadequate systemic perfusion and coronary blood flow. In a recent report by Meyers et al.,[2] 1308 patients underwent cardiac surgery for acquired heart disease. Eighty-seven patients (6.7%) could not be weaned from CPB and were treated with an IAB. Ultimately, 19 patients (1.45%) could not be separated from CPB following their open heart procedure.[2] These results correlate well with an earlier series by Koffsky and co-workers,[3] in which 19 patients could not be weaned from CPB. This represented less than 2% of the population undergoing intracardiac surgery in their institution during the same period. Thus, despite recent advances in all aspects of perioperative care and management of the cardiotomy patient, the problem of low cardiac output remains a significant one.

One promising solution to this problem is the use of some form of mechanical circulatory support that is capable of decompressing the hypokinetic ventricle and decreasing myocardial work and oxygen demand while maintaining adequate systemic perfusion and coronary blood flow. Moreover, a temporary ventricular assist device provides time for the metabolic recovery of injured myocardium. Laboratory and early clinical studies delineated a number of fairly specific requirements which must be fulfilled by any ventricular assist device if it is to serve its intended function.

REQUIREMENTS FOR LEFT VENTRICULAR ASSIST DEVICE (LVAD)

1. Insertion of the device should be simple, utilizing existing exposure during implantation, thereby allowing rapid institution when necessary.
2. The device should be able to assume the cardiac workload, thereby providing (for hours or days) sufficient blood flow to maintain organ function.
3. The device should produce only a minimum of damage to the heart and blood components.
4. The materials of construction must be biocompatible, with little or no potential for thromboembolic complications.[3-5]

Attempts have been made to support or substitute for the function of the right and left ventricles by intra- or paracorporeal pumps since the late 1950s. Liotta et al.[6] reported the first clinical use of a left heart assist device in 1963. Two years later, Spencer et al.[7] described the first successful use of a left heart assist device in a patient who underwent left atrial-to-femoral bypass for 6 hours postoperatively. DeBakey[8] subsequently reported on two additional survivors in 1971. Since that time groups in Boston, New York, Hershey, Cleveland, Tokyo, Vienna, and Zurich have all reported use of pneumatic pumps for left and right heart support in patients with severe ventricular failure following cardiac surgery.

VENTRICULAR FAILURE AND DECISION TO USE AN ASSIST PUMP

Etiology of Ventricular Failure

The precise etiology of ventricular failure following a cardiac operation is often unknown. In all probability, there is no single cause but rather a number of minor insults, which combine to prevent the successful separation of a patient from CPB. Preoperative risk factors include pre-existing ventricular dysfunction, advanced age, and extensive cardiovascular disease.[9] Depression of ventricular function in the perioperative period may be due to air or calcific debris embolization of the coronary arteries, coronary artery spasm, ventricular distension, ventricular fibrillation, myocardial infarction, and incomplete myocardial protection.[12,10,11] Most groups now use similar techniques for myocardial protection, including cold potassium cardioplegia, topical myocardial hypothermia, and systemic hypothermia. However, the difficulty in obtaining adequate myocardial protection in a patient with diffuse coronary artery disease secondary to the maldistribution of cardioplegia is well described.[12]

The common pathway in most forms of perioperative injury is ischemia, and ischemia may progress to infarction. Ischemia, infarction, and even CPB all lead to myocardial edema with decreased ventricular compliance.[13,14] The noncompliant ventricle exhibits poor contractility and, if progressive, leads to ventricular failure. Ultrastructural changes, including intermyofibrillar edema and mitochondrial swelling, are seen on electron microscopic examination of right and left ventricular myocardium in patients with postcardiotomy and ventricular failure. These changes are felt to be ischemic in origin and potentially reversible, provided they are not permitted to progress to infarction.[15]

Conventional Therapy

The patient who cannot be weaned from CPB following a technically successful open heart procedure is initially treated by conventional means. Adequate correction of all hemodynamically significant lesions must be verified; myocardial revascularization must be as complete as is technically feasible. Inadequate circulating blood volume is detected by low right and left atrial pressures (RAP, LAP) and is easily overcome by infusing blood from the pump-oxygenator. Inotropic support consists of the administration of such agents as calcium chloride and the pressor amines: dopamine, dobutamine, and isoproterenol. Vasodilators and cardiac pacing are utilized as indicated.

Patients who exhibit severe myocardial dysfunction despite volume loading and pharmacological support are eligible for IAB counterpulsation. In left ventricular failure (LVF), the IAB serves to reduce afterload and augment coronary blood flow. As a result, the IAB is capable of providing a modest degree of circulatory support in acute heart failure (up to 0.8 liters/min/m^2).[16] It is important to note that the IAB is also helpful in treating right ventricular failure (RVF). In this condition, the IAB serves to lower the LAP, and accordingly, pulmonary artery pressure, but also improves right ventricular function by increasing coronary blood flow.[17] The percutaneous technique of IAB implantation has greatly reduced the time required to evaluate the efficacy of conventional therapy in the postcardiotomy patient in cardiogenic shock. This is important because the successful use of mechanical cardiac support is dependent upon the speed with which such support is instituted. With the percutaneous implantation technique, an individual's response to conventional therapy can often be determined within 30 minutes, and always within 1 hour, of his initial failure to wean from CPB.

Indications for Left Ventricular Assist Device Implantation

Successful use of a ventricular assist device depends upon careful patient selection. The indications include a number of specific hemodynamic criteria. Following a technically successful operation, a patient who cannot be weaned from CPB is first treated by conventional means. According to Pierce et al.[10] and Turina et al.,[18] patients who fail conventional therapy, have corrected pH and electrolytes, a mean LAP > 25 mm Hg, arterial systolic pressure < 90 mm Hg, and a cardiac output index (C.I.) $\leq$ 1.8 liters/min/m^2 are considered candidates for insertion of an LVAD.[2, 18]

Indications for Right Ventricular Assist Device (RVAD) Implantation

Cardiogenic shock following an open heart procedure may also be due to RVF. Profound RVF may be equally unresponsive to conventional therapy. An RVAD is indicated when conventional therapy fails in the presence of a C.I. $\leq$ 1.8 liters/min/m^2, and there is an inability to volume load the left ventricle despite an RAP > 20 mm Hg.

Contraindications to Ventricular Assist Device (VAD) Use

Implantation of an assist device should not be considered in a cardiotomy patient who has had a technically imperfect procedure. For instance, a VAD should not be used in a patient who has a residual hemodynamically significant lesion such as a paravalvular leak or residual ventricular septal defect, or who has obviously incomplete myocardial revascularization. Moreover, a successful outcome is unlikely in a patient who has well-documented preoperative organ dysfunction such as renal failure, or other intercurrent condition such as bacterial endocarditis. Evidence suggests that advanced age serves as a relative contraindi-

cation; most series report no survivors in patients over age 70.[10, 11, 16]

Prolonged cardiopulmonary bypass was one problem addressed by the panel conference on Cardiac Support at the American Society for Artificial Internal Organs meeting in 1980.[5] Most groups represented felt that the sequelae of a protracted period of CPB, specifically, elevated plasma hemoglobin levels and bleeding diatheses secondary to damage of blood components, significantly reduced the chance of success with ventricular assistance, but do not serve as a definite contraindication.

Preparation for Assist Device Implantation

Once the decision has been made to utilize a VAD, several items must be considered prior to its implantation. Accurate hemodynamic monitoring, including RAP, pulmonary artery pressure, LAP, and aortic pressures, as well as a means by which to determine cardiac output, is mandatory. Adequate monitoring is essential to differentiate between RVF and LVF, either or both of which may lead to heart failure in the postcardiotomy patient.[19] It is important to recognize the existence of isolated RVF. Intraoperative differentiation between RVF and LVF is possible by first volume loading the patient to raise the LAP to 15–20 mm Hg. If the C.I. remains below 1.8 liters/min/m^2, LVF exists. If efforts to increase the patient's C.I. by additional volume augmentation succeed only in raising the RAP, then RVF exists. In more profound RVF it may be impossible to load the left heart despite an RAP > 20 mm Hg.

Prior to implanting an LVAD, a decision must be made regarding the use of atrial vs. ventricular cannulation. Considerable controversy exists regarding the optimum inflow cannulation technique. Cannulation of the left ventricle results in total capture of the cardiac output with maximum reduction of both pressure and volume during ventricular filling and ejection.[20] By providing complete ventricular decompression, apical cannulation can maximally reduce myocardial oxygen consumption, left ventricular work, and may even decrease infarct size.[21, 22] However, left ventricular cannulation through the apex immobilizes the heart, thereby making it difficult if not impossible to lift the heart while looking for sites of bleeding. Ventricular apex cannulation in a small-chambered ventricle may result in inflow cannula obstruction, which has resulted in decreased C.I. and subsequent high mortality.[2] In addition, avoidance of apical cannulation in a patient with poor ventricular function to avoid causing further myocardial damage would appear wise, particularly in a patient with an apical myocardial infarction.

Left atrial cannulation, on the other hand, is technically simpler to perform, less susceptible to inflow cannula obstruction, less likely to result in insertion site bleeding, and far easier to remove than the ventricular apex cannula.[10, 11] The major disadvantages are that assisted circulation (via atrial cannulation) results in smaller reductions in left ventricular pressure and volume, and thus, myocardial oxygen consumption. Moreover, the atrial cannulation technique may result in capture of only a fraction of the cardiac output. Total capture of the cardiac output only occurs in patients in whom the left ventricle is severely depressed. In spite of these concerns, most groups now prefer atrial cannulation.[3, 10, 11]

If left atrial cannulation is chosen, closure of the foramen ovale is mandatory. During left ventricular assist pumping, the LAP is usually < 10 mm Hg while the RAP is often 15 to 20 mm Hg. With these atrial pressure relationships, a patent foramen ovale can result in right-to-left shunting, and fatal systemic hypoxemia.[2]

TYPES OF PUMPS

Attempts to support the ventricular function have led to the development of a number of assist devices of unique design. Their construction, insertion technique, method of removal, and the clinical experience with each device are well documented (Table 6.1). This section includes a description of the four major types of assist pumps currently employed and provides a summary of the results of their use in patients with refractory cardiogenic shock following cardiac operations.

Roller Pump

Litwak's group[3] from the Mount Sinai Medical Center (New York City) developed a LVAD consisting of a pair of cannulae connected to an external roller pump by a single loop of tubing (Fig. 6.1). The cannulae are constructed of silicone elastomer with a polyester fabric skirt proximally (Fig. 6.2). The skirts are designed in two layers such that the vascular tissue at the anastomotic site is sandwiched between the layers. The blood-fabric interface of the most proximal layer of the skirt is coated with silicone elastomer to decrease its thrombogenicity. The inflow cannula is inserted into the left atrium at its junction with the right superior pulmonary vein, while the aortic cannula is anastomosed to the ascending aorta. The cannulae are 6.4 mm internal diameter (ID)

Table 6.1
Clinical Results of Ventricular Assist Pumping

Group (Principal Investigator)	Number of Patients	Duration of Support (hours)	Weaned	Survived	References
New York (Litwak)	19	2–500	13	7	3
New York (Spencer)	16	2.5–92	9	8	11
Cleveland (Golding)	6	72–168	5	2	27
St. Louis (Pennington)	16	10–432	4	2	28
Boston (Bernhard)	21	2–190	7	3	33
Hershey (Pierce)	11 (LV-Ao)*	1–192	1	1	34
	14 (LA-Ao)†	3–264	11	7	2, 10, 35

* LV-Ao = left ventricular to aortic.
† LA-Ao = left atrial to aortic.

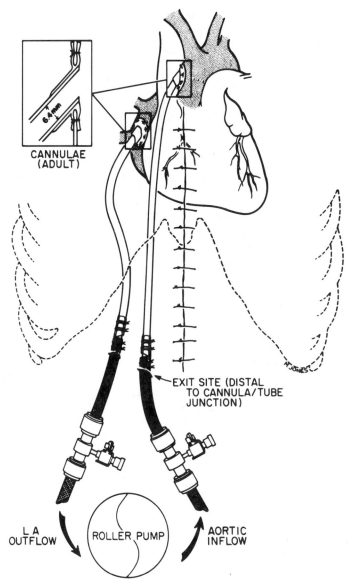

Figure 6.1. A schematic of the roller pump and cannulae employed by Litwak and co-workers is depicted. For left ventricular assistance, the pump inflow cannula is inserted into the left atrium at its junction with the right superior pulmonary vein. The pump outflow cannula is anastomosed to the ascending aorta. Both cannulae traverse the diaphragm and connect to the silicone elastomer roller tube in a subcutaneous position in the right upper quadrant of the patient's abdomen. Reproduced with permission from R. S. Litwak.

× 25 cm in length, and connect to a 9.5 mm diameter × 3 m long silicone elastomer pump tube. The latter tube provides sufficient length to allow the roller contacting surface to be changed every 72 hours, thereby preventing stress-induced tube failure. The roller pump is reported to be capable of producing a maximum flow rate of

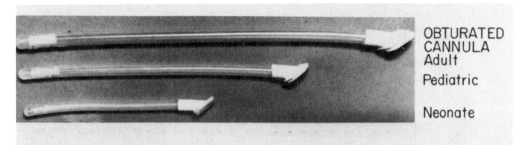

Figure 6.2. These cannulae were utilized by Litwak and associates for left atrial-to-aortic bypass. The proximal end of each cannula (*right*) is covered with a polyester fabric skirt. The skirt is designed in two layers such that the vascular tissue at the anastomotic site is sandwiched between the leaves. The distal end of each cannula (*left*) is fitted with a removable obturator which can be inserted upon completion of mechanical cardiac support. This obviates the need for cannula removal and, hence, repeat sternotomy. Reproduced with permission from R. S. Litwak.

7.5 liters/min. Heparin is administered to keep the activated clotting time (ACT) 110 to 140 seconds while pumping.

The cannula-roller tube junctions are located in a subcutaneous position in the right upper quadrant of the patient's abdomen. Exposure at the termination of left ventricular assistance is obtained by isolating these connections at the bedside using local anesthesia. The roller pump tube is removed and obturators are placed in both cannulae, which are subsequently returned to the subcutaneous pocket. This technique obviates the need for a repeat sternotomy. At the time of Litwak's most recent review,[3] this pump had been utilized in 19 patients. Duration of use varied from 2 to 500 hours. Thirteen patients were weaned from the assist device, while seven were eventually discharged from the hospital.

Spencer and colleagues[11] from the New York University School of Medicine recently reviewed their experience with another roller pump left heart assist in 16 patients who could not be weaned from CPB with inotropic agents and the IAB. Their technique utilizes equipment which is readily available to any cardiac surgical team. Left atrial-to-ascending aortic bypass is accomplished using a 28 to 32 French venous cannula, a 5 to 6 mm outer diameter (OD)

pediatric endotracheal tube as an arterial cannula, and 9.5 mm ID × 14.3 mm OD diameter silicone rubber medical tubing. A maximum flow rate of 3.5 liters/min is obtained using a Sarns battery-operated portable roller pump. The inflow cannula is inserted through the left atrial appendage and exits the left chest parasternally by way of the second or third intercostal space. The aortic cannula is brought out through the sternal incision (Fig. 6.3). Heparin is required to maintain an ACT of one and one-half to twice normal values (120 to 250 seconds). Again, to avoid excessive tubing wear, it is necessary to move the tubing within the pump head every 6 to 12 hours depending upon the flow rate. Failure to do this may result in tubing perforation.

Pump removal requires reopening of the sternotomy incision. A purse-string, previously placed in the left atrial appendage, is tied as the inflow cannula is removed. The aortic cannula is removed in a similar manner. During a period of 2 and ½ years, Spencer and his colleagues[11] utilized this assist device in 16 patients. The duration of left heart bypass varied from 2.5 to 92 hours with the average duration of implantation being 34 hours. Nine patients were weaned from bypass, while eight went on to become long-term survivors.

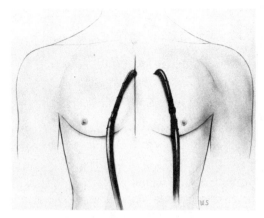

Figure 6.3. Cannulae positions utilized in left heart assistance by Spencer and colleagues are depicted. Roller pump inflow is obtained from the left atrium by a 28 to 32 F cannula which exits the chest through the second or third intercostal space. Pump outflow is through a 5 to 6 mm OD pediatric endotracheal tube which enters the chest through the sternal incision and is inserted into the ascending aorta. Reproduced with permission from F. C. Spencer.

Impeller Pump

A compact impeller pump has been used by several groups to provide circulatory support. The pump consists of a cylindrical housing containing an impeller-rotor assembly[23,24] (Fig. 6.4). The impeller is constructed of pyrolytic carbon and is driven by a rotating electromagnetic coupling. The pump is capable of a maximum flow rate of 5 liters/min and can be combined with an IAB to produce pulsatile perfusion. The pressure generated by the impeller is proportional to its rotational speed, while 50 to 80 mm Hg of pulse pressure may be provided by continuous IAB counterpulsation. The cannulae utilized with this pump are thin-walled polyurethane tubes reinforced with stainless steel wire and coated internally and externally with either Kontrathane or the segmented polyurethane, Biomer (Fig. 6.5). Pump inflow is obtained from the left ventricle either by way of a 9.9 mm ID polyurethane apical cannula or by insertion of a 7.2 mm OD cannula into the ascending aorta, retrograde across the aortic valve.[25] The return cannula from the pump directs

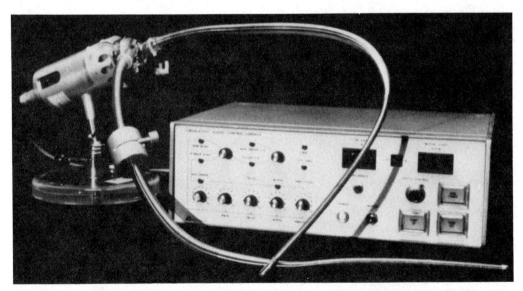

Figure 6.4. This centrifugal pump and control unit were utilized by Golding and associates. Blood enters the pump from the left ventricle through the inflow cannula, which in this photograph is extended above the control unit. Nonpulsatile blood flow is produced by a rotating impeller and is returned to the ascending aorta through the pump outflow cannula, seen lying in front of the control unit. Pulsatile perfusion is possible with continuous IAB counterpulsation. Reproduced with permission from L. A. R. Golding and A. N. Brest.

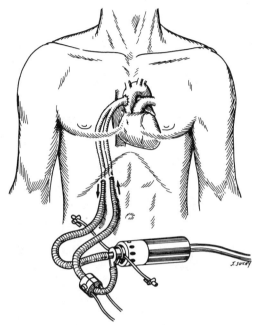

Figure 6.5. The cannulae placement utilized by Golding and co-workers for left ventricular assistance is presented. A 12-mm biolized Dacron prosthesis is anastomosed to the ascending aorta. Pump inflow is obtained by passing a 7.2-mm (OD) polyurethane cannula through this graft, retrograde across the aortic valve into the left ventricle. The pump outflow occurs through the second limb of the bifurcated prosthesis, with blood return being directed into the ascending aorta. An alternate form of pump inflow utilized by this group employs a 9.9-mm (ID) polyurethane cannula inserted into the left ventricular apex. Reproduced with permission of L. A. R. Golding.

the flow of blood into a 12 mm biolized Dacron graft anastomosed end-to-side to the ascending aorta. Heparin is administered during pumping to maintain the ACT at twice normal values.

Pump removal is performed during repeat sternotomy. The apical cannula is removed while the aortic graft is divided and oversewn. The centrifugal pump has been employed at two institutions. Golding and associates[26,27] in Cleveland and Pennington et al.[28] in St. Louis have utilized this pump in a total of 22 patients. Of these, nine were

weaned from the assist devices while four survived. In Golding's series, the duration of assist pumping varied from 72 to 168 hours, the average being 115 hours.

Concentric Tube Pump

Bernhard and co-workers[16,29-31] have designed and utilized a pneumatically driven, axisymmetric assist device to provide circulatory support in 21 patients with intractable cardiogenic shock after cardiac operations. The pump consists of a titanium housing enclosing a cylindrical polyurethane bladder capable of producing a maximum stroke volume of 75 cc and a maximum blood flow rate of 7.0 liters/min (Fig. 6.6). The polyurethane and titanium blood-contacting components are lined with a firmly adherent layer of polyester fibrils which attract a thin fibrin coagulum upon contact with blood. The paracorporeal pump is interposed between the left ventricle and ascending aorta and lies on the right anterior chest wall (Fig. 6.7). Inflow and outflow conduits consist of woven Dacron grafts 20 mm in diameter and 15 cm in length, each containing a glutaraldehyde preserved porcine xenograft valve. The inflow conduit exits from the chest beneath the sternum while the outflow conduit passes through a space created by a 4-cm resection of the third or fourth rib to the right of the sternotomy incision. The pneumatic power and control system can provide either synchronized counterpulsation or fixed rate pumping. Heparin is only required during the end stages of the weaning process just prior to pump removal.

Removal of the pump requires a repeat sternotomy. The conduits are divided 0.5 cm beyond their cardiovascular connections and the stumps are oversewn. An alternate method is the division of the conduits at skin level under local anesthesia. The advantage of this latter technique is that the chest need not be reopened. However, prosthetic material remains between the subcutaneous tissue and the cardiovascular system and presents a constant risk of infection.[32] As of December 1981, this LVAD had been implanted in 21 patients for a range of 2 to 190 hours.[33] Of these, seven were weaned from the pump and three were long-term survivors.

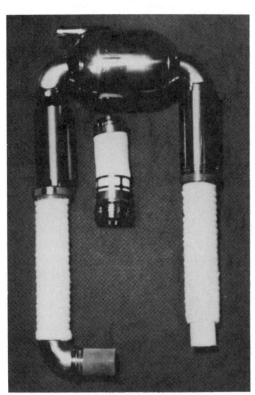

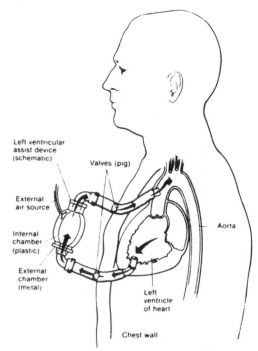

Left ventricular
assist device
(schematic)

Valves (pig)

External
air source

Internal
chamber
(plastic)

External
chamber
(metal)

Aorta

Left
ventricle
of heart

Chest wall

Figure 6.7. The positioning of the axisymmetric assist device as employed by Bernhard and co-workers is depicted. The paracorporeal pump is interposed between the left ventricle and ascending aorta and lies on the right anterior chest wall. The pump inflow conduit exits from the chest beneath the sternum, while the outflow conduit passes through a space created by a 4 cm resection of the third or fourth rib to the right of the sternotomy incision. Reproduced with permission of W. F. Bernhard.

Figure 6.6. The assembled concentric tube LVAD was utilized by Bernhard and associates. The inflow conduit (*left*) is inserted into the left ventricular apex, while the outflow conduit (*right*) is anastomosed to the ascending aorta. The conduits consist of woven Dacron prostheses, 20 mm in diameter and 15 cm in length, and each contains a glutaraldehyde preserved porcine xenograft valve. The pneumatic drive line exits from the titanium housing (*upper left corner* of this photograph). Reproduced with permission from W. F. Bernhard.

Sac Pump

Pierce and associates[2, 10] at The Pennsylvania State University have designed and implanted a sac-type ventricular assist pump in 25 patients. The pump consists of a highly smooth, segmented polyurethane inner sac enclosed in a rigid polysulfone case (Fig. 6.8). Björk-Shiley inlet and outlet valves are used to provide unidirectional flow. The assist device can be implanted as a right atrial-to-pulmonary artery RVAD, a left atrial (appendage)-to-ascending aortic LVAD, or both pumps can be implanted for biventricular assistance as needed. For left

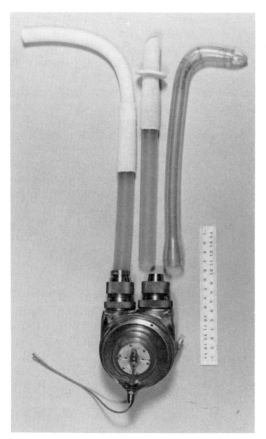

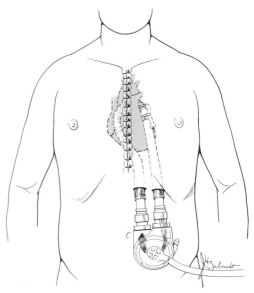

Figure 6.9. Left ventricular assistance as employed by Pierce and colleagues is presented. Blood is taken from the left atrial appendage by a 51 F lighthouse tip segmented polyurethane coated cannula. Blood return is through a composite segmented polyurethane-woven Dacron prosthesis which is anastomosed to the ascending aorta. Both cannulae exit the chest below the left costal margin, while the pump lies on the anterior abdominal wall.

Figure 6.8. Sac-type VAD utilized by Pierce and associates is shown. The inflow cannula (*right*) is inserted into the left atrium in order to perform left atrial-to-aortic bypass. Alternatively, a second inflow cannula (*middle*) allows apical ventricular cannulation for left ventricular-to-aortic bypass if atrial cannulation is technically impossible. The wire exiting the polysulfone case is attached to the Hall-effect switch utilized in the "full to empty" mode.

ventricular assistance, blood is taken from the left atrial appendage using a 51 F cannula and returned to the ascending aorta through a composite segmented polyurethane-woven 14 mm Dacron prosthesis (Fig. 6.9). The two cannulae exit the chest below the costal margin while the pump itself lies on the anterior abdominal wall. The pump is tethered to a control console by a 2-m long vinyl tube. The pneumatic drive unit will function in a synchronous mode, coupling the pump to either a Hall-effect fill switch or an EKG signal, or an asynchronous fixed rate mode. Dynamic stroke volume is 65 cc while the maximum blood flow is 6.5 liters/min. Anticoagulants are not required, although drug therapy to reduce platelet adhesiveness is recommended. Pump removal is accomplished through the sternotomy incision. The atrial cannula is removed as a previously placed purse-string is tied. The Dacron prosthesis is divided just above its anastomosis and the stump oversewn.

In Pierce's series,[34] before 1979, blood flow to the LVAD was obtained from the left ventricular apex. Eleven patients were included in this series with one long-term survivor. Since then, a left atrial cannulation technique has been employed. To date, 14 additional patients have received left ventricular assistance with seven long-term survivors.[2,10,35] Duration of implantation has varied from 1 hour to 11 days.

THE WEANING PROCESS AND MECHANISMS OF LEFT VENTRICULAR RECOVERY

The Weaning Process

As can be expected, there are numerous techniques to wean a patient from an assist device. Bernhard et al.[16] recommend that weaning be attempted only when the cardiovascular dynamics have improved sufficiently to maintain a C.I. of 2.0 liters/min/m² with no concomitant rise in left atrial or pulmonary capillary wedge pressure, while the assist pump flow rate is reduced by 50% (2 liters/min). Mean aortic, left atrial, and pulmonary capillary wedge pressures as well as the C.I. are checked at 15-minute intervals and, if unchanged after several hours, LVAD output is reduced by an additional 25%. If there is any indication of LVF, such as a drop in C.I. or systemic pressure or rise in left atrial or pulmonary capillary wedge pressure, full LVAD support is reinstituted for an additional 8 to 12 hours.

Litwak and his associates[3] have employed the concept of the percentage of left ventricular contribution to total systemic blood flow (TBSF) to guide the weaning process. The percentage of left ventricular contribution to flow is defined as:

$$\frac{TSBF - LHADF}{TSBF} \times 100$$

where LHADF is the flow produced solely by the left heart assist device. With their techniques, flow from the assist device is slowly decreased until the left ventricular contribution to the TBSF is >90% with a stable mean LAP $\leq$ 20 mm Hg. The device can then be removed. Spencer and associates[34] use a similar technique in discontinuing roller pump support but further state that a flow rate of 400 to 600 ml/min

should be maintained for 6 to 12 hours prior to pump removal.

Pierce and associates[2] discontinue the pump daily for periods up to 60 seconds in order to permit a sequential evaluation of the patient's ventricular function. When the patient's left ventricle is capable of maintaining an LAP $\leq$ 20 mm Hg, systolic aortic pressure $\geq$ 100 mm Hg, and C.I. > 2.0 liters/min/m² with the pump off for 60 seconds, the assist device output is progressively decreased at 6-hour intervals to permit the patient's left ventricle to assume complete circulatory support gradually. Adequate left ventricular function as defined by the criteria above, must be demonstrated four times over 24 hours prior to assist pump removal.

Left Ventricular Recovery

The mechanism by which the left ventricle fails is poorly understood. Thus, it is not surprising that our understanding of left ventricular recovery is incomplete. It has been proposed that ventricular dysfunction may be due, in part, to ischemia and resultant myocardial edema. Myocardial ultrastructural studies have been reported in one patient who could not be weaned from CPB following a double valve replacement, and who eventually required cardiac allografting following a trial with an LVAD. Microscopic changes observed included loss of normal A-band and Z-band patterns, mitochondrial swelling with fusion of cristae, interfibrillar edema, and glycogen depletion.[15] The significance of this case report becomes apparent when the ultrastructural features of this irreversible myocardial injury are compared with those described by Kloner et al.[36]

In the study by Kloner et al.[36], anesthetized dogs each underwent a 15-minute period of occlusion of the left anterior descending coronary artery, followed by reperfusion. Significant hemodynamic abnormalities were not encountered; nonetheless, myocardial biopsies showed early mitochondrial edema, occasional mild intermyofibrillar edema, wide I-bands, and depletion of glycogen granules. Three days later, these cells showed a reduction in the severity of these abnormalities, indicating progressive resolution of the myocardial injury. Dogs subjected to periods of myocardial ischemia longer than 20 minutes, however, developed areas of necrosis in the severely ischemic subendocardium, suggesting that there is a point in time at which ischemic myocardial cells pass through a reversible stage of injury, and become irreversibly damaged. No one has yet been able to define "the point of no return" in terms of criteria for cell death. It has been suggested, however, that in the event of a reversible myocardial injury, cardiac support may provide the time required to permit resorption of both intracelllar and interstitial water from the injured myocardium.[2] A reduction in myocardial water content would certainly improve ventricular function by increasing ventricular compliance.[13]

Considerable work has also been done in an effort to understand better the biochemical derangements associated with reversible myocardial ischemia. In one such study, Reimer et al.[37] occluded the circumflex artery for 15 minutes in a group of dogs. This period of ischemia was shown to result in a 65% reduction in tissue adenosine triphosphate (ATP) content. Furthermore, adenine nucleotide catabolism resulted in an accumulation of nucleotide precursors. Ischemic myocardium is permeable to such metabolites, which are lost via the venous effluent during reperfusion. This loss was shown to constitute 50% of the total adenine nucleotide pool in the ischemic myocardium. The importance of such a loss becomes apparent during reperfusion, when ATP resynthesis is limited by the availability of nucleotide precursors. In fact, ATP content was markedly depressed for as long as 3 to 4 days following the ischemic insult.[36,37] These findings correlate well with the clinical observation that the depressed ventricle may require days of assistance to regain adequate function and again support the circulation.[10,28]

PROBLEMS AND COMPLICATIONS ASSOCIATED WITH THE USE OF A VENTRICULAR ASSIST DEVICE

Delay in application of a VAD while futile attempts are made to save a patient's life by conventional therapeutic measures is the major cause of postoperative morbidity and mortality in patients with cardiac assist pumps. Agonizing over the decision to employ mechanical cardiac support only prolongs CPB time. In Bernhard's early series,[5] a mean CPB time in excess of 5 hours appeared to correlate with serious postoperative bleeding. Postoperative bleeding is a result of the length of the operative procedure and the associated coagulation defects rather than to the use of an assist device.[20,27] In one series, there were no survivors among patients who developed diffuse postoperative bleeding.[2] Rapid evaluation of patients who fail to come off bypass utilizing established implantation criteria will minimize CPB time and reduce the incidence of postoperative bleeding.

RVF may be the primary cause of an inability to wean from CPB. However, RVF frequently accompanies profound LVF and is difficult to recognize prior to implantation of an LVAD. In one series of six patients who received LVADs, all six showed varying degrees of RVF as evidenced by high RAPs (>20 mm Hg) and distention of the right ventricle.[27] A reasonable explanation for this association is that myocardial injury may have been of a global nature manifested by biventricular failure rather than a process confined entirely to the left ventricular myocardium.

Since the right and left ventricles are in series, poor right ventricular function will prevent an LVAD from achieving an adequate flow rate. Failure will result from a low cardiac output or high RAP. Elevated RAP (>20 to 25 mm Hg) will lead to generalized edema, splanchnic congestion, and renal failure. Accordingly, some provision to provide right ventricular support is mandatory. Volume loading with elevation of RAP to 20 mm Hg may be helpful in producing passive flow through the pulmonary bed. Pharmacological support includes the use of pressor amines. Isoproterenol is the drug of choice in RVF in that it will not only enhance right ventricular contractile force, but will also act as a pulmonary vasodilator to reduce right ventricular afterload. When dopamine is used for inotropic support of the right ventricle, dosages greater than those usually employed for the left ventricle may be needed. At equal doses of dopamine, the contractile response in the left ventricle has been shown to be greater than that of the right ventricle.[38] This difference in inotropic response is thought to be related to an unequal distribution of myocardial beta-receptors in the two ventricles.

Catecholamine infusion combined with volume loading provides sufficient support for mild RVF. Shumway's group[39] has proposed pulmonary artery balloon counterpulsation to provide moderate right ventricular support. However, if more severe right ventricular dysfunction exists, as indicated by an RAP > 20 mm Hg, LAP < 20 mm Hg, and C.I. < 1.8 liters/min/m^2, biventricular mechanical support is indicated to ensure adequate left assist pump filling and a C.I. > 1.8 liters/min/m^2.

As with mechanical ventilation and IAB counterpulsation, an occasional patient may not tolerate separation from the assist device. The incidence of such device dependency is not known at present, however, as patients who cannot be weaned from cardiac support usually die from multisystem failure. To date, death in patients with VADs has usually been due to bleeding, improper pumping, renal failure, or sepsis.

Sepsis is a significant problem in cardiac assist patients because of invasive monitoring, prolonged initial operative time, mediastinal clot, and repeat sternotomies. Bernhard and his associates[32] have presented two patients who developed graft infections in the remnant of a left ventricular apex cannula. One patient died of sepsis, while the other required several operations for a chronic draining sinus and hemorrhage from a left ventricular cutaneous fistula. The problem can be prevented by complete removal of LVAD conduits.

There are a number of unique, but interesting, complications that have been encountered during clinical application of VADs. Fibrinous fusion of the free edges of a prosthetic aortic valve during left ventricular-to-aortic bypass has been described.[40] In this patient, cardiac ejection occurred entirely by way of the ventricular apex both actively during assist pump function and

passively while assist pumping was discontinued to check on the patient's hemodynamic status. Avoiding tissue and ball valves, and ensuring that the valves open and close periodically, can obviate this problem. Assist pump use in patients with transmural myocardial injury, either in the recent past or in the perioperative period, has led to mural thrombi in three patients.[35] Anticoagulation is required to prevent mural thrombus formation within the depressed ventricle.

SUMMARY

Clinical experience in several institutions has shown the VAD to be an important adjunct in the care of patients with postcardiotomy cardiogenic shock. Improved pump design, development of implantation criteria with rapid utilization of such devices when indicated, as well as a better understanding of the problems associated with the use of mechanical circulatory assistance have resulted in 50% survival rates in several recent series. This is a remarkable accomplishment considering the critically ill patient population involved.

Future accomplishments must include identification of perioperative factors that indicate which patients will benefit from the assist device and simplification of implantation techniques. Consideration must also be given to the application of ventricular support in patients presenting with cardiogenic shock secondary to acute myocardial infarction or reversible cardiomyopathy. Finally, the equipment, instrumentation, and techniques for long-term ventricular assistance are in an advanced stage of development and, when available, will do much to improve longevity and quality of life in patients suffering from irreversible cardiomyopathy.

Acknowledgment. This work was supported, in part, by USPHS Grant RO1-HL-13426; the Robert J. Kleberg, Jr. and Helen C. Kleberg Foundation; the H. G. Barsumian, M.D., Trust Fund; and the McKean County Cardiac Committee.

References

1. McEnany MT, Kay HR, Buckley MJ, et al: Clinical experience with intra-aortic balloon pump support in 728 patients. *Circulation* 58(Suppl):124, 1978.
2. Myers JL, Parr GVS, Pae WE Jr, et al: The role of the ventricular assist pump for postcardiotomy cardiogenic shock: A four and one-half year experience. Proceedings of the Third Meeting of ISAO. *Artif Organs* 5(Suppl):244, 1981.
3. Koffsky RM, Litwak RS, Mitchell BL, et al: A simple left heart assist device for use after intracardiac surgery: Development, deployment and clinical experience. *Artif Organs* 2:257, 1978.
4. Wolner E: Cardiac function: Assist devices. Proceedings of the Third Meeting of ISAO. *Artif Organs* 5(Suppl):29, 1981.
5. Pierce WS, Chairman: Panel Conference: Cardiac Support. *Trans Am Soc Artif Intern Organs* 26:625, 1980.
6. Liotta D, Hall CW, Walter SH, et al: Prolonged assisted circulation during and after cardiac or aortic surgery. Prolonged partial left ventricular bypass by means of intracorporeal circulation. *Am J Cardiol* 12:399, 1963.
7. Spencer FC, Eiseman B, Trinkle JK, et al: Assisted circulation for cardiac failure following intracardiac surgery with cardiopulmonary bypass. *J Thorac Cardiovasc Surg* 49:56, 1965.
8. DeBakey ME: Left ventricular bypass pump for cardiac assistance. Clinical experience. *Am J Cardiol* 27:3, 1971.
9. Kennedy JW, Kaiser GC, Fisher LD, et al: Multivariate discriminant analysis of the clinical and angiographic predictors of operative mortality from the Collaborative Study in Coronary Artery Surgery (CASS). *J Thorac Cardiovasc Surg* 80:876, 1980.
10. Pierce WS, Parr GVS, Myers JL, et al: Ventricular-assist pumping in patients with cardiogenic shock after cardiac operations. *N Engl J Med* 305:1606, 1981.
11. Rose DM, Colvin SB, Cullliford AT, et al: Long-term survival with partial left heart bypass following perioperative myocardial infarction and shock. *J Thorac Cardiovasc Surg* 83:483, 1982.
12. Hilton CJ, Teubl W, Acker M, et al: Inadequate cardioplegic protection with obstructed coronary arteries. *Ann Thorac Surg* 28:323, 1979.
13. Foglia RP, Lazar HL, Steed DL, et al: Iatrogenic myocardial edema with crystalloid primes: Effects on left ventricular compliance, performance, and perfusion. *Surg Forum* 29:312, 1978.
14. Powell WJ Jr, Dibona DR, Flores J, et al: The protective effect of hyperosmotic mannitol in myocardial ischemia and necrosis. *Circulation* 54:603, 1976.
15. Sturm JT, Bossart MI, Holub DA, et al: Ultrastructural analyses of stone heart syndrome at onset and six days later following total support of the circulation with a partial artificial heart or left ventricular assist device (ALVAD). *Cardiovasc Dis Bull Texas Heart Inst* 6:29, 1979.
16. Bernhard WF, Berger RL, Stetz JP, et al: Temporary left ventricular bypass: Factors affecting patient survival. *Circulation* 60(Suppl 1):131, 1979.
17. Kopman EA, Ramirez-Inawat RC: Intra-aortic balloon counterpulsation for right heart failure. *Anesth Analg* 59:74, 1980.
18. Turina MT, Bosio R, Senning A: Paracorporeal artificial heart in postoperative heart failure. *Artif Organs* 2:273, 1978.
19. Pierce WS: Clinical left ventricular bypass: Problems of pump inflow obstruction and right ventricular failure. *ASAIO J* 2:1, 1979.
20. Norman JC, Duncan JM, Frazier OH, et al: Intracorporeal (abdominal) left ventricular assist devices or partial artificial hearts. A five year clinical experience. *Arch Surg* 116:1441, 1981.
21. Laks H, Oh RA, Standeven JW, et al: Effect of left atrial to aortic assistance on infarct size. *Circulation* 56(Suppl 2):38, 1977.
22. Pennock JL, Pae WE, Pierce WS, et al: Reduction of myocardial infarct size: Comparison between left atrial and left ventricular bypass. *Circulation* 59:275, 1979.
23. Bernstein EF, DeLaria GA, Johansen KH, et al: Twenty-four hour left ventricular bypass with a centrifugal blood pump. *Ann Surg* 181:412, 1975.
24. Johnston GC, Hammill FS, Johansen KH, et al: Prolonged pulsatile and nonpulsatile LV bypass with a centrifugal pump. *Trans Am Soc Artif Intern Organs* 22:323, 1976.
25. Golding L: A simplified blood access method for a temporary left ventricular assist system in humans. *Artif Organs* 2:317, 1978.
26. Golding LR, Loop FD, Sandberg GW, et al: Left ventricular assist device support. Twenty-one month survival. *Cleve Clin Q* 48:373, 1981.
27. Golding LR, Jacobs G, Groves LK, et al: Clinical results of mechanical support of the failing left ventricle. *J Thorac Cardiovasc Surg* 83:597, 1982.
28. Pennington DG, Merjavy JP, Swartz MT, et al: Clinical experience with a centrifugal pump ventricular assist device. *Trans Am Soc Artif Intern Organs* 28:93, 1982.
29. Bernhard WF, Poirier V, LaFarge CG, et al: A new method for left ventricular bypass. *J Thorac Cardiovasc Surg* 70:880, 1975.
30. Berger RL, McCormick JR, Stetz JD, et al: Successful use of a paracorporeal left ventricular assist device in man. *JAMA* 243:46, 1980.
31. Berger RL, Merin G, Carr J, et al: Successful use of a left ventricular assist device in cardiogenic shock from massive postoperative myocardial infarction. *J Thorac Cardiovasc Surg* 78:626, 1979.
32. McCormick JR, Berger RL, Davis Z, et al: Infection in remnant of left ventricular assist device after successful separation from assisted circulation. *J Thorac Cardiovasc Surg* 81:727, 1981.
33. Bernhard WF: Clinical evaluation of ventricular assist devices: Report from Children's Hospital Medical Center Cardiovascular Surgical Research Laboratory, Boston, Mass. Devices and Technology Branch (NHLBI) Contractors Meeting, p. 23, 1981.
34. Pae WE, Rosenberg G, Donachy JH, et al: Mechanical circulatory assistance for postoperative cardiogenic shock: A three year experience. *Trans Am Soc Artif Intern Organs* 26:256, 1980.

35. Pierce WS: Unpublished data, November 1982.
36. Kloner RA, DeBoer LWV, Dansee JR, et al: Prolonged abnormalities of myocardium salvaged by reperfusion. *Am J Physiol* 240:H591, 1981.
37. Reimer KA, Hill ML, Jennings RB: Prolonged depletion of ATP and of the adenine nucleotide pool due to delayed resynthesis of adenine nucleotides following reversible myocardial ischemic injury in dogs. *J Mol Cell Cardiol* 13:229, 1981.
38. Trigt PV, Spray TL, Peyton RB, et al: Right ventricular mechanics: A quantitative comparison of the biventricular contractile response to inotropic stimulation in the conscious dog. *Surg Forum* 33:326, 1982.
39. Miller DC, Moreno-Cabral RJ, Stinson EB, et al: Pulmonary artery balloon counterpulsation for acute right ventricular failure. *J Thorac Cardiovasc Surg* 80:760, 1980.
40. Myers JL, Bull A, Kastl DG, et al: Fusion of prosthetic aortic valve during left heart bypass. *J Thorac Cardiovasc Surg* 82:263, 1981.

CHAPTER 7

ANESTHETIC CONSIDERATIONS IN CORONARY ARTERY DISEASE

THOMAS J. CONAHAN III, M.D.

PREOPERATIVE EVALUATION

Anesthetic care begins with the preanesthetic visit. Several studies have demonstrated the value of the preanesthetic visit in contributing to the patient's calmness in the immediate preoperative period.[1] Of all the physicians participating in the patient's care, the anesthesiologist has the briefest period of time to establish rapport with the patient. If the operation has been planned and scheduled long in advance, the patient has had the opportunity to adjust to the concept of harboring a life-threatening disease which requires surgical therapy. The poorly prepared patient, or the patient who is involved in the rapid progression from onset of angina to cardiac catheterization to surgery is likely to be terrified. Consider this situation: one day a perfectly healthy individual leading his normal life; 24 hours later, a patient in the hospital, told that his/her previously "perfect" body is in great danger of not existing much longer, and that in order to survive his/her sick heart must be stopped, repaired, and restarted. With little time to absorb the facts, let alone adjust to them, the patient is often frightened, confused, perhaps even overwhelmed. The emotional responses may range from anger to withdrawal. The anesthesiologist often finds himself/herself thrust into this situation.

Taking a brief history serves two purposes. It allows the patient to talk about familiar events, providing time to dissipate some of the anxiety generated by meeting another new physician. The history, of course, is important is assessing the extent of the patient's coronary artery disease, as well as in uncovering previous untoward anesthetic experiences. Clues to difficult intubation, malignant hyperthermia, pseudocholinesterase deficiency or a myriad of other anesthesia or surgery-related complications may be elicited.

ANESTHESIA-DRUG INTERACTION

Beta-Adrenergic Blockers

Specific questioning about recent medication is mandatory. The coronary artery patient is often taking a beta-adrenergic blocker. This class of drugs acts to decrease myocardial contractility, to reduce resting heart rate, and to block the tachycardic and a portion of the hypertensive responses to stress. Propranolol is the most widely used beta-blocker and is nonselective, blocking both beta$_1$ and beta$_2$ receptors. Drugs such as atenolol, metoprolol and practolol are being used which selectively block the cardiac (beta$_1$) receptors.[2]

At the very least, beta-blockers will blunt expected responses to manipulations under anesthesia. Other effects to be observed and compensated for include the profound bradycardia possible when high vagal tone is combined with beta-blockade; hypotension and low cardiac output when anesthetic-included myocardial depression is superimposed upon contractility already lowered by beta-blockade.

Calcium Channel Blockers

Calcium antagonists are commonly administered to patients with coronary artery disease—either alone or in combination with beta-adrenergic blocking drugs. Nifedipine acts directly to reduce both peripheral and coronary vascular resistance, as well as to decrease contractility.[3,4]

Combined with the depressive and vasodilatory effects of some anesthetic agents, the cardiovascular effects of the calcium channel blockers may become devastating. The interaction among anesthetic agent, beta-blocker, and calcium blocker must be carefully monitored for negative inotropism, bradycardia, heart block, and hypotension.

Antihypertensive Drugs

Medication used to control hypertension may interact with anesthetics in several ways. Diuretic agents deplete both circulating blood volume and potassium stores. Hypovolemia may be unmasked by anesthetic agents which cause vasodilation. Hypokalemic myocardial irritability and arrhythmias are well known. The vasoactive and neuroactive antihypertensives act by interfering with normal homeostatic mechanisms. Direct vasodilators such as hydralazine and diazoxide may have their effects amplified by general anesthetic agents. The alpha- and β-adrenergic blocking antihypertensives also block the effector limb of many protective cardiovascular reflexes. Reflex arcs and effector activation are also affected by guanethidine and reserpine, occasionally leading to protracted hypotension under anesthesia.

The preceding paragraph catalogs a sample of the possible untoward interactions between antihypertensive medications and anesthetics. Years ago, conventional wisdom dictated that these interactions be prevented by withdrawing the patient from antihypertensive medication 2 to 3 weeks prior to surgery. Current thinking is that the patient needs antihypertensives to control disease and the anesthetic can be selected and administered so as to minimize detrimental interactions.[5]

Anticoagulants

Platelet inhibitors such as aspirin are usually discontinued 5 days prior to surgery. Oral anticoagulants may be continued until 2 to 3 days preoperatively and either stopped completely or replaced with heparin.

PHYSICAL EXAMINATION

Pertinent points in the physican examination include the usual concerns about head and neck mobility, airway patency, cardiac and pulmonary signs and sounds, Allen's test for ulnar artery flow, and inspection of other monitoring sites. The period of the physical exam is often a convenient time to explain to the patient what is being examined and why—and to describe the procedure and sensations associated with introduction of each of the monitoring cannulae in the immediate preoperative period.

CARDIAC CATHETERIZATION DATA

Cardiac catheterizations are often performed after the patient has been in the hospital for several days. Rest and therapy tend to contract the blood volume prior to the examination, reducing intracardiac pressures. By the time the patient gets to the operating room, intracardiac pressures may well have risen again. We attempt to relate cardiac catheterization data to the values determined in the operating room, but unless discrepancies between the two sets of data are unusually large, we do not suspect an acute change in the patient's condition. More likely, the patient has become rehydrated and his/her cardiac function is closer to its usual state.

Ejection fraction (EF) provides some index of global myocardial function. A high EF (>0.60) is reassuring—but is no guarantee that the heart will continue to function well.

A low EF (<0.35) suggests disrupted contraction patterns and minimal myocardial reserve. Those patients (the vast majority) who fall between these values, typically do well, but the exception occurs often enough to remind us of the unpredictability of this determinant.

Left ventricular end-diastolic pressure (LVEDP) has been suggested as an index of myocardial function and reserve. By itself, the number means little unless it is markedly elevated. Precatheterization preparation often reduces LVEDP to within the normal range, only to have the pressure return to its usually elevated value between cardiac catheterization and operation. The change in LVEDP in response to coronary angiography is used by some anesthesiologists as an indicator of myocardial reserve. The marginal heart responds to contrast material by failing briefly. The robust heart tolerates the insult. Such an approximation is an oversimplification—not a hard and fast rule; but it does seem to predict problem patients with some reliability.

MONITORING

The premedicated patient is made as comfortable as possible in the operating room. Blood pressure (cuff) and electrocardiographic monitoring, including a lead V_5 (or any other surface lead known to demonstrate ischemic changes in that particular patient) are established immediately. One or two large (14- or 16-gauge) intravenous cannulae are inserted, and additional sedation (fentanyl, lorazepam) administered if needed.

Patients premedicated with morphine (0.1 to 0.15 mg/kg) and scopolamine (0.4 to 0.6 mg) an hour before arriving in the operating room typically do not need supplemental sedation. They appear (and state that they feel) calm and tranquil, and display little apprehension. When questioned postoperatively, they often have no memories of the preoperative period.

A 20-gauge arterial cannula is placed percutaneously into a radial artery. In the absence of a definitive study disproving its utility, we continue to employ a modification of Allen's test for collateral circulation to the hand before cannulating a radial artery.

We introduce a flow-directed pulmonary artery (PA) catheter into most of our patients being operated upon for coronary artery disease. As we have gained experience with the intraoperative interpretation (and manipulation) of cardiac output and pulmonary artery and wedge pressures, the PA catheter has become more and more useful. PA catheterization is probably not indicated in every coronary artery bypass graft (CABG) patient, but it is difficult to identify with certainty those patients who appear relatively "healthy" preoperatively but who develop intraoperative problems with myocardial ischemia or cardiac failure. Because of this uncertainty, we place a PA catheter in *most* of our CABG patients. All patients with a history of cardiac failure, elevated left or right ventricular diastolic pressure, pulmonary hypertension, concomitant cardiac valvular disease or abnormal heart wall motion are candidates for a PA catheter.

The right external jugular vein is our preferred catheter entry site. The incidence of complications (carotid puncture, hematoma, A-V fistula) is lower than with an internal jugular vein approach—but so is the success rate. If the external jugular vein is inadequate or if the catheter cannot be passed into the central venous circulation, the right internal jugular vein is cannulated.

The induction of anesthesia is the time of greatest physiological change and poses the greatest threat to the patient's well-being. We believe that it is in the patient's best interest for the anesthesiologist to have as much data as possible to aid in maintaining circulatory stability, and for this reason establish all of our cardiovascular monitoring lines prior to anesthetic induction. Preinduction studies of CABG patients have yielded conflicting interpretations. Some groups believe that establishing monitoring lines while the patient is awake creates unnecessary stress. Others have demonstrated that there appear to be no unfavorable hemodynamic consequences of awake cannulation in the adequately premedicated patient.[6]

ANESTHESIA AND MYOCARDIAL OXYGENATION

The major concern in anesthetizing a patient with coronary artery disease is maintaining adequate oxygen supply to the myocardium. Myocardial oxygen consumption is determined largely by heart rate, contractility, and ventricular wall tension. The oxygen supply depends on coronary artery pressure (primarily on diastolic pressure) and the oxygen content of arterial blood. The classic advice, "avoid hypoxia and hypotension" remains valid—but oversimplified.

The vessels in the myocardium beyond a stenosed coronary artery may be maximally dilated and receiving all the blood which can pass the stenosis. Maneuvers to increase flow through a fixed stenosis are likely to fail. In fact, actions which dilate those coronary arteries capable of dilating may actually induce a "coronary steal" and *reduce* blood flow to the area beyond the arterial lesion. Consequently, most anesthetic decisions are based on the concept of reducing oxygen demand, or at least preventing those events which increase it, rather than attempting to increase myocardial oxygen supply.

PHARMACOLOGY OF ANESTHETICS

Volatile Agents

The volatile anesthetic agents, enflurane, halothane, and isoflurane, all decrease myocardial contractility directly. These agents are also potent vasodilators. The combination of decreased contractility and afterload reduction, in controlled circumstances, can decrease myocardial oxygen consumption by 40 to 60%.[7] Table 7.1 summarizes hemodynamic effects of the volatile anesthetics.

Narcotics

Narcotic analgesics (morphine, fentanyl) are the other major group of drugs used for cardiac anesthesia. Neither agent has a significant direct effect on the myocardium (Table 7.2). Morphine acts (at least in part

**Table 7.1
Hemodynamic Effects of Volatile Anesthetics***

	Halothane	Enflurane	Isoflurane
ABP	↓	↓	↓↓
CO	↓	↓	±
SVR	↓	↓	↓↓
HR	↓	↑	↑
Myocardial function	↓	↓	↓
MV̇O₂	↓	↓?	↓

* Abbreviations used are: ABP, arterial blood pressure; CO, cardiac ouput; SVR, systemic vascular resistance; HR, heart rate; MV̇O₂, myocardial oxygen consumption.

**Table 7.2
Hemodynamic Effects of Narcotic Agents***

	Morphine	Fentanyl
ABP	↓ ↑	? slight ↓
CO	0	0
SVR	↓ ↑	usually 0
HR	↓	↓
Myocardial function	0	0
MV̇O₂	0	0

* Abbreviations as in Table 7.1.

through histamine release) as a peripheral vasodilator. The initial attraction of narcotic anesthesia for cardiac surgery was the striking cardiovascular stability in patients with severe valvular disease.[8,9] The absence of myocardial depression has become less of an aspect in caring for patients with coronary artery disease.

Anesthetic Agents and Coronary Artery Disease

There have been only a few comparative studies of anesthetic agents in patients with coronary artery disease. Reves et al.[10] compared halothane and enflurane for their effects on hemodynamic parameters and myocardial damage in patients undergoing CABG. Sonntag et al.[11] reported on the effects of high dose fentanyl on myocardial blood flow and oxygen consumption, as well as on the hemodynamic effects of the technique. Zurick and his colleagues[12] compared hemodynamic and hormonal effects of high dose fentanyl and halothane anesthesia for coronary artery surgery. Wilkinson et al.[13] compared the effects of halothane and morphine on intraoperative ischemia as well as on hemodynamic parameters. Table 7.3 summarizes the conditions under which each study was performed. Measurements were made at some awake control period, after all monitoring lines had been inserted but before the induction of anesthesia. Measurements were repeated after tracheal intubation, prior to surgical incision, and during or shortly after sternotomy. The study conditions are not identical, but they are similar enough to allow comparison of anesthetic agents under actual surgical conditions. Selected hemodynamic data from these studies are presented in Tables 7.4 and 7.5.

Table 7.3
Studies Comparing Anesthetic Agents

	No. of Patients	Dose	Measurements	Interventions
Zurick et al. (1982)[12]	12 Halothane 10 Fentanyl	150 μg/kg	5 minutes after event	Nitroglycerine, propranolol
Sonntag et al. (1982)[11]	9 Fentanyl	100 μg/kg	During sternotomy	Etomidate, additional fentanyl, nitroglycerine
Reves et al. (1980)[10]	25 Halothane 25 Enflurane		Maximum or minimum during interval	Tracheal lidocaine, pressors, vasodilators, propranolol
Wilkinson et al. (1981)[13]	14 Halothane 12 Morphine	2 mg/kg	10 minutes after event	Tracheal lidocaine

Table 7.4
Heart Rate during Anesthesia for Coronary Artery Surgery

Study	Anesthetic Agent	No. of Patients	Control	Intubation	Prep	Sternotomy
Zurick et al.[12]	Halothane	12	67	80		69
	Fentanyl	10	66	83		80
Sonntag et al.[11]	Fentanyl	9	76		82	98
Reves et al.[10]	Enflurane	25	72	91	79	76
	Halothane	25	72	96	78	74
Wilkinson et al.[13]	Halothane	14	65	67		70
	Morphine	12	63	62		72

Table 7.5
Systolic Blood Pressure during Anesthesia for Coronary Artery Surgery

Study	Anesthetic Agent	No. of Patients	Control	Intubation	Prep	Sternotomy
Zurick et al.[12]	Halothane	12	132	110		109
	Fentanyl	10	141	133		132
Sonntag et al.[11]	Fentanyl	9	141		124	152
Reves et al.[10]	Enflurane	25	132	163	116	140
	Halothane	25	133	177	124	128
Wilkinson et al.[13]	Halothane	14	148	95		110
	Morphine	12	144	118		160

Zurick et al.,[12] comparing large, single dose fentanyl/O_2 anesthesia with halothane/N_2O, found that heart rate was elevated after intubation and after sternotomy in patients anesthetized with fentanyl. A decrease in systolic blood pressure was measured after intubation and again after sternotomy in halothane-anesthetized patients. A second portion of this study sought to detect changing biochemical markers of stress: blood levels of epinephrine and norepinephrine; plasma renin activity; and blood growth hormone levels. Only growth hormone levels were demonstrably different. Halothane did not block the intubation- or surgery-induced rise as completely as fentanyl did. Zurick et al.[12] concluded that they could not demonstrate significant hormonal or hemodynamic advantages of one agent over the other.[12]

Sonntag et al.[11] administered high dose fentanyl/O_2 anesthesia in stages (first 10 μg/kg, then 90 μg/kg more) with etomidate supplementation. Standard hemodynamic variables as well as myocardial blood flow and oxygen consumption were measured several times during the start of the anesthetic and operation. Large doses of fentanyl produced slight decreases in heart rate and blood pressure. Myocardial blood flow and myocardial oxygen consumption paralleled these values. During sternotomy, heart rate and blood pressure increased, as did both myocardial blood flow and oxygen consumption. Measurement of lactate production indicated myocardial ischemia even before surgical stimulus in five of the nine patients studied. Sternotomy increased the incidence of biochemical evidence of ischemia to seven of nine. This study concluded that fentanyl was inadequate as the sole anesthetic agent.[11]

Reves et al[10] compared two inhalation agents, halothane and enflurane, administered with N_2O. The usual pre- and intraoperative hemodynamic measurements were made. Evidence of myocardial damage was also sought through serial intra- and postoperative EKGs and creatine phosphokinase MB fraction (CK MB) determinations. An elaborate protocol for pharmacological intervention was established. They found no difference between halothane and enflurane. Both agents allowed a transient increase in heart rate and blood pressure in response to tracheal intubation, with no EKG evidence of ischemia. They detected no difference between the agents in need for pharmacological intervention, nor in the pattern or magnitude of CK MB release. They concluded that what myocardial damage occurred apparently did so during cardiopulmonary bypass (CPB).[10]

Wilkinson et al.[13] measured systemic and coronary hemodynamics in patients anesthetized with N_2O and either halothane or morphine (2 mg/kg). They found that morphine anesthesia allowed a hypertensive response to sternotomy which was not seen with halothane. Intraoperative myocardial ischemia (detected by either ST-segment depression or myocardial lactate production) occurred in about 70% of anesthetics with either agent.[13]

Several inconsistencies arise—the hypertensive response to intubation in the study by Reves et al.[10] is absent from the patients of Zurick et al.[12] The patients of Sonntag et al.[11] became hypertensive after sternotomy—none of the others receiving fentanyl did. Heart rates also increased after sternotomy in the patients in the study by Sonntag et al.[11] These data are confusing. They suggest that there are factors other than choice of primary anesthetic agent which influence the patient's response to anesthesia and surgery. None of these studies was performed using the primary anesthetic as the only agent. Vasopressors and vasodilators, additional sedatives, and beta-adrenergic blocking agents were added to the milieu as necessary.

ANESTHETIC TECHNIQUE

The lack of clear distinction among agents underscores that there is no ideal cardiac anesthetic agent. The volatile agents produce myocardial depression and some hypotension—which may be good, if controlled, because myocardial oxygen demand is reduced. Properly administered and supplemented, the volatile agents are capable of suppressing potentially harmful responses to such stimuli as tracheal intubation and sternotomy. Excess myocardial depression from these agents may lead to hypotension and myocardial ischemia.

The narcotic analgesics are easy to administer. Fentanyl has replaced morphine as the more popular drug because of its shorter duration of action and decreased tendency toward hypotension. The incidence of tachycardia and hypertension in response to surgical stimuli seems greater with fentanyl than with volatile agents, but judicious use of beta-blockers and vasodilators can overcome these disadvantages.

No anesthetic is administered in a vacuum. A drug is administered, its effect assessed, and an adjustment made. This is the secret of successful cardiac anesthesia. There are many ways to approach the goal of a stable, pain-free, ischemia-free intraoperative course. The combination of a base of narcotic with supplemental inhalation agent is becoming increasingly popular. Fentanyl (20 to 100 mg/kg) is supplemented by 0.2 to 1% halothane to maintain filling pressures and arterial pressure near preoperative levels. Vasodilators like nitroglycerin or nitroprusside are added for severe hypertension or elevated filling pressures.

Sedation on Cardiopulmonary Bypass

Sedation on bypass is aided by reduced blood flow and decreased temperature. Additional volatile agents may be administered via a vaporizer in the fresh gas line to the oxygenator. Fixed agents such as diazepam or lorazepam, barbiturates, or additional narcotics may be added to the blood in the pump. Muscle relaxants are used to control unwanted muscular activity (e.g., flipping of the diaphragm) after ascertaining that gas exchange and sedation are adequate.

Termination of Cardiopulmonary Bypass

Termination of CPB is a complex event. The patient's heart has not yet regained full ability to function. The work of circulation must be transferred slowly and carefully from the pump-oxygenator to the heart. There are many variations to this technique. One commonly used method of weaning transfuses the patient from the pump until

barely adequate filling pressures and cardiac output are achieved. Output from the pump is decreased slowly until only blood loss is being replaced. Typically, myocardial function improves rapidly in the first 5 to 10 minutes after bypass, and as it does, additional volume may be translocated from the pump to the patient. Vasodilators are often administered at this point to decrease both arteriolar and capacitance vessel tone. Transfusion is continued and vascular resistance and inotropic support manipulated to optimize cardiac output. Preparations for weaning the patient from bypass include:

1. discontinuing any volatile anesthetic agent to pump;
2. checking hematocrit, blood gases, electrolytes, and acid base status and correcting as necessary;
3. initiating ventilation with 100% O_2;
4. determining that the patient has been rewarmed adequately;
5. confirming that vasopressor, inotropic, and vasodilator infusions are ready for administration;
6. confirming that there is adequate volume in pump reservoir system to transfuse patient as necessary while discontinuing CPB;
7. confirming that blood is available for transfusion;
8. confirming that antiarrhythmic drugs are available.

The Postbypass Period

Patients vary widely in their pharmacological needs in the postbypass period. The most common course is continually improving myocardial function. Deepening anesthesia and vasodilator therapy are often required to block hypertension and tachycardia. Other patients may require little anesthesia, but a significant level of pharmacological support of a failing heart. Epinephrine, dopamine, and dobutamine are the inotropes most commonly employed. Concomitant vasodilator therapy and/or balloon assist devices may be necessary.

Some anesthesiologists believe that administration of N_2O in the postbypass period risks enlarging any air emboli which may have entered the systemic circulation during bypass. Others believe that if N_2O is the agent of choice in the postbypass period, it may be administered with impunity if the inspired concentration is kept under 50%. Few data exist to support either position.

Transition to Intensive Care Unit

The availability of battery-powered monitors and infusion pumps has improved patient safety during the transition from the operating room to the recovery or intensive care area. Physical movement of a patient with an unstable cardiovascular system risks severe hypotension. Protective reflexes may be nonfunctional; blood volume may be marginally replaced. The situation is one of potential disaster. The ability to monitor vascular pressures and EKG during this period has reduced the incidence of untoward events.

If a volatile anesthetic agent has been a major contributor to post-CPB sedation, the transition to postoperative care and ventilator support may be smoothed by the administration of morphine. A small dose (0.05 to 0.10 mg/kg) given intravenously during closure of the wound also provides some postoperative analgesia.

CONCLUSION

This chapter has reviewed the perioperative course of the patient undergoing coronary artery surgery. Interactions between antihypertensive and antianginal medication and anesthetic agents were discussed, and the necessity for continuing most medication into the immediate preoperative period was examined.

The discussion of assessment of the patient and selection of an appropriate anesthetic technique summarized the cardiovascular effects of volatile and narcotic anesthetic agents, and concluded that there is no one ideal anesthetic agent or technique. The narcotics provide cardiovascular stability but do not reliably block hypertensive and tachycardic responses to surgical stimuli. Volatile agents depress myocardial contractility and blood pressure, but also decrease myocardial oxygen demand. However, the risks of excessive myocardial depression,

hypotension, and myocardial ischemia are real. Care in the administration of the chosen agents, thoughtful monitoring, and meticulous attention to detail appear to be more important factors in ensuring a successful outcome than is the actual selection of anesthetic agents.

References

1. Egbert LD, Battit GE, Turndorf H, et al: The value of the preoperative visit by an anesthetist. *JAMA* 185:553, 1963.
2. Weiner N: Drugs that inhibit adrenergic nerves and block adrenergic receptors. In Gilman AJ, Goodman LS, Gilman M (eds): *Pharmacological Basis of Therapeutics*, 6th ed., New York, McMillan Publishing Company, Inc., 1980.
3. Antman EM, Stone PH, Muller JE, et al: Calcium channel blocking agents in the treatment of cardiovascular disorders. Part I: Basic and clinical electrophysiologic effects. *Ann Intern Med* 93:875, 1980.
4. Stone PH, Antman EM, Muller JE, et al: Calcium channel blocking agents in the treatment of cardiovascular disorders. Part II: Hemodynamic effects and clinical applications. *Ann Intern Med* 93:886, 1980.
5. Prys-Roberts C, Meloche R: Management of anesthesia in patients with hypertension or ischemic heart disese. *Int Anesth Clin* 18:181, 1980.
6. Waller JL, Zaiden JR, Kaplan JA, et al: Hemodynamic responses to preoperative vascular cannulation in patients with coronary artery disease. *Anesthesiology* 56:219, 1982.
7. Hickey RF, Eger EI, II: Circulatory pharmacology of inhaled anesthetics. In Miller RD (ed): *Anesthesia*. New York, Churchill Livingstone, 1981.
8. Bailey P, Gerbode F, Garlington L: An anesthetic technique which utilizes 100% oxygen as the only inhalant. *Arch Surg* 76:437, 1958.
9. Lowenstein E, Hallowell P, Levine F, et al: Cardiovascular response to large doses of intravenous morphine in man. *N Engl J Med* 281:1389, 1969.
10. Reves JG, Samuelson PN, Lell WA, et al: Myocardial damage in coronary artery bypass surgical patients anesthetized with two anesthetic techniques: A random comparison of halothane and enflurane. *Can Anaesth Soc J* 27:238, 1980.
11. Sonntag H, Larsen R, Hilfiker O, et al: Myocardial blood flow and oxygen consumption during high dose fentanyl anesthesia in patients with coronary artery disease. *Anesthesiology* 56:417, 1982.
12. Zurick AM, Urzua G, Yared J-P, et al: Comparison of hemodynamic and hormonal effects of large single-dose fentanyl anesthesia and halothane/nitrous oxide anesthesia for coronary artery surgery. *Anesth Analg* 61:521, 1982.
13. Wilkinson PL, Hamilton WK, Moyers JR, et al: Halothane and morphine-nitrous oxide anesthesia in patients undergoing coronary artery bypass operation; patterns of intraoperative ischemia. *J Thorac Cardiovasc Surg* 82:372, 1981.

CHAPTER 8

INTRAOPERATIVE PROTECTION OF THE MYOCARDIUM

RENEE S. HARTZ, M.D.
LAWRENCE L. MICHAELIS, M.D.

By strictest definition, myocardial protection includes therapeutic manipulations made during the entire perioperative period. The preoperative preparation of the patient, especially regarding drug management of myocardial ischemia and/or cardiac failure, has profound influence on the condition of the patient's heart following operation. Decisions to maintain, discontinue, or taper such drugs as propranolol, calcium blocking agents, nitroglycerin, and other vasoactive drugs are good examples of this principle. Similarly, the timing of surgical intervention has direct influence on the outcome of operation, especially in patients with unstable angina, recent or evolving myocardial injury, bacterial endocarditis, etc.

In the operating room, prior to the institution of cardiopulmonary bypass (CPB), pharmacological manipulation continues to be crucial, as does implementation of appropriate hemodynamic monitoring and choice of anesthetic agents. During this period hemodynamic instability secondary to high levels of circulating catecholamines and the myocardial depressant effects of the anesthetic must be controlled as carefully as possible. Cardiac operative techniques, such as the methodology of extracorporeal circulatory support, blood temperature, degree of hemodilution, and the decision whether

to decompress the left ventricle all play roles in the recovery of the patient. Finally, and most importantly, the intellectual and technical skill of the entire operating team (surgeon, anesthesiologist, perfusionist, and nursing staff) contributes to the end result.

Postbypass considerations also influence myocardial recovery; techniques of weaning from CPB, maintenance of the coronary perfusion pressure within an acceptable range, discontinuation of drugs postoperatively, avoidance of coronary spasm, and the decision to institute inotropic support, pharmacological unloading, or mechanical assist devices.

For the purpose of this presentation, we will limit our discussion to actual intraoperative protection of the myocardium while the heart is undergoing operative repair. This, of course, refers mainly to the use of hypothermic cardioplegic techniques.

The student of myocardial protection is referred to the proceedings of four symposia, an editorial, and two book chapters (listed as *Additional Reading* following the references) which give an excellent overview of the present "state of the art." It is to be emphasized that the principles and theories presented herein, and our particular approach to intraoperative protection of the myocardium, are prejudiced by personal experiences. The practice of surgery remains an art as well as a science; nowhere is this more evident than in a surgeon's choice of myocardial protective techniques. Cardiac surgeons differ greatly in their approaches to myocardial protection. In spite of these differences, however, results are usually excellent when the surgical team makes decisions based on sound physiological and pharmacological principles. This essay will provide a brief historical review, an outline of basic physiological principles involved, a discussion of cardioplegic solutions and additives, and a detailed description of our own operative technique using cold blood cardioplegia.

HISTORICAL REVIEW

The 1970s will be remembered as the decade when cardiac surgeons became aware that good myocardial protection was responsible for good surgical results. During these years, attention to the details of myocardial protection, both in the laboratory and clinical environment, resulted in profoundly positive results on the outcome of cardiac surgical operations. This was the decade when the mortality for elective coronary surgery fell beneath that of most other major surgical procedures.

In 1955, chemical cardioplegia was first used by Melrose et al.[1] with a potassium citrate arrest; other surgeons immersed the heart in an iced slush. For a variety of reasons, both of these techniques were abandoned and efforts were directed to the use of continuous coronary artery perfusion,[2] either by maintenance of continuous, nonpulsatile retrograde coronary flow during CPB (when the aortic valve was competent), or in operations performed on the aortic root and outflow tract, by direct cannulation of the coronary arteries. In theory, this should have provided uniformly excellent protection, but a number of factors contributed to the still too-frequent occurrence of death or profound morbidity. These included inadequate perfusion because of low flow or pressure of unrecognized coronary disease, subendocardial necrosis related to prolonged ventricular fibrillation,

direct injury to the coronary arteries, and the numerous technical difficulties associated with working on a beating or fibrillating heart.[2]

Shumway et al.[3] introduced hypothermic myocardial protection by advocating continuous aortic crossclamping with continuous cold saline lavage. Bretschneider et al.[4] and Kirsch et al.[5] in Europe persisted in the use of chemical cardioplegia, but it was the work of Gay and Ebert[6] in the early 1970s which brought renewed interest to the use of potassium-induced hypothermic cardioplegic arrest. At about the same time, Reitz and his associates,[7] in our laboratory, were preserving hearts for transplantation. We were successful in storing excised canine hearts for periods of up to 24 hours in a potassium-rich hypothermic solution.

During the last 12 years, hypothermic cardioplegia has been a subject of intense clinical and laboratory interest. Gerald Buckberg and his associates at UCLA and Braimbridge and Hearse at St. Thomas' hospital in London have been among the leading contributors in these studies. In 1980, McGoon published an editorial outlining many of the difficulties in assessing cardioplegic techniques.[8] In essence, there are now so many variables that it is impossible to analyze independently every proposed additive. Intraoperative protection of the myocardium is still not perfect, but the progress made has been spectacular, and this single intervention, the use of hypothermic cardioplegic solution, is probably most responsible for the widespread excellent cardiac surgical results existing today.

BASIC PHYSIOLOGICAL PRINCIPLES

The basic physiological and biochemical principles which have influenced the current state of the art in cardioplegia are fully explained in the *Additional Readings*. Some of the more important principles (in the authors' opinion) are the following:

In order to avoid global or regional myocardial cellular injury, *energy supply* (whether from aerobic or anaerobic metabolism) *must equal energy demand*. Anerobic metabolism is far less efficient than aerobic.

Anoxia, hypoxia, and *ischemia* have different metabolic consequences. When flow is normal, but oxygen content is absent (anoxia) or decreased (hypoxia), the unwanted results of anaerobic metabolism are washed out and carried away. In *ischemia*, with a reduction in both coronary flow and oxygen content, the waste metabolites (acidic in nature) remain and accumulate. Therefore, ischemia is much more dangerous to the myocardium than anoxia or hypoxia.

When the aorta is crossclamped, *ischemia* (rather than anoxia) occurs. This is because *noncoronary collaterals* pass through the pericardial attachments and pulmonary venous walls. These collaterals, which are more abundant in patients with coronary artery obstructive disease, left ventricular hypertrophy, and certain forms of congenital heart disease not only create the ischemic environment but wash away cardioplegic solution.

▷ Soon after the onset of *ischemia*, there is a gradual development of: (a) depletion of myocardial high-energy phosphates, (b) inhibition of necessary enzymes, (c) intracellular (and eventually extracellular) acidosis, (d) intracellular edema, (e) damage and disruption of the cellular membrane with movement of calcium into the cell.

▷ Prolonged *ventricular fibrillation*, even in the presence of normal coronary flow, causes subendocardial ischemia, and eventually necrosis. This pathological process is potentiated when fibrillation is electrically induced and maintained and in the presence of left ventricular hypertrophy or significant coronary artery obstructive disease. Increasing the coronary perfusion pressure of oxygenated blood may delay or inhibit this unwanted effect of ventricular fibrillation. Myocardial energy demands are reduced, but not eliminated, by *hypothermia*. This reduction is greatly enhanced in the arrested heart. At 5°C, myocardial oxygen consumption is about one-tenth the level occurring at 37°. But *even at low temperatures, oxygen consumption continues*. The addition of oxygen to cardioplegic solution therefore improves its protective capabilities and seems to explain the advantage of cold blood as compared to nonoxygenated crystalloid solutions.

Besides the obvious technical difficulties involved (especially in coronary revascularization) there are clear experimental data that *intermittent* perfusion of cardioplegic solution is more effective than *continuous*.

CARDIOPLEGIA COMPONENTS AND ADDITIVES

The perfect cardioplegic solution would preserve all myocardial function and cellular integrity during a period of global ischemia (aortic crossclamping) long enough to perform even the most complicated cardiac operation. Realistically, finite myocardial cellular damage always occurs, even if unmeasurable by today's methods. The composition of an ideal cardioplegic solution remains controversial. The authors' have been greatly influenced by our own experience and experimentation, and by the laboratory and clinical efforts directed by Buckberg, Levitsky, and Spencer.

Potassium

The introduction of potassium into the coronary circulation depolarizes the cell membrane resulting in diastolic arrest which persists until the potassium is washed out. Early solutions contained potassium citrate, but since citrate itself is an end-product of glycolysis, most investigators have switched to the more physiological potassium chloride (KCl). The most appropriate concentration of potassium is unknown and its effects are related to temperature. It is doubtful that concentrations greater than 20 to 30 mEq/liter are necessary; they may even be detrimental. Some investigators believe that potassium may not be necessary at all.[9]

Comment: Our routine is to assure immediate diastolic arrest with 20 mEq KCl in the first dose of cardioplegia, and decrease the amount in subsequent doses (10 mEq, then none) to maximize potential for electrical recovery and minimize systemic hyperkalemia.

Hypothermia

Between 10 and 20°C there is a dramatic reduction in myocardial oxygen consumption. Experimentally, both myocardial energy levels and left ventricular function are better preserved in hearts arrested with hypothermia and potassium, than with potassium alone.[10, 11]

Comment: We routinely employ hypothermia in three ways: systemic cooling (28 to

30°C for routine bypass surgery), topical cooling with intermittent iced saline in the pericardial well, and cooling of our blood cardioplegic solution to 8°C. Methods to assure maximal and uniform myocardial cooling are discussed below.

Oxygen

Although the blood-crystalloid controversy continues, the theoretical advantages of adding oxygen and substrate (blood) to a cardioplegic solution are compelling and recent clinical work is providing convincing data favoring the use of blood.[12] Besides the obvious capacity of blood to exchange oxygen and carbon dioxide in the myocardium, it can serve as a buffer and it already contains physiological amounts of many of the ingredients currently being added to crystalloid solutions. In the last few years, several clinical studies have suggested better postoperative myocardial contractility and cardiac output, plus less mortality, perioperative infarction, and need for circulatory support using blood rather than crystalloid cardioplegia.[13–15]

Comment: Although the clinical data must still be considered preliminary, the theoretical and technical advantages of cold blood cardioplegia are so obvious to us that its use is routine in our institution. A detailed description of its application and advantages (Table 8.1) will follow.

Table 8.1
Crystalloid versus Blood Cardioplegia

	Crystalloid	Blood
Ease of preparation	Yes	No
Widely available	Yes	Yes
Potential for labeling error*	Yes	No
Potential for pre-O.R. processing contamination	Yes	No
Oxygen delivery	No	Yes
Delivery postobstruction†	No	Yes
Volume load	Yes	No
Easier surgical technique	No	Yes
Strict temperature control	No	Yes
Advantages	1/9	7/9

* The authors are aware of at least two deaths secondary to this complication.
† Cold blood is better distributed past coronary stenosis than is crystalloid solution.[25]

Buffer

Based on early studies showing better energy levels in hearts arrested with slightly alkalotic solutions, there is essentially uniform agreement that an alkaline cardioplegia solution provides an appropriate climate for any metabolic activity which may be occurring and combats ischemia-generated acidosis. Although the pH of a physiological solution increases as the temperature is lowered, some cardioplegic solutions require the addition of a buffer to maintain a pH greater than 7.6.

Comment: With our cold blood system, the temperature corrected pH is routinely 7.70 to 7.85 without buffering.

Osmolarity and Oncotic Pressure

Ideally, cardioplegic solutions should be slightly hypertonic and hyperosmolar to prevent the development of myocardial edema and keep the solution within the coronary vascular compartment.

Comment: Because the blood used in our cardioplegia is altered by hemodilution, we readjust the osmolarity of the cold blood solution to 320–360 mosm/liter by adding mannitol and we raise the oncotic pressure to 17–20 mm Hg with albumin.

Calcium and Magnesium

Hearts arrested with calcium-free solution are subjected to the danger of extensive myocardial damage when reperfused with calcium-containing solutions, especially after prolonged global ischemia (the "calcium-paradox" or "stone-heart" phenomenon). It is probably fair to say that crystalloid solutions should contain 1 to 2 mEq Ca^{++}/liter. Magnesium may also be important since it is the second most prevalent intracellular cation.

Comment: It is unnecessary to add these cations to blood cardioplegia which already contains physiological amounts.

Calcium Antagonists

Although several experimental studies and some early clinical work[16–19] lend support to the use of calcium channel blockers in cardioplegic solutions, it is undoubtedly too early to recommend their routine use. Not only has the experimental work been diluted by the fact that several different drugs have been used (which are not pharmacologically identical) but the clinical work is also suspect because of the uncertain relationship between preoperative calcium blocker therapy and intraoperative response to these drugs. Although *routine* use is not recommended, an exception *may* be the very high-risk patient in whom a prolonged ischemic period is anticipated. Clark et al.[18] have suggested, in a controlled clinical study, that mortality and the need for postoperative mechanical support are significantly lowered in these patients when nifedipine was added to the cardioplegia.

Comment: We have not added calcium blockers to our blood cardioplegia and wonder if there would have been any differences in Clark's patients had blood been the vehicle for cardioplegia delivery.

Other Additives

Numerous other additives have been suggested and employed in cardioplegic solutions: coronary vasodilators, corticosteroids, propranolol, procaine or xylocaine for membrane stabilization, etc.

Comment: We add 200 mg nitroglycerine to our first dose of cardioplegia for its vasodilatory effect. Xylocaine is added to the first dose to potentiate immediate arrest (it has less systemic toxicity than procaine and has also been shown experimentally to reduce infarct size after coronary occlusion) and to the last dose to lessen the degree of electrical activity while rewarming systemically. We have the distinct clinical impression that its addition has increased the incidence of spontaneous return to normal sinus rhythm after removing the aortic crossclamp.

OPERATIVE CONSIDERATIONS

Several operative interventions are necessary to enhance myocardial protection. The technical goals of these maneuvers are much more straightforward than the complex physiological requirements of myocardial protection already discussed. The objective is to minimize the period of global and regional ischemia through the following interventions: the heart must be kept cold and empty, the operative field must be quiet and

relatively dry, cardioplegia should be delivered easily and without manipulation of cumbersome apparatus or prolongation of operative time, and above all, the methods of myocardial protection should not, in themselves, be injurious to the heart.

Venous Decompression

Recently, much attention has been directed to the relationship of venous return cannulae and cardiac decompression. Bicaval cannulation seems to be unnecessary for optimal decompression and cooling,[20, 21] and more surgeons are employing a single, two-staged, right atriocaval cannula for routine coronary bypass procedures. Depending on the size of the patient and the amount of work to be done with the heart elevated for exposure of its posterior aspect, a 40- to 50-French cannula is effective. Using this approach, we have not had problems with distension of the heart or rising central venous pressure (even when grafting the circumflex artery in the atrioventricular groove) despite the fact that we have vented only the aortic root for our last 1200 cases.

Left Ventricular Venting

Although Roberts demonstrated that left ventricular function is not different in vented versus unvented patients,[20] most surgeons agree that some measure must be taken to guard against ventricular distention. In a survey performed by Utley,[22] only 30% of coronary surgeons used a no-vent technique in 1980. Most were using aortic or pulmonary artery venting or a combination of the two. We prefer an ascending aortic vent, on suction, because of its effectiveness and simplicity. Techniques used to avoid and correct for distention are discussed below.

Cold Blood Cardioplegia System

Although our blood cardioplegia system requires a separate reservoir and pump circuit, it offers tremendous advantages to the patient and surgeon; the blood can be rapidly cooled and filtered, its delivery (flow and pressure) can be tightly controlled, and it can be made up and delivered without need of an additional perfusionist. The cost, approximately $100/case, is offset by the rapid functional recovery of the arrested heart.

As soon as CPB is established, 1 liter of blood is diverted from the pump oxygenator to a separate cardiotomy reservoir where the additives are introduced (Table 8.2). The solution is then passed through a Travenol Miniprime heat exchanger attached to a Thermatrol heater-cooler with a water temperature of 7°C, and is circulated through the cardioplegia tubing itself (Fig. 8.1).

The cardioplegia tubing is attached to a 14-gauge DLP aortic root cardioplegia cannula with a side arm for venting (Fig. 8.2). A simple adventitial suture is used to maintain traction on the aorta while the cannula is inserted (thus avoiding injury to the back wall of the aorta) and to hold the cannula

Table 8.2
Cardioplegia Additives—1000 cc of Cold Blood

KCl dose
   1st, 20 mEq
   2nd, 10 mEq
   3rd, None
200 μg nitroglycerin
3 gm mannitol
12.5 gm albumin
Lidocaine, 50 mg (first and last dose)

in place. The site of cannulation is generally used for a proximal anastomosis after the crossclamp is removed.

The aorta is then clamped and the cold blood solution is infused into the aortic root by simply moving a tubing clamp from position A to B on the cardioplegia tubing (Fig. 8.1). The line pressure in the cardioplegia tubing is constantly displayed and kept *below 150 mm Hg* (there is a 30-mm drop across the cannula itself) resulting in a coronary blood flow of *200 to 300 cc/minute*. Sudden rises in line pressure indicate kinking in the tubing or ventricular distention. Sudden drops (or inability to achieve an adequate pressure initially) indicate aortic valve incompetence. The surgeon must check for the presence of aortic insufficiency by manually palpating the heart several times during each cardioplegia delivery. A small amount is frequently present and can be dealt with simply by decompressing the heart via the vent line on the cardioplegia cannula after partial delivery of the solution. Rarely, the aortic valve cannot be made competent at all, even by rapidly removing and reapplying the aortic crossclamp. In these instances, consideration should be given to performing an aortotomy and delivering the cardioplegic solution directly into the coronary ostia (just as in aortic valve

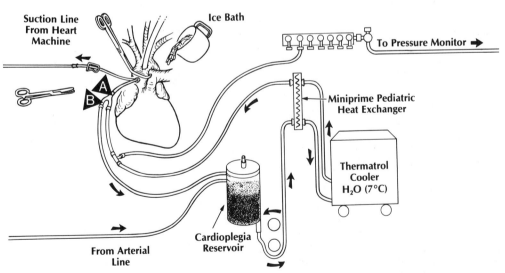

Figure 8.1. The diagram represents the cold blood cardioplegia system developed at Northwestern Memorial Hospital.

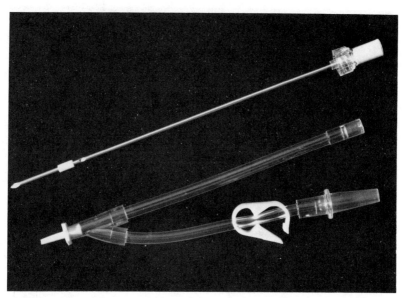

Figure 8.2. The DLP cardioplegic cannula and trocar are shown.

replacement procedures) especially in high-risk patients requiring multiple grafts. We prefer a hand-held metal cannula with a swivel ball tip (Fig. 8.3*A* and *B*) for this purpose because it is so maneuverable and atraumatic.

Cardioplegia delivery is repeated every 25 to 30 minutes unless there is earlier reappearance of electrical activity. The atrial appendages are frequently observed as they usually contract before ventricular activity occurs. The temperature of the cardioplegia is approximately 8°C. This resulted in a myocardial temperature of 10 to 15°C in perfused areas of the myocardium in several hundred patients tested. We have now abandoned routine myocardial temperature monitoring since we found that nonperfused myocardium did not cool readily, and have turned our attention instead to early proximal and distal grafting of the most ischemic myocardial segments.

Conduct of the Operation

Although the protection afforded by cold blood cardioplegia is good enough to afford an unhurried approach to operation, physiological objectives must be constantly kept in mind and *regional* ischemia should not defeat the overall goal of *global* protection.

We routinely bypass first the artery supplying the myocardium which we think is responsible for symptoms. After the distal anastomosis is completed, the proximal is done with the aortic crossclamp in place (Fig. 8.4) so that the cold blood cardioplegia can be immediately delivered to this ischemic territory. This approach has been exceedingly useful in urgent and emergency operations for unstable and postinfarction angina, cardiogenic shock, and acute dissection of the coronary arteries. Once the most crucial vessels are grafted distally and proximally, the approach to the rest of the operation is more straightforward and anatomic, although very tight obstructions (greater than 90%) are similarly treated.

Performance of a proximal anastomosis with the crossclamp on is rapid and easy because of the "open" technique. The graft is sized by distending the aorta with about 100 cc of blood cardioplegia and the heart is distended by partially occluding venous drainage for a moment. Air enters the aortic root with the open technique but is easily removed via the vent line and by aspirating the vein graft before flow to the myocardium is established. The cardioplegia needle is left in place, with the vent on suction, until the crossclamp is removed and the

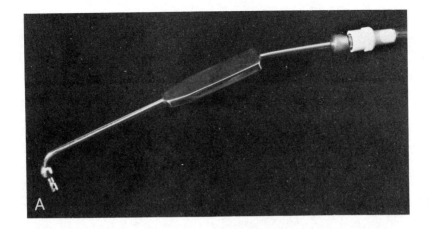

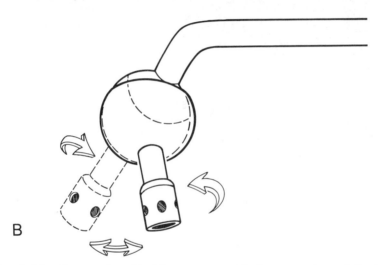

Figure 8.3. *A.* The Permco hand-held coronary perfusion cannula and *B.* swivel tip are shown.

heart is beating. Formal de-airing procedures have been unnecessary.

Alternative Techniques

The use of cold blood cardioplegia technique in our hands has provided a pleasant and unhurried operation with excellent results; mortality is under 1% in elective coronary revascularization. Even in high-risk or emergency patients with recent infarction, cardiogenic shock, acute septal rupture or mitral regurgitation, arrhythmia with aneurysmectomy, and/or endocardial resection, our overall operative mortality is less than 5%.

Nonetheless, no currently available technique affords perfect protection of the myocardium and there exists an extremely high-risk group of patients for whom any additional refinements in technique may be significant. In this regard, the work currently being conducted with warm cardioplegia induction and glutamate-rich solution[23] is impressive and may be a direction for the near future.

Lastly, synthetic blood substitutes (fluorocarbons) became commercially available in 1983 and provide better capillary to tissue oxygen gradients than does blood. Experimentally, they seem to protect the myocar-

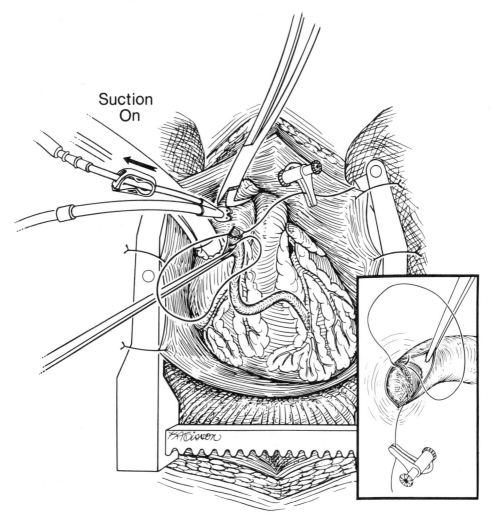

Figure 8.4. The open technique for proximal aortocoronary anastamosis is depicted.

dial cell better early in the crossclamp period, but after prolonged ischemia, and with recovery, appear quite similar to cold blood cardioplegia.[24] We watch with interest developments in this field but cannot subscribe to the theory that fluorocarbons will result in decreased disease transmission, since none of the cardioplegia systems currently in use involve homologous blood infusions.

Acknowledgment. The authors wish to thank Arthur J. Roberts, MD; John H. Sanders, Jr., MD; and Richard Wade, CCP for their innovative contributions in the de-velopment of the technique of cold blood cardioplegia presented herein.

velopment of the technique of cold blood cardioplegia presented herein.

References

1. Melrose DG, Dreyer B, Nentall HH, et al: Elective cardiac arrest. *Lancet* 2:21, 1955.
2. Michaelis LL: Coronary artery perfusion. *Ann Thorac Surg* 20:72, 1975.
3. Shumway NE, Lower RR, Stofer RC: Selective hypothermia of the heart in anoxic cardiac arrest. *Surg Gynecol Obstet* 109:750, 1959.
4. Bretschneider H, Hubner G, Knoll D, et al: Myocardial resistance and tolerance to ischemia. Physiological and biochemical basis. *J Cardiovasc Surg* 16:241, 1975.
5. Kirsch U, Rodewald G, Kalmer P: Induced ischemic

arrest. Clinical experience with cardioplegia in open-heart surgery. *J Thorac Surg* 63:121, 1972.

6. Gay WA, Ebert PA: Functional, metabolic, and morphologic effects of potassium-induced cardioplegia. *Surgery* 74:284, 1973.

7. Reitz BA, Brody WR, Hickey RP, et al: Protection of the heart for 24 hours with intracellular (high K$^+$) solution and hypothermia. *Surg Forum* 25:149, 1974.

8. McGoon DC: The quest for ideal myocardial protection—editorial. *J Thorac Cardiovasc Surg* 79:150, 1980.

9. Jacocks MA, Fowler BN, Chaffin JS, et al: Hypothermic ischemic arrest versus hypothermic potassium cardioplegia in man. *Circulation* 62(Suppl III):324, 1980.

10. Schaff HV, Dombroff R, Flaherty JT, et al: Effect of potassium cardioplegia on myocardial ischemia and post-arrest ventricular function. *Circulation* 58:240, 1978.

11. Gott VL, Bartlett M, Johnson JA, et al: High energy phosphate levels in the human heart during potassium citrate arrest. *Surg Forum* 10:544, 1960.

12. Cunningham JN, Catinalla FP, Spencer FC. Blood cardioplegia—experience with prolonged crossclamping. In Engleman RM, Levitsky S (eds): *A Textbook of Clinical Cardioplegia.* Mt. Kisko, NY, Futura Publishing Company, 1982.

13. Follette D, Fey K, Becker H, et al: Superiority of blood cardioplegia over asanguinous cardioplegia: experimental and clinical study. *Circulation* 60(Suppl II):36, 1979.

14. Barner HB, Kaiser GC, Codd JE, et al: Clinical experience with cold blood as the vehicle for hypothermic cardioplegia. *Ann Thorac Surg* 29:224, 1980.

15. Shapiro N, Behrendt D, Kirsch M, et al: Comparison of the effect of blood cardioplegia to crystalloid cardioplegia on human myocardial contractility. *J Thorac Cardiovasc Surg* 80:647, 1980.

16. Clark RE, Christilieb IY, Henry PD, et al: Nifedipine: A myocardial protective agent. *Am J Cardiol* 44:825, 1979.

17. Prinsky WH, Lewis RM, McMillan-Wood JB, et al: Myocardial protection from ischemic arrest: Potassium and verapamil cardioplegia. *Am J Physiol* 240:H326, 1981.

18. Clark RE, Christlieb IY, Ferguson TB, et al: The first American clinical trial of nifedipine in cardioplegia. *J Thorac Cardiovasc Surg* 82:848, 1981.

19. Yamamoto F, Manning AS, Braimbridge MV, et al: Cardioplegia and slow calcium-channel blockers.

Studies with verapamil. *J Thorac Cardiovasc Surg* 86:252, 1983.

20. Roberts AJ: Efficacy of intraoperative myocardial protection in coronary artery bypass graft surgery. In Roberts AJ (ed): *Coronary Artery Surgery: Application of New Techniques.* Chicago, Year Book Medical Publishers Inc., 1983.

21. Bennett EV, Fervel JG, Grover FL, et al: Myocardial preservation: Effect of venous drainage. *Ann Thorac Surg* 36:132, 1983.

22. Utley JR: Venting during cardiopulmonary bypass. *Pathophysiology and techniques of cardiopulmonary bypass III.* Cardiothoracic Surgery Series, Williams & Wilkins, 1983.

23. Rosenkranz ER, Buckberg GD, Laks H, et al: Warm induction of cardioplegia with glutamate-enriched blood in coronary patients with cardiogenic shock who are dependent on inotropic drugs and intraaortic balloon support. *J Thorac Cardiovasc Surg* 86:507, 1983.

24. Hicks GL, Arnold W, DeWall RA: Fluorocarbon cardioplegia and myocardial protection. *Ann Thorac Surg* 35:200, 1983.

25. Robertson JM, Buckberg GD, Vinten-Johansen J, et al: Comparison of distribution beyond coronary stenoses of blood and asanguineous cardioplegic solutions. *J Thorac Cardiovasc Surg* 86:80, 1983.

Additional Reading

Buckberg GD: A proposed "solution" to the cardioplegic controversy. An editorial. *J Thorac Cardiovasc Surg* 77:803, 1979.

Buckberg GD: Progress in myocardial protection during cardiac operations. In McGoon DC (ed): *Cardiac Surgery.* Philadelphia, F. A. Davis Co., 1982.

Engleman RM, Levitsky S: *A Textbook of Clinical Cardioplegia.* Mt. Kisko, New York, Futura Publishing Company, 1982.

Longmore DB: *Towards Safer Cardiac Surgery.* Boston, G. K. Hall Medical Publishers, 1981.

Michaelis LL, Behrendt DM: Intraoperative Protection of the Myocardium. A Symposium. *Ann Thorac Surg* 20, 1975.

Moran JM, Michaelis LL: *Surgery for the Complications of Myocardial Infarction.* New York, Grune & Stratton, Inc., 1980.

Roberts AJ: Efficacy of intraoperative myocardial protection in coronary artery bypass graft surgery. In Roberts AJ (ed): *Coronary Artery Surgery: Application of New Techniques.* Chicago, Year Book Medical Publishers, Inc., 1983.

CHAPTER 9

PERIOPERATIVE MYOCARDIAL INFARCTION IN OPEN HEART SURGERY

ARTHUR J. ROBERTS, M.D.

The incidence of perioperative myocardial infarction (POMI) is variable depending upon patient selection, the skill and availability of the operating room team, as well as experienced application of newer diagnostic methods used in defining this event.[1,2] The recent coronary artery surgery study (CASS) found POMI in 5%,[3] while studies using broader definitions find an incidence of from 10 to 40%.[4,5] The mechanism responsible for myocardial necrosis is often multifactorial[6,7] involving such considerations as technical misadventure, graft occlusion, reperfusion injury in the presence of patent bypass grafts, coronary artery spasm, or subendocardial necrosis resulting from an unfavorable balance between myocardial oxygen supply and demand with or without fixed coronary obstruction. This last-mentioned imbalance may be due to inappropriate mechanical, hemodynamic, or metabolic responses during cardiac surgery. Most of the available information related to POMI emanates from studies in coronary artery bypass graft (CABG) patients, but a few studies in patients undergoing valvular surgery have documented the importance of POMI in patients with either normal coronary arteries or combined valvular and coronary disease.[8,9] The presence of POMI presumes that myocardial necrosis has occurred during the immediate perioperative period. Although the quantity of myocardial cell loss may be large in patients dying during cardiac surgery,[10] it is often difficult to be quantitative in situations where lesser amounts of damage have occurred. In fact, the differentiation between severe myocardial ischemia and cell death may be impossible to note on clinical grounds and difficult to make by direct microscopic examination of heart muscle. Since most patients who suffer POMI survive, we are forced to use clinically available indirect estimates of myocardial cell death. Although each cardiac operation probably causes some amount of cell injury, there is difficulty in defining substantial myocardial necrosis. Fortunately, most (but not all) patients who survive POMI have been selected for a reasonably favorable prognosis.[2,6] At least, compared to patients with naturally-occurring myocardial infarction,[11] subsequent left ventricular performance and survival appear superior in patients surviving POMI.[2,3]

CLINICAL ASSOCIATIONS

There are several preoperative factors which predispose patients to POMI (Table 9.1). Similarly, intraoperative events also influence the occurrence of POMI (Table 9.2). We arbitrarily define the time-frame during which POMI can occur as beginning with the preoperative medications and ending some 12 hours postoperatively. During

Table 9.1

Preoperative Factors which Predispose to POMI

Preoperative factors
  Severe myocardial ischemia
  Recent myocardial necrosis
  Severe depression of left ventricular function
  Left ventricular hypertrophy
  Abrupt withdrawal of propranolol or nitrates
  Severe diffuse multiple-vessel coronary disease

Table 9.2

Intraoperative Events which Influence the Development of POMI

Intraoperative events
  Anesthetic-related difficulties
  Incomplete revascularization
  Technical complications
  Duration of aortic crossclamp time
  Duration of CPB
  Inadequate myocardial protection

this time, we can identify several periods during which myocardial necrosis can occur (Table 9.3). Not uncommonly, the final level of myocardial injury may reflect abnormalities occurring at several points in time with a resulting cumulative effect. Unfortunately, in any given case of POMI, we cannot always precisely define the reason for the outcome. Consequently, the available data can be used to characterize the risk of POMI in groups of patients while the individual case of POMI may occur as an apparent random event.

CLINICAL PRESENTATION

The clinical syndrome related to POMI may present in several ways. Intraoperative identification may become apparent prior to or at the termination of cardiopulmonary bypass (CPB). Severe left ventricular dysfunction, coronary spasm, primary right ventricular failure, or biventricular failure may become noticeable. This syndrome carries a high mortality despite the judicious use of inotropic support, intra-aortic balloon pumping, calcium channel blockers, sec-

Table 9.3

Intervals during the Perioperative Period when Myocardial Necrosis can Occur

Periods when damage may evolve
  Preoperative (unrecognized necrosis)
  Induction of general anesthesia
  Pre-CPB
  CPB (aortic crossclamping)
  Early reperfusion (after global ischemia)
  Initial postoperative recovery

ondary cardioplegia, and additional coronary bypass grafting. In a few cases, this drastic situation has been salvaged by the application of mechanical assist devices and/or heart transplant.

A more favorable form of POMI involves a low cardiac output syndrome which responds favorably to additional CPB support, inotropic support, or a combination of inotropic support and systemic afterload reduction.

Additional situations suggesting POMI are seen in patients with serious ventricular arrhythmias including ventricular tachycardia or fibrillation in the early postoperative period. Although this syndrome may occur unrelated to myocardial necrosis, when associated with clinical evidence for left ventricular dysfunction, this combination of events has a poor prognosis. Finally, the patient may have an uncomplicated clinical course but during postoperative evaluation EKG, enzymatic, scintigraphic, or echocardiographic data suggest a perioperative event. This distinct group of patients has a favorable prognosis but remains a diagnostic dilemma.

EFFECT OF MYOCARDIAL PROTECTION ON POMI

There are several methods of myocardial protection currently in use during coronary artery surgery (Table 9.4). In addition, the use of calcium antagonists, warm cardioplegic induction, cardioplegic substrate enhancement, secondary cardioplegia, or fluorocarbons may improve upon the level of myocardial protection in the future. While the CASS investigation suggests that the use of hypothermic potassium cardioplegia has

Table 9.4
Methods of Myocardial Production Currently Employed in Coronary Artery Surgery

Continuous aortic crossclamping
    Profound cardiac hypothermia (10–15°C)
    and
    Cold potassium cardioplegia

Intermittent aortic crossclamping
    Moderate systemic hypothermia (32°C)
    and/or
    Cold potassium cardioplegia

Ventricular fibrillation with local coronary sharing
    Systemic hypothermia (25–32°C)
    High perfusion pressure (>70 mm Hg)

decreased the incidence of POMI, we and others have found that under appropriate conditions the other forms of myocardial protection may be more than adequate. While potassium cardioplegic arrest may provide a greater margin of safety during cardiac surgery, the well-conceived and carefully applied method of protection may be more important than the protective effects of a particular method itself. In addition, the positioning of catheters for intracardiac venous drainage and the placing of a left ventricular vent are variables which should not adversely affect clinical results provided that left ventricular distention is avoided.[12] Furthermore, while inhomogenous myocardial cooling and cardioplegic distribution have been reported in the application of clinical cardioplegia,[13] it appears that operative mortality, the level of ventricular performance, and evidence for myocardial damage are similar whether proximal aortic anastomoses or distal coronary anastomoses are performed first in CABG surgery. The adequacy of myocardial cooling may be the most important factor in successful myocardial protection.[15] The usage of adjunctive measures to maintain a cold myocardium (< 15°C) and overcome factors related to myocardial rewarming include large volume, topical hypothermia, multidose cardioplegia, decreased CPB flow rates, decreased systemic perfusate temperatures, and surgical maneuvers to distribute

cold solutions distal to high-grade proximal coronary obstructions.[14]

TECHNIQUES USEFUL IN THE DIAGNOSIS OF PERIOPERATIVE MYOCARDIAL INFARCTION

Electrocardiogram

The reported incidence of POMI using the EKG as the diagnostic standard has varied from 2 to 40%.[4, 5] At the present time, the incidence in terms of new Q waves is about 5% in our experience. Although many variables associated with patient selection and surgical experience are involved, certain limitations in the diagnostic accuracy of the EKG are also important in this wide variability. When the EKG is obtained preoperatively and daily for several days after operation, the following criteria may be used to identify POMI. Myocardial infarction is very likely with the postoperative appearance of new, persistent Q waves of 0.04 seconds' or longer duration, or new QS deflections associated with characteristic evolutionary changes in the ST segment and T waves. Myocardial ischemic injury is probable with the development of (a) flat ST-segment depression >2 mm in left ventricular leads, lasting more than 48 hours; (b) deep T-wave inversions persisting for more than 48 hours; (c) serious ventricular arrhythmias such as ventricular tachycardia or fibrillation; and (d) the appearance of a shift in electrical axis or new left bundle branch block.

During open heart surgery, transient abnormal Q waves have been observed.[16] These Q waves were thought to be caused by temporary alterations in ventricular depolarization and/or local changes in metabolism, oxygenation, or temperature. The surface EKG has also been shown to underestimate the prevalence of epicardial Q waves obtained during cardiac surgery.[17] Postoperative ventriculographic studies have shown that new Q waves are usually, but not always, associated with new areas of ventricular asynergy, implying a POMI.[18–20] Conversely, some investigators[21] have suggested that these new Q waves may, in fact, be pre-existent and unmasked by improved contraction of the contralateral ventricular segment. Furthermore, there are a few patients in whom either new Q waves develop, in association with improved postoperative ventriculograms and patent grafts,[22] or in whom the disappearance of preoperative abnormal Q waves is manifest within a few days after CABG surgery.[23] The explanation for these occurrences is uncertain at the present time. In addition, changes in the postoperative ventriculogram may not accurately reflect differences related to the surgical procedure itself. For instance, relatively minor amounts of necrosis may not alter the appearance of the ventriculogram. Also, the late postoperative occurrence of myocardial necrosis (after hospital discharge) might falsely suggest a perioperative origin for resultant abnormalities seen on a late postoperative ventriculographic study.

The appearance of postoperative EKG abnormalities consisting of changes in the T waves, the ST segments, or severe ventricular arrhythmias with or without axis shift or bundle branch block have been considered "nondiagnostic" but suggestive of findings consistent with acute ischemic myocardial injury. Such changes may reflect pericarditis, minor surgical trauma, localized ventricular conduction delays or blocks, electrolyte imbalances, hypothermia, hypoglycemia, or pancreatitis.[2] However, some investigators have concluded that approximately 50% of such episodes may indicate acute myocardial necrosis,[24] especially when serum enzymes are also abnormally elevated. Furthermore, postoperative ventriculograms in patients with so-called nonspecific perioperative ST-segment changes or T-wave changes show a definite new regional wall motion abnormality in a considerable number.[19]

Serum Enzymes and Isoenzymes

Serial serum enzyme analysis has long been used as an adjunct in the diagnosis of acute myocardial infarction. In fact, the diagnosis of a subendocardial infarction is made when the EKG shows abnormal ST-T wave changes, but no new Q waves, in the presence of abnormal elevations in certain serum enzymes that may be released from damaged myocardium.[25] Traditionally, levels of the standard serum enzymes serum glutamic oxaloacetic transaminase, creatine phosphokinase (CK), and lactic dehydrogenase have been used to indicate the presence and extent of POMI. These serum enzyme levels have lacked sensitivity and specificity, however, because of a multiplicity of factors contributing to increased enzyme values after cardiac surgery.[26–28]

In recent years, the myocardial-specific isoenzyme CK (CK MB) has proved useful in the diagnosis of acute myocardial infarction in the coronary care unit.[29] In the first published surgical series, serum CK MB was detected in 51% of patients after CABG surgery.[30] Of these 51 patients, 21 were considered to show EKG signs of POMI. Transient postoperative serum CK MB elevations occurred in the remaining 30 patients and were attributed to varying degrees of myocardial damage from intraoperative cardiac manipulations including defibrillation. With more frequent intraoperative serum sampling by the same group in a subsequent series of 39 patients, serum CK MB was demonstrated in 77%. Further studies by other investigators[31] showed that in some patients serum CK MB rose before CPB. Fortunately, careful hemodynamic monitoring and specific pharmacological treatment of early myocardial ischemia may decrease the incidence of isoenzyme release during the critical induction and pre-CPP periods. Nevertheless, using a more sensitive biochemical assay for serum CK MB, other investigators have found that the serum CK MB fraction is elevated postoperatively in practically all patients undergoing CABG surgery.[32] Methodology, therefore, can alter the usefulness of results obtained from studies depicting changes in serum levels of CK MB during and after CABG surgery. Consequently, absolute values of serum CK MB found in one study may not necessarily be comparable to values obtained in another study.

Positive arterial-coronary sinus CK MB gradients have been demonstrated in patients undergoing CABG surgery, with the peak gradient occurring within 2 hours after completion of aortic crossclamping.[33] Additionally, peak enzyme levels in the serum have been found to occur at various times, including the end of the operation,[34] 3 hours postoperatively, or 6 hours postoperatively.[35] Several studies have also shown that serum CK MB, when used in conjunction with scintigraphic methods for detecting POMI, provides additional diagnostic accuracy[36] (Fig. 9.1). However, the relationship between the magnitude of serum CK MB release postoperatively and the duration

Correlation between ⁹⁹ᵐ*Tc-Glucoheptonate Scans and Other Evidence of Perioperative Myocardial Damage*

Factor	Positive Scan[a] (N = 7)	Negative Scan (N = 20)
MB-CPK > 40 mIU/ml	7	1
MB-CPK < 40 mIU/ml[b]	0	19
Positive ECG[c]	4	0
Negative ECG	3	20

[a]New localized increased uptake seen after operation.
[b]Marked elevation is > 40 mIU/ml and slight elevation is 6–40 mIU/ml postoperatively.
[c]Evolving transmural electrocardiographic changes.

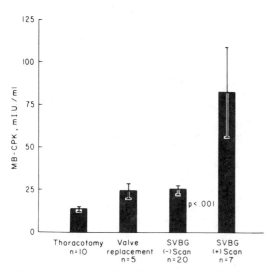

Figure 9.1. Relationship between the serum level of CK MB and myocardial infarct scintigraphy is shown. Reproduced by permission of *Ann Thorac Surg*, 1979.[91]

of aortic crossclamping intraoperatively is variable.[37] This relationship is probably influenced by the adequacy of myocardial protection.

The analysis of serum enzyme time-activity curves has proved to be a useful technique in the diagnosis of POMI after CABG surgery.[34, 38] Besides manipulations directly related to surgical trauma, general anesthesia may contribute to elevations in serum CK MB by decreasing its disappearance rate,[39] and hypothermia and/or hemodilution may alter the release and local destruction of this isoenzyme.[40] In patients with an EKG suggestive of myocardial damage, the total amount of serum CK MB released per unit of time is greater than that observed in patients with normal postoperative EKGs. In addition, the serum CK MB curve often shows a delayed peak or a long plateau. A profile of serum CK MB activity based on frequent perioperative blood samples may prove to be a most discriminating technique in separating "abnormal" liberation of isoenzyme secondary to myocardial infarction from the ordinary elevation observed secondary to general surgical trauma.

At the present time, the diagnostic and prognostic significance of the postoperative levels of serum CK MB has not been firmly established. Initial attempts at correlating myocardial infarct size with peak or total release of serum CK MB have not been convincing.[33, 34] In addition to release of CK MB into the bloodstream, there is some degradation of the enzyme locally in the heart and loss and destruction of it in the lymphatic system.[41] Thus, it appears that only about 15% of the total CK MB in the injured area of the heart appears in the plasma after a myocardial infarction.[42] Furthermore, occlusion of a coronary artery, followed by reperfusion, is associated with a larger percentage of isoenzyme in the plasma.[43] Consequently, efforts at establishing absolute levels of abnormal elevations of serum CK MB after CABG surgery have shown consistent overlap between normal and abnormal values.[34, 35]

Serum CK MB analysis has also been useful in excluding acute myocardial infarction in patients with unstable angina[44] and in the evaluation of new techniques for intraoperative myocardial protection.[45] One study[18] showed that 1 year after CABG surgery EKG evidence for myocardial necrosis was 100% specific, and serum CK MB appearance was 78% specific for new asynergy on postoperative contrast ventriculograms. However, these tests were only 20% and 54% sensitive, respectively. Indeed, they showed that 46% of patients with new asynergy, unrelated to apical left ventricular venting, had neither QRS changes nor serum CK MB appearance in the perioperative period.

Infarct-Avid Myocardial Imaging

In recent years, there has been a great deal of interest in attempts to visualize areas of myocardial necrosis by radiopharmaceutical uptake.[46, 47] The most commonly used hot-spot imaging agent has been technetium-99m pyrophosphate (^{99mm}Tc-PYP) which complexes with calcium in mitochondria such that the myocardial uptake of the radionuclide can be detected by a gamma camera.[48] At least 3 gm of myocardial necrosis must be present to identify acute myocardial infarcts scintigraphically,[49] and ^{99mm}Tc-PYP myocardial uptake is greatest in myocardial regions where coronary blood flow is reduced to levels of 20 to 40% of normal following coronary occlusion.[50] The timing between the onset of myocardial infarction and acquisition of the ^{99mm}TC-PYP myocardial scintigram is also of critical importance. Scintigrams using ^{99mm}TC-PYP become positive approximately 12 hours after acute myocardial infarcts and become increasingly positive during the first 24 and 72 hours after the event.[51] Most positive scintigrams fade and/or become negative approximately 6 to 10 days after acute myocardial infarction, but a small percentage of patients maintain a persistently positive scintigram for long periods of time.[52]

In 1976, an initial clinical study[53] showed that ^{99mm}Tc-PYP scintigrams identified 30% of patients undergoing CABG surgery in whom scintigraphic evidence of myocardial infarction developed 3 to 5 days postoperatively. This same surgical group later showed that by altering both surgical tech-

nique and myocardial protection, this incidence could be lowered to 14%.[54] This incidence is nearly identical to the 15% of level of positive scans which we find at the present time. Using a different radionuclide agent, ^{99mm}TC-glucoheptonate, we showed that scintigraphic identification of POMI has been possible as early as 6 hours postoperatively.[36] Such a positive scintigram following CABG surgery is shown in Figure 9.2.

Several investigators[36, 55] have shown the importance of obtaining a preoperative myocardial scintigram. The preoperative image may identify some patients with acute myocardial necrosis in whom surgery should be delayed if clinically possible. In fact, as many as one-third of all patients with unstable angina and angiographic proof of coronary artery disease have positive scans but absence of EKG or enzymatic evidence of myocardial necrosis.[56] Furthermore, increased myocardial uptake of ^{99mm}Tc-PYP may be noted in other conditions unrelated to acute myocardial necrosis. Examples of these situations include remote myocardial infarction,[57] ventricular aneurysm,[58] and cardioversion.[59] Whether the ^{99mm}Tc-PYP scan is positive in severe but reversible ischemia or whether the scintigram is more sensitive than the EKG or isoenzymes in detecting small areas of myocardial necrosis remains to be determined.

Since some patients have abnormal scintigrams preoperatively (as many as 30%), a comparison of preoperative and postoperative scintigrams is necessary before POMI can be diagnosed on the basis of hot-spot imaging. POMI seems likely in cases of well-defined or localized postoperative uptake of radionuclide without similar uptake in intensity or location preoperatively. The new onset of diffuse uptake postoperatively is suggestive but not diagnostic of myocardial necrosis, but the significance of its presence preoperatively and its disappearance or persistence postoperatively has not yet been clarified.[60] In addition, the lack of sensitivity of ^{99mm}Tc-PYP scintigraphy in the diagnosis of subendocardial infarction (characteristically showing diffuse patchy uptake) has been disappointing.[60, 61] This observation

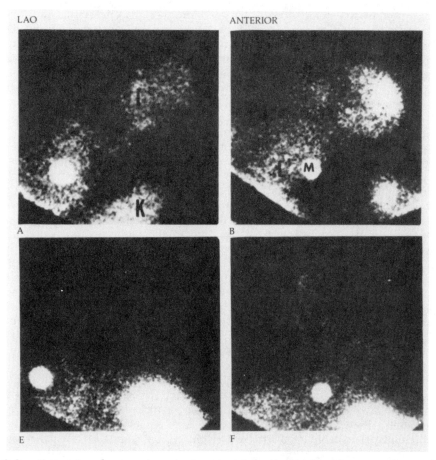

Figure 9.2. Example of normal and abnormal infarct-avid imaging are shown in the postoperative period. Reproduced by permission of *Ann Thorac Surg*, 1983.[12]

has considerable importance, since a significant number of POMIs are subendocardial.[62]

Myocardial scintigraphy clearly yields a higher incidence of POMI than that indicated by EKG alone.[63] The concordant use of myocardial scintigraphy and serum levels of CK MB may improve diagnostic accuracy, and the correlation between focal increased uptake of radionuclide and abnormal elevations of serum CK MB has been reasonably good.[36]

Myocardial Perfusion Imaging

Myocardial perfusion imaging (cold-spot imaging) has found wide application in the clinical evaluation of patients with ischemic heart disease.[64] A monovalent cationic radionuclide thallium-201 (^{201}Tl) has biological properties similar to potassium,[65] and over a wide physiological range of myocardial blood flow the uptake of ^{201}Tl by the heart is proportional to such flow.[66] This imaging technique has found wide use in the coronary care unit[67] for the detection of acute myocardial infarction.

Perfusion imaging at rest and with exercise is useful in detecting exercise-induced ischemia[68] and is sometimes helpful in deciding the necessity of CABG surgery in certain patients who have marginally severe anatomic obstructions of the coronary arterial system. Since symptomatic improvement following CABG surgery is not always related to improved coronary blood flow but may result from a placebo effect[69] or

POMI,[70] a noninvasive means for assessing myocardial blood flow and graft patency would be useful. Cardiac catheterization can be used to determine graft patency, but its invasiveness and risk prohibit large-scale serial studies. In addition, during catheterization, myocardial perfusion is usually assessed only in the resting state such that exercise-related changes remain uncertain. Consequently, postoperative evaluation of myocardial perfusion with ^{201}Tl has considerable potential value.

Symptomatology alone does not clearly predict successful CABG surgery. For example, one group of investigators[71] reported relief of angina in five patients with asymptomatic perioperative myocardial infarction in which all bypass grafts were occluded. Another group[72] also reported on 12 patients in whom all grafts had occluded, but symptomatic improvement occurred in each case, and POMI could be identified in only four of the 12 patients. The relationship between POMI, saphenous vein bypass graft patency, and effective myocardial perfusion is not clearly understood. Although some authors[19] have suggested that POMI is associated with a high incidence of graft closure, others[73] have shown by postoperative catheterization data that patients with POMI have an equal chance of having the graft supplying the area of infarction open or occluded. Furthermore, in one study, approximately 20% of patients had early postoperative graft angiograms showing at least one graft occluded and yet no evidence of transmural infarction.[20] In an autopsy report,[74] necrosis in the distribution of widely patent vessels occurred in 82% of cases. At the present time, early graft patency is approximately 90% and initial symptomatic relief nearly the same. Further evaluation is necessary to clarify such myocardial perfusion relationships.

Recent studies utilizing ^{201}Tl have shown that patients with no new perfusion defects during rest and exercise postoperatively have a high graft patency (approximately 86%).[75] An example of a perioperative ^{201}Tl image is shown in Figure 9.3. Conversely, patients with new perfusion defects at rest or a defect that develops with exercise have fewer patent grafts (approximately 50%).

Moreover, it appears that improvement in myocardial perfusion occurs in most cases following CABG surgery.[75] Whether increases in myocardial perfusion are associated with improvement in regional left ventricular wall motion after myocardial revascularization remain to be proven.

Scintigraphic Evaluation of Left Ventricular Function

Radionuclide blood-pool scintigrams involve the use of either a first-pass[76] or equilibrium multigated scintigraphic technique.[77] Either technique allows the determination of global ejection fraction (EF), left ventricular volume, and regional wall motion.[78] The equilibrium radiopharmaceutical technique permits multiple assessment of ventricular performance over a 6-hour period after a single isotope injection. A computer-based, time-activity curve is generated, and ventricular contractions may be observed in real-time cine format.[79] Normal and abnormal left ventricular contractions are depicted in Figure 9.4.

Serial radionuclide ventriculograms permit the accurate assessment of changes in left ventricular performance related to CABG surgery.[80] Most reports have shown that global resting EF remains unchanged at both 1 week[81] and several months[82] after CABG surgery. Nevertheless, a postoperative increase in EF with exercise appears to be a hallmark of successful CABG surgery.[83] Our initial experience demonstrated that resting global EF was increased 1 week after CABG surgery, despite immediate (within 2 hours) postoperative depression.[84-86] The initial 2-hour postoperative depression in EF occurred in more than 90% of patients, was transient, and not associated with hemodynamic instability. Presently, we observe no early decrease in cardiac output but no significant increase from baseline EF at 1 week postoperatively.[12] We believe that changes in perioperative management including a change in anesthetic technique from halothane to fentanyl and more vigorous postoperative intravenous and oral afterload reduction are related to the observed difference in the pattern of EF. In addition, this difference in resting EF is small in terms of absolute values. Furthermore, the resting

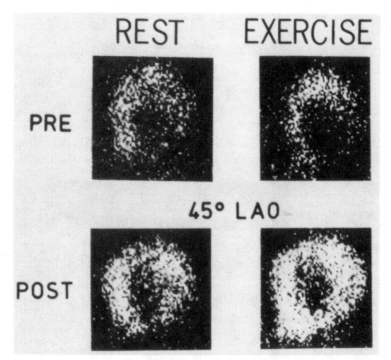

Figure 9.3. Perfusion imaging with Thallium-201 preoperatively and postoperatively is shown in a patient undergoing coronary artery surgery. Reproduced by permission of *Ann Thorac Surg*, 1983.[12]

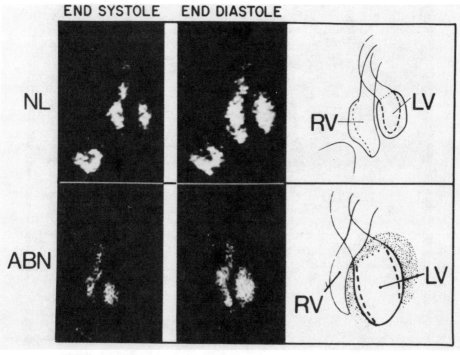

Figure 9.4. Equilibrium-gated blood pool scintigraphy in the perioperative period. Illustrations of normal and abnormal contraction patterns. Reproduced by permission of *Ann Thorac Surg*, 1983.[12]

value of EF is maintained 8 months postoperatively, while the exercise-related EF increases significantly at this time.[87]

Newer Techniques in the Evaluation of Myocardial Performance

The M-mode and two-dimensional echocardiogram have been used intraoperatively to describe dimension and rate of shortening changes.[88,89] An example of this modality which we have used intraoperatively is shown in Figure 9.5. This technique may help noninvasively in the assessment of changes in diastolic compliance related to cardiac surgery. This dynamic relationship reflecting ventricular distensibility is often

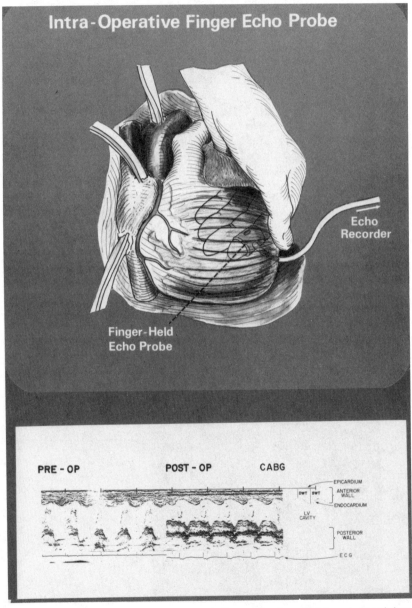

Figure 9.5. Intraoperative hand-held echocardiography is used for determining changes in regional wall motion. Echocardiogram recordings prior to and following myocardial revascularization are shown.

difficult to distinguish from changes in systolic performance when attempting to assess global ventricular performance perioperatively.[90] Implantable ultrasonic crystals have also been employed clinically to determine serial changes in left ventricular dimensions postoperatively.[91] Perhaps less hazardous for clinical use is the availability of special epicardial metal clips placed on the surface of the heart during open heart surgery.[92] With proper alignment of these clips, postoperative computer-based evaluations of ventricular geometry can be obtained by cinefluoroscopic techniques.[93] Preliminary clinical perioperative evaluations using digital subtraction ventriculography[94] and nuclear magnetic resonance[95] may offer additional information related to ventricular performance after initial problems with new technology and methodology are overcome.

PROGNOSIS IN PERIOPERATIVE MYOCARDIAL INFARCTION

While the current mortality of acute myocardial infarction treated in the coronary care unit is approximately 10%,[11] we believe that the entire spectrum of POMI has a 30-day mortality of approximately 3 to 4%. These medical and surgical estimates are selective, however, since many patients with naturally-occurring myocardial infarction die before reaching the hospital and left ventricular pump failure secondary to massive subendocardial necrosis remains the most common cause of death within the first 24 hours after technically satisfactory open heart surgery. We would argue that most survivors of POMI recover without major complications, but the early mortality is still greater than the expected 1 to 2% for elective CABG surgery. The long-term prognosis in patients surviving POMI is uncertain at the present time. Several groups have observed no detrimental effects on survival[2, 96] or resting left ventricular performance,[97] while others have found impaired survival[3, 98, 99] and decreased exercise performance.[100] The CASS group is presently evaluating the long-term effects of POMI and the outcome of this analysis may offer additional information. We recently concluded a study[100] relating the influence of the EKG, serum CK MB, and myocardial infarct images to early and late radionuclide-determined EF. We found that neither short-term (1 week) nor long-term (8 months) depression in resting EF occurred subsequent to any index of POMI, except for severe low cardiac output syndrome postoperatively. However, new Q waves were associated with markedly decreased immediate (2 to 24 hours) EF. Similarly, but to a lesser extent, abnormal elevation of serum CK MB was associated with a decreased immediate (2 to 24 hours) EF. Abnormal ^{99mm}Tc-PYP images were least important in this regard since changes in perioperative EFs were similar to those observed in patients who did not suffer a POMI. Finally, 8 months postoperatively, the exercise-related increase in EF seen in revascularized patients without POMI was not observed in survivors who had POMI (Fig. 9.6).

CONCLUSION

The importance of POMI is described in this report. Although its incidence may have decreased in recent years due to many concurrent improvements, the occasional intraoperative death or postoperative patient

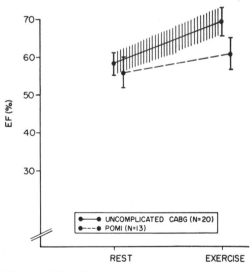

Figure 9.6. Comparison of resting and exercise-related to EF in two groups of patients; those who had suffered POMI and those who had uncomplicated postoperative courses.

with persistent heart failure highlight our lack of understanding of cellular events which give rise to myocardial necrosis. Until we better understand these subcellular mechanisms, we will be unable to prevent periodic and often unpredictable myocardial damage. Improvements in diagnostic techniques useful in the diagnosis of POMI must be followed by more accurate assessments of myocardial infarct size. Further evaluations of long-term morbidity and survival following POMI are still needed.

References

1. Roberts AJ: Perioperative myocardial infarction and changes in left ventricular performance related to coronary artery bypass graft surgery. *Ann Thorac Surg* 35:208, 1983.
2. Roberts AJ: Perioperative myocardial infarction associated with coronary artery bypass graft surgery. *Cardiovasc Rev Rep* 3:1760, 1982.
3. Chaitman BR, Alderman EL, Sheffield LT, et al: Use of survival analysis to determine the clinical significance of new Q waves after coronary bypass surgery. *Circulation* 67:302, 1983.
4. Kouchoukos NT, Oberman A, Kirklin JW, et al: Coronary bypass surgery: Analysis of factors affecting hospital mortality. *Circulation* 62:84, 1980.
5. Schrank JP, Stabaugh TK, Beckwith JR: The incidence and clinical significance of ECG-VCG changes of myocardial infarction following aortocoronary saphenous vein bypass surgery. *Am Heart J* 87:46–54, 1974.
6. Roberts AJ, Lichtenthal PR, Spies SM, et al: Perioperative myocardial damage in coronary artery bypass graft surgery: Analysis of multifactorial etiology and evaluation of diagnostic techniques. In Moran JM, Michaelis LL (eds): *Surgery for the Complications of Myocardial Infarction*. New York, Grune & Stratton, pp. 67–92, 1980.
7. Baur HR, Peterson TA, Arnar O, et al: Predictors of perioperative myocardial infarction in coronary artery operation. *Ann Thorac Surg* 31:36, 1981.
8. Cheung D, Flemma RJ, Mullen DC, et al: Ten-year follow-up in aortic valve replacement using the Björk-Shiley prosthesis. *Ann Thorac Surg* 32:138, 1981.
9. Nunley DL, Grunkemeier GL, Starr A: Aortic valve replacement with coronary bypass grafting: Significant determinants of ten-year survival. *J Thorac Cardiovasc Surg* 85:705, 1983.
10. Najafi H, Henson D, Dye WS, et al: Left ventricular hemorrhagic necrosis. *Ann Thorac Surg* 7:550, 1969.
11. Davis HT, DeCamilla J, Bayer LW, et al: Survivorship patterns in the posthospital phase of myocardial infarction. *Circulation* 60:1252, 1979.
12. Roberts AJ, Faro RS, Williams LA, et al: Relative efficacy of left ventricular venting and venous drainage techniques commonly used during coronary artery bypass graft surgery. *Ann Thorac Surg* 35:71, 1983.
13. Guyton RA, Jacobs ML, Fowler BN, et al: Regional myocardial protection: Use of a new method to compare cold potassium cardioplegia with hypothermic coronary perfusion. *Circulation* 62:I-62, 1980.
14. Roberts AJ, Faro RS, Watson WD, et al: Coronary artery bypass graft surgery: Relative efficacy of initial proximal versus distal anastomoses. *Ann Thorac Surg* 38:15, 1984.
15. Jacocks MA, Fowler BN, Chaffin JS, et al: Hypothermic ischemic arrest versus hypothermic potassium cardioplegia in human beings. *Ann Thorac Surg* 34:157, 1981.
16. Klein HO, Gross H, Rubin IL: Transient electrocardiographic changes simulating myocardial infarction during open-heart surgery. *Am Heart J* 79:463, 1968.
17. Bodenheimer MM, Banka VS, Troute RG, et al: Pathophysiologic significance of S-T and T wave abnormalities in patients with intermediate coronary syndrome. *Am J Cardiol* 39:153, 1977.
18. Warren SG, Wagner GS, Bethea CF, et al: Diagnostic and prognostic significance of electrocardiographic and CPK isoenzyme changes following coronary bypass surgery: Correlation with findings at one year. *Am Heart J* 93:189, 1977.
19. Achuff SC, Griffith LSC, Conti CR, et al: The "angina-producing" myocardial segment: An approach to the interpretation of results of coronary bypass surgery. *Am J Cardiol* 36:723, 1975.
20. Wolf NM, Kruelen TH, Bove AA, et al: Left ventricular function following coronary bypass surgery. *Circulation* 58:63, 1978.
21. Bassan MD, Oatfield R, Hoffman I, et al: New Q waves after aortocoronary bypass surgery. *N Engl J Med* 290:349, 1974.
22. Berger BC, Watson DD, Burwell LR, et al: Redistribution of thallium at rest in patients with stable and unstable angina and the effect of coronary artery bypass surgery. *Circulation* 60:1114, 1979.
23. Conde CA, Meller J, Espinoza J, et al: Disappearance of abnormal Q waves after aortocoronary bypass surgery. *Am J Cardiol* 36:889, 1975.
24. Hultgren HN, Shettigar UR, Pfeifer JF, et al: Acute myocardial infarction and ischemic injury surgery for coronary artery disease. *Am Heart J* 94:146, 1977.
25. Madigan NP, Rutherford BD, Frye RL: The clinical course, early prognosis and coronary anatomy of subendocardial infarction. *Am J Med* 60:634, 1976.
26. Galen RS: Myocardial injury during open heart surgery. *Lancet* 1:1085, 1976.
27. Hultgren HN, Miyagawa M, Buck W, et al: Ischemic myocardial injury during coronary artery surgery. *Am Heart J* 82:624, 1971.
28. Klein MS, Shell WE, Sobel BE: Serum creatine phosphokinase (CPK) isoenzymes following intramuscular injection, surgery, and myocardial infarction: Experimental and clinical studies. *Cardiovasc Res* 7:412, 1972.

29. Roberts R, Sobel BE: Creatine kinase isoenzymes in the assessment of heart disease. *Am Heart J* 95:521, 1978.

30. Dixon SH Jr, Limbird LE, Roe CR, et al: Recognition of postoperative acute myocardial infarction: Application of isoenzymes techniques. *Circulation* 48:137, 1973.

31. Isom WO, Spencer FC, Feigenbaum H, et al: Prebypass myocardial damage in patients undergoing coronary revascularization: An unrecognized vulnerable period. *Circulation* 52:119, 1975.

32. Klein MS, Coleman E, Weldon CS, et al: Concordance of electrocardiographic and scintigraphic criteria of myocardial injury after cardiac surgery. *J Thorac Cardiovasc Surg* 71:934, 1976.

33. Gray RJ, Whell WE, Conklin C, et al: Quantification of myocardial injury during coronary artery bypass graft. *Circulation* 58:38, 1978.

34. Delva E, Maille J-G, Solymoss BC, et al: Evaluation of myocardial damage during coronary artery grafting with serial determinations of serum CPK-MB isoenzyme. *J Thorac Cardiovasc Surg* 75:467, 1978.

35. Roberts AJ, Combes JR, Jacobstein JG, et al: Perioperative myocardial infarction associated with coronary artery bypass graft surgery: Improved sensitivity in the diagnosis with 6 hours after operation with ^{99m}Tc-glucoheptonate myocardial imaging and myocardial-specific isoenzymes. *Ann Thorac Surg* 27:42, 1979.

36. Roberts AJ, Jocobstein JG, Combes JR, et al: ^{99m}Tc-labeled glucoheptonate myocardial infarct imaging in patients undergoing coronary artery revascularization. *J Surg Res* 25:83, 1978.

37. Roberts AJ, Combes JR, Alonso DR, et al: Technetium-99m, glucoheptonate myocardial scintigrams in the early recognition of myocardial infarction after saphenous vein bypass graft operations. *Circulation* 54:II-64, 1976.

38. Klausner SG, Botvnick EH, Shames D, et al: The application of radionuclide infarct scintigraphy to diagnose perioperative myocardial infarction following revascularization. *Circulation* 56:173, 1977.

39. Roberts R, Sobel BE: Effect of selected drugs and myocardial infarction on the disappearance of creatine kinase from the circulation in conscious dogs. *Cardiovasc Res* 2:103, 1977.

40. Roe C, Wagner G, Young W, et al: Correlation of creatine kinase isoenzyme MB to postoperative electrocardiographic diagnosis in patients undergoing coronary artery bypass surgery. *Clin Chem* 25:93, 1979.

41. Gervin C, Hackal D, Roe C: Enzyme content of canine cardiac lymph during acute myocardial infarction. *Surg Forum* 25:175, 1974.

42. Cairns J, Missirlis E, Fallen E: Myocardial infarction size from serial CPK: Variability of CPK serum entry ratio with size and model of infarction. *Circulation* 58:1143, 1978.

43. Jarmakani J, Limbird L, Graham T, et al: Effect of reperfusion on myocardial infarct, and the accuracy of estimating infarct size from serum creatine phosphokinase in the dog. *Cardiovasc Res* 10:245, 1976.

44. Klein MS, Ludbrook PA, Mimbs JW, et al: Perioperative mortality rate in patients with unstable angina selected by exclusion of myocardial infarction. *J Thorac Cardiovasc Surg* 73:253, 1977.

45. McDaniel HC, Reves JG, Kouchoukos NT, et al: Detection of myocardial injury after coronary artery bypass grafting using a hypothermic, cardioplegic technique. *Ann Thorac Surg* 33:139, 1982.

46. Crowley MJ, Mantle JA, Rogers WJ, et al: Technetium-99m stannous pyrophosphate myocardial scintigraphy: Reliability and limitations in assessment of acute myocardial infarction. *Circulation* 56:192, 1977.

47. Lowenthal IS, Parisi AF, Tow DE, et al: Diagnosis of acute myocardial infarction in patients undergoing open heart surgery: A comparison of serial myocardial imaging with cardiac enzymes, electrocardiography, and vectorcardiography. *J Nucl Med* 18:770, 1977.

48. Bonte FJ, Parkey RW, Graham KD, et al: A new method for radionuclide imaging of acute myocardial infarcts. *Cardiology* 110:473, 1974.

49. Stokely EM, Buja LM, Tenis SE, et al: Measurement of acute myocardial infarcts in dogs with technetium-99m stannous pyrophosphate scintigrams. *J Nucl Med* 17:1, 1976.

50. Buja LM, Parkey RW, Stokely EM, et al: Pathophysiology of technetium-99m stannous pyrophosphate and thallium-201 scintigraphy of acute anterior myocardial infarcts in dogs. *J Clin Invest* 57:1508, 1976.

51. Buja LM, Parkey RW, Dees JH, et al: Morphologic correlates of technetium-99m stannous pyrophosphate imaging of acute myocardial infarcts in dogs. *Circulation* 52:596, 1975.

52. Parkey RW, Bonte FJ, Meyer SL, et al: A new method for radionuclide imaging of acute myocardial infarction in humans. *Circulation* 50:540, 1974.

53. Platt MR, Parkey RW, Willerson JT, et al: Technetium stannous pyrophosphate myocardial scintigrams in the recognition of myocardial infarction in patients undergoing coronary artery revascularization. *Ann Thorac Surg* 21:311, 1976.

54. Platt MR, Mills LJ, Parkey RW, et al: Perioperative myocardial infarction diagnosed by technetium-99m stannous pyrophosphate myocardial scintigrams. *Circulation* 54:24, 1976.

55. Rucker CM, Dugall JC, Ganter EL, et al: The detection of perioperative myocardial infarction in aortocoronary bypass surgery. *Chest* 75:300, 1979.

56. Donsky MS, Curry GC, Parkey RW, et al: Unstable angina pectoris: Clinical, angiographic, and myocardial scintigraphic observations. *Br Heart J* 38:257, 1976.

57. Olson HG, Lyons KP, Aronow WS, et al: Prognostic value of a persistently positive technetium-99m stannous pyrophosphate myocardial scinti-

gram after myocardial infarction. *Am J Cardiol* 43:889, 1979.

58. Ahmad M, Dubiel J, Verdon TA, et al: Technetium-99m stannous pyrophosphate myocardial imaging in patients with and without left ventricular aneurysm. *Circulation* 53:833, 1976.

59. Pugh BR, Buja LM, Parkey RW, et al: Cardioversion and "false positive" technetium-99m stannous pyrophosphate myocardial scintigrams. *Circulation* 54:399, 1976.

60. Moore CH, Gordon FT, Allums JA, et al: Diagnosis of perioperative myocardial infarction after coronary artery bypass. *Ann Thorac Surg* 24:323, 1977.

61. O'Rourke RA, Righetti A, Schelbert H, et al: Usefulness of preoperative and postoperative Tc-99n(SN) pyrophosphate scans in patients with ischemic and valvular heart disease. *Am J Cardiol* 39:43, 1977.

62. Buckberg GD, Towers B, Paglia DE, et al: Subendocardial ischemia after cardiopulmonary bypass. *J Thorac Cardiovasc Surg* 64:669, 1972.

63. Hung J, Kelly DT, McLaughlin AF, et al: Preoperative and postoperative technetium-99m pyrophosphate myocardial scintigraphy in the assessment of operative infarction in coronary artery surgery. *J Thorac Cardiovasc Surg* 78:68, 1979.

64. Hamilton GW: Myocardial imaging with thallium-201: The controversy over its clinical usefulness in ischemic heart disease. *J Nucl Med* 20:1201, 1979.

65. Nishlyama H, Sodd VJ, Adolph RJ, et al: Intercomparison of myocardial imaging agents: ^{201}Tl, ^{129}Cs, ^{43}K, and ^{81}Rb. *J Nucl Med* 17:880, 1976.

66. Strauss HW, Harrison K, Lagan JK, et al: Thallium-201 for myocardial imaging: Relation of thallium-201 to regional myocardial perfusion. *Circulation* 51:541, 1975.

67. Smitherman TC, Osborn RC, Harahara KA: Serial myocardial scintigraphy after a single dose of thallium-201 in men after acute myocardial infarction. *Am J Cardiol* 42:177, 1978.

68. Bailey IK, Griffith LSC, Roueau J, et al: Thallium-201 myocardial perfusion imaging at rest and during exercise: Comparative sensitivity to electrocardiography in coronary artery disease. *Circulation* 55:79, 1977.

69. Winer HE, Glassman E, Spencer FC: Mechanism of relief of angina after coronary bypass surgery: An angiographic study. *Am J Cardiol* 44:202, 1979.

70. Lim JS, Proudfit WL, Sheldon WC, et al: Perioperative myocardial infarction related to coronary bypass surgery. *Am Heart J* 96:463, 1978.

71. DiLuzio V, Roy PR, Sowton E: Angina in patients with occluded aortocoronary vein grafts. *Br Heart J* 36:139, 1974.

72. Benchimol S, dos Santos A, Desser KB: Relief of angina pectoris in patients with occluded coronary bypass grafts. *Am J Med* 60:339, 1976.

73. Assad-Morell JL, Frye RL, Connolly DC, et al: Relation of intraoperative or early postoperative transmural myocardial infarction to patency of aorto-coronary bypass grafts and to diseased underlying coronary arteries. *Am J Cardiol* 35:767, 1975.

74. Bulkley BH, Hutchins GM: Myocardial consequences of coronary artery bypass graft surgery: The paradox of necrosis in areas of revascularization. *Circulation* 56:906, 1977.

75. Ritchie JL, Narahara KA, Trobaugh GB, et al: Thallium-201 myocardial imaging before and after coronary revascularization: Assessment of regional myocardial blood flow and graft patency. *Circulation* 56:830, 1977.

76. Berger HJ, Mathay RA, Pytik LM, et al: First-pass radionuclide assessment of right and left ventricular performance in patients with cardiac and pulmonary disease. *Semin Nucl Med* 9:275, 1979.

77. Borer JS, Bacharach SL, Green MV, et al: Real-time radionuclide cineangiography in the noninvasive evaluation of global and regional left ventricular function at rest and during exercise in patients with coronary artery disease. *N Engl J Med* 296:839, 1977.

78. Okada RD, Kirshenbaum HD, Kushner FG, et al: Observer variance in the qualitative evaluation of left ventricular wall motion and the quantitation of left ventricular ejection fraction using rest and exercise multigated blood pool imaging. *Circulation* 61:118, 1980.

79. Kent KM, Borer JS, Green MV, et al: Effects of coronary artery bypass on global and regional left ventricular function during exercise. *N Engl J Med* 298:1434, 1978.

80. Gray R, Maddahi J, Berman D, et al: Scintigraphic and hemodynamic demonstration of transient left ventricular dysfunction immediately after uncomplicated coronary artery bypass grafting. *J Thorac Cardiovasc Surg* 77:504, 1979.

81. Lawrie GM, Reid JW, Young JB, et al: Sequential assessment of left ventricular performance following coronary artery bypass surgery with gated cardiac blood pool imaging. *Circulation* 59,60:238, 1979.

82. Righetti A, Crawford MH, O'Rourke RA, et al: Interventricular septal motion and left ventricular function after coronary bypass surgery: Evaluation with echocardiography and radionuclide angiography. *Am J Cardiol* 39:372, 1977.

83. Kamath ML, Hellman CK, Schmidt DH, et al: Improvement of left ventricular function after myocardial revascularization. *J Thorac Cardiovasc Surg* 79:645, 1980.

84. Roberts AJ, Spies SM, Sanders JH, et al: Serial assessment of left ventricular performance following coronary artery bypass grafting. *J Thorac Cardiovasc Surg* 81:69, 1981.

85. Roberts AJ, Sanders JH Jr, Moran JM, et al: Nonrandomized matched pair analysis of intermittent ischemic arrest versus potassium crystalloid cardioplegia during myocardial revascularization. *Ann Thorac Surg* 31:502, 1981.

86. Roberts AJ, Moran JM, Sanders JH, et al: Clinical evaluation of the relative effectiveness of multidose crystalloid and cold blood potassium cardioplegia in coronary artery bypass graft surgery:

A nonrandomized matched-pair analysis. *Ann Thorac Surg* 33:421, 1982.

87. Roberts AJ, Spies SM, Meyers SN, et al: Early and long-term improvement in left ventricular performance following coronary bypass surgery. *Surgery* 88:467, 1980.

88. Spotnitz HM, Bergman D, Bowman FO, et al: Effects of open heart surgery on end-diastolic pressure-diameter relations of the human left ventricle. *Circulation* 59:662, 1979.

89. Macoviak JA, Likoff M, Reichek N, et al: Delmeation of contractile heterogeneity by high frequency epicardial echo mapping in man. *Surg Forum* 32:276, 1981.

90. Ellis RJ, Mangano DT, Van Dyke DC, et al: Hypothermic potassium cardioplegia preserves myocardial compliance. *Surgery* 86:810, 1979.

91. Van Trigt P, Spray TL, Pasque MK, et al: The influence of time on the response to dopamine after coronary artery bypass grafting: Assessment of left ventricular performance and contractility using pressure/dimension analyses. *Ann Thorac Surg* 35:3, 1983.

92. Ingels NB, Daughters GT, Stinson EB, et al: Measurement of midwall myocardial dynamics in intact man by radiography of surgically implanted markers. *Circulation* 52:859, 1975.

93. Mintz LJ, Ingels NB, Daughters GT, et al: Sequential studies of left ventricular function and wall motion after coronary arterial bypass surgery. *Am J Cardiol* 45:210, 1980.

94. Myerowitz PD, Swanson DK, Turnipseed WD, et al: The role of digital subtraction angiography in the evaluation and management of patients with coronary artery disease. In Roberts AJ (ed): *Coronary Artery Surgery: Application of New Technologies.* Chicago, Year Book Medical Publishers, 1983, pp. 129–139.

95. Kaufman L, Crooks L, Sheldon P, et al: The potential impact of nuclear magnetic resonance imaging on cardiovascular diagnosis. *Circulation* 67:251, 1983.

96. Gray RJ, Matloff JM, Conklin CM, et al: Perioperative myocardial infarction: Late clinical course after coronary artery bypass surgery. *Circulation* 66:1185, 1982.

97. Codd JE, Wiens RD, Kaiser GC, et al: Late sequelae of perioperative myocardial infarction. *Ann Thorac Surg* 26:208, 1978.

98. Oberman A, Cutter G, Kouchoukos N, et al: Survival following perioperative myocardial infarction. *Circulation* 62:94, 1980.

99. Namay DL, Hammermeister KE, Zia MS, et al: Effect of perioperative myocardial infarction on late survival in patients undergoing coronary artery bypass graft surgery. *Circulation* 65:1066, 1982.

100. Roberts AJ, Spies SM, Lichtenthal PR, et al: Changes in left ventricular performance related to perioperative myocardial infarction in coronary artery bypass graft surgery. *Ann Thorac Surg* 35:516, 1983.

CHAPTER 10

REANIMATION OF THE HEART

FRANCIS ROBICSEK, M.D.

Before the advent of modern methods of myocardial protection, inability to restore forceful heartbeat following artificially induced ischemic arrest was commonplace. Nowadays such difficulties are less frequent, but they do occur, and when they do, serious, sometimes life-threatening situations can easily develop. Under such conditions, one or more of the three basic properties of the heart muscle, i.e., *automaticity*, *conduction*, and *excitability* may be significantly altered. While disturbances in automaticity and conduction can be usually easily countermanded by pacing, abnormal excitability (either too low or exceedingly high) may require measures of greater complexity.

Such "problem situations" in connection with intraoperative cardiac resuscitation can be roughly divided into the following groups: Asystole refractory to pacing; sustained ventricular contraction; ventricular fibrillation resistant to electroshock; and recurrent ventricular fibrillation. The purpose of this chapter is to recommend measures of possible remedy but not to discuss in detail the prevention of development of any or all of the above situations. Similarly, the scope of this discussion is limited to enumerate steps one may take to initiate effective heartbeat, but it also recommends how to treat the failure of the beating heart which may occur during the course of or immediately after cardiac surgery.

At the beginning, it should be emphasized that if the patient is on well-controlled cardiopulmonary bypass (CPB) extended measures of cardiac resuscitation should not be done in haste, but only after a reasonable effort to identify and to eliminate factors which may have precipitated the existing difficulty. In this endeavor the surgeon should comply with the following "checklist":

1. The heart should not be overdistended. Opinions regarding the necessity of venting the left heart vary among cardiac surgeons. While the majority of the profession believes that the left ventricle should be vented during most operations in induced arrest, others utilize cardiac decompression selectively, and again others vent the left ventricle only exceptionally. While the merit of these opinions is debatable, the necessity of decompression is readily evident if overdistention already occurred, especially if there are difficulties in restarting heartbeat. In such cases, venting of the left ventricle should be carried out with speed, because overstretching of the myocardial fibers for even a limited period could cause severe, sometimes irreversible, damage.

If a left ventricular drain has not been previously inserted, venting in emergency situations should be done preferably through the apex instead of the commonly used transatrial approach because it readily assures the operator that the tip of the vent is indeed in the left ventricular cavity, even if the heart is in asystole or in fibrillation.

It should not be forgotten that left heart overdistention can also occur even in the presence of left ventricular vent. The first corrective step in such a situation is to confirm the patency of the catheter and the proper position of its tip. If the vent was inserted through the left atrium utilizing the confluence of the pulmonary veins as the point of entry, its proper position can usually be confirmed by lifting the heart and by palpating the drain through the posterior left atrial wall to verify its passage through the mitral orifice. If doubt persists, the venting catheter should be either removed or clamped and another vent should be inserted through the cardiac apex.

Persistent left ventricular overdistention in the presence of a properly positioned and well-functioning vent indicates discrepancy between the performance of the drainage system and the volume of blood entering the left heart. The former may be improved by exchanging the drainage catheter for one with a larger caliber and/or placing it on mechanical suction instead of relying on gravity drainage alone. The amount of blood entering the heart may be diminished by snaring the vena cavae around the venous catheters.

Especially dangerous overdistention may occur in the presence of uncorrected aortic regurgitation when the perfusion pressure generated by the pump-oxygenator is readily transmitted to the left ventricular cavity. Such a situation may develop from several causes:

(a) The otherwise normal aortic orifice is made incompetent by the position in which the heart is held, such as elevating it by hand or with a posteriorly placed sponge. Incompetence is usually readily corrected by restoring the heart's normal posture.

(b) The second possibility is that the patient's aortic valvular abnormality was known preoperatively but was judged to be moderate enough to leave uncorrected in the course of a procedure intended to remedy another, more significant, anomaly. While such a mild aortic valve disease may not influence a clinical course appreciably after the otherwise successful operation, it could indeed create a most difficult situation during cardiac resuscitation, especially if, after the removal of the aortic crossclamp, heartbeat is not rapidly restored. Such distention, which is caused by "moderate" aortic valve disease, should be first managed with measures of improved venting. Some may even try to insert a Foley-bag catheter retrograde through the aortic root to seal off the left ventricular outflow tract to eliminate reflux temporarily from the aorta into the heart. If increased venting does not relieve ventricular overdistention or the excessive syphonage creates an unacceptable drop in perfusion pressure, then it should become evident that the degree of aortic valvular incompetence has been preoperatively underestimated and the aortic valve needs to be replaced.

(c) Another situation may develop if overdistention is caused by overlooked aortic regurgitation or incompetence created or left uncorrected by the operation itself, such as an improperly inserted or malfunctioning aortic valve prosthesis. Whatever the case, it is evident that if the aortic regurgitation is significant, it needs to be eliminated before effective resuscitation can be undertaken.

It has to be realized, however, that such a "delayed" correction of aortic regurgitation requires the extension of operative time as well as additional aortic crossclamping and myocardial ischemia, which may further damage the already injured myocardium. As a result of this, the surgeon who begins with a heart he cannot resuscitate because of aortic reflux may end up with a heart he cannot restart because of myocardial damage. To prevent this, one should use every available means of myocardial protection. Among other methods this should include interim myocardial perfusion before the aortic valve is explored. To minimize further overdistention, this "interim" perfusion should be done in an alternating manner with the right hand of the surgeon placed over the vented left ventricle to observe its state of fullness while his other hand applies and removes the aortic crossclamp, in a way, to allow as much coronary perfusion time as possible without permitting significant overdistention.

Isolated right heart overdistention is rare, but occasionally may also confront the surgeon, especially if there is impediment to the blood flow through the lungs, such as the case of advanced obstructive pulmonary vascular disease. Right heart distention can usually be relieved by snaring the caval veins to prevent all blood but the coronary flow to enter the right atrium. If right heart distention occurs in the presence of caval snares, paradoxically enough, the opposite approach may also work. The release of the snares may allow the caval catheters to drain the blood from the right atrium as well. If neither method is effective, the problem should be solved by withdrawing one of the caval catheters into the right atrium and then forwarding it into the chamber of the right ventricle. A vent placed in the pulmonary artery may be helpful.

2. Perfusion hemodynamics should be appropriate. The word "appropriate" instead of "normal" was chosen because the state of CPB during which the primary perfusion of most vital organs are either replaced with or supported by mechanical means can be called anything but normal. Based on practical experience, however, it is believed that a mean arterial pressure of 60 to 70 mm Hg and a blood flow of 4 to 5 cc/kg is adequate to maintain circulatory support in a normothermic adult. The surgeon should indeed confirm during the process of difficult cardiac resuscitation that the perfusionist indeed maintains flows within (and preferably in the upper range of) these parameters.

3. The patient should have acceptable blood gases as well as an optimal concentration of electrolytes and metabolites. If the equipment is functioning correctly and the perfusionist is attentive, perfusion hypoxia or hypercarbia is virtually nonexistent. In case of some unexpected or unrecognized mishap, however, it is indeed possible that difficulties in restarting the heart may be traced back to deficiency in blood gas exchange. Therefore, it is advisable to monitor blood gases and blood pH during the entire period of CPB either continuously or by periodic sampling, even if there are no evident difficulties. It is especially important to confirm electrolyte balance and presence of proper blood gas values shortly before the expected termination of bypass. If blood gas and/or electrolyte values are grossly abnormal and/or difficulties in restarting the heartbeat arise, their close monitoring should be continued well into the postbypass period.

Abnormally low arterial PO_2 and O_2 saturation levels should be immediately corrected by increasing the flow of oxygen to the oxygenator. Excessively high arterial oxygen levels have not yet been proven to cause either standstill or continued ventricular fibrillation; however, knowing as little as we do of the mysterious syndrome of "oxygen poisoning," it appears reasonable to maintain PO_2 levels not exceeding 250 torr.

Moderately low venous PO_2 and O_2 saturation levels could be either "good news or bad news" and should be evaluated within the context of other data monitored. If the arterial PO_2 level is normal and the blood flow is sufficient, moderately low venous oxygen levels may indicate adequate oxygen utilization by the tissues. Very low (<20 torr of <30% saturation venous PO_2 and O_2 saturation levels, however, certainly indicate the presence of either arterial hypoxia and/or inadequate perfusion rate and requires immediate correction.

The significance of abnormally high venous PO_2 and O_2 saturation levels are poorly understood. They may indicate either oversupply of oxygen to the blood, or just the contrary, the inability of the tissues to utilize the same. The latter may occur in the presence of excessive arteriovenous shunting but also when the ability of hemoglobin to release oxygen to the tissues is impaired. Therefore, it is fair to state that while abnormally high venous oxygen content certainly indicates adequate oxygen supply to the oxygenator, it neither proves nor disproves adequate tissue perfusion. It should be regarded as information which is somewhat reassuring but is not especially helpful in charting the course of cardiac resuscitation.

As far as the CO_2 content of the arterial blood is concerned, it seems desirable to maintain the partial pressure of CO_2 within 25 to 35 torr. This could be regulated by the amount of CO_2 added to the gas mixture of the oxygenator.

What one may say of the importance of the value of pH measurements is roughly the same that was stated regarding the blood gases: abnormally low values strongly indicate underperfusion; however, normal blood pH may suggest, but certainly does not prove, that "everything is in order." In cases of dysrhythmias, a serious effort should be made toward the normalization of low arterial pH by assuring more than optimal blood flow rate and—if the P_{CO_2} level is elevated as well—by decreasing the proportion of CO_2 in the gas mixture to the oxygenator and by the administration of sodium bicarbonate. In the course of cardiac resuscitation alkalosis, unless excessive, it is not regarded as dangerous and is even seen as advisable by some. Very high (>7.55) pH levels, however, would be detrimental and treated accordingly, especially if they are associated with hypokalemia.

The importance of sodium, chloride, and magnesium homeostasis in the treatment of either refractory standstill or ventricular fibrillation resistant to electroshock is not entirely clear. It is ample clinical evidence, however, implicating potassium imbalance as a primary factor in the development of intraoperative dysrhythmias of wide variety, including those which may hinder or preclude the restoration of effective heartbeat. For this reason, blood samples for potassium determination should be obtained regularly during CPB including the time period immediately before cardiac resuscitation. This sampling should be frequent, the technique of determination simple and immediate, preferably using equipment adjacent to the operating theater. Serum potassium levels should be especially carefully monitored if the patient was on digitalis or received diuretics before the operation. Similarly, special attention should be given to the matter if there was either a previous history of potassium imbalance,

marginal values were obtained preoperatively, or urinary output was either abnormally low or excessively high during the operation.

If significantly abnormal potassium imbalance is detected during cardiac resuscitation, the surgeon should temporarily suspend excessive efforts to restore heartbeat until steps to restore normal potassium levels are initiated. Low potassium levels can usually be easily corrected by adding potassium chloride to the perfusate and by correction of alkalosis which often accompanies potassium deficit. Abnormally high potassium concentration in the blood, however, could create a more serious problem. Levels above 5.2 but not exceeding 6.0 mEq/liter may not require special action but continued close monitoring if the heart is resuscitated with ease, but it should be treated energetically if dysrhythmias occur. Potassium concentrations above those values should be treated actively even if normal heartbeat can readily be restored.

The first step in treating hyperpotassemia is the rapid and simultaneous infusion of 0.25 I.U./kg regular insulin in 2 cc/kg 20% glucose solution, a measure which usually restores acceptable potassium levels. Calcium chloride, sodium bicarbonate, and furosemide may be useful in managing hyperkalemia during CPB. If these measures fail and the heart cannot be restarted, emergency hemodialysis should be instituted using either one of the conventional models of the artificial kidney, or preferably, the Corning hemofiltration device. Needless to say, while using any of these devices, extremely close monitoring of the entire electrolyte spectrum is mandatory.

Other laboratory data which may deserve laboratory monitoring under special circumstances are the digoxin levels if digoxin intoxication is suspected and the serum glucose level in diabetics. It should be emphasized that although a surgeon must rely heavily on laboratory analysis, one should also be aware of nonlaboratory signs of blood gas and electrolyte imbalance. These are: the color of the heart and the blood entering and leaving via the extracorporeal circuits, general cyanosis of the tissues, the tone of the heart muscle, and bizarre changes in the EKG.

CARDIAC ASYSTOLE REFRACTORY TO PACING

True systole, which does not respond to ventricular pacing of appropriate amplitude and frequency, is very rare. If the color of the heart is good, its temperature normal, and it does not appear overdistended, the first assumption should be not that the heart is unresponsive but that the pacing system is faulty. The pacing current may be interrupted at any part of the pulse generator-pacing wire system. First the appropriate position of the intramyocardial part of the electrodes should be ascertained. It should be confirmed that their "bare" part lies indeed within the heart muscle and does not touch either the pericardium nor the opposite electrode and that it does not bathe in blood or in saline solution. The optimal position of the two pacing electrodes is the midanterior surface of the right ventricle, about 1 cm distance from each other. We have observed, however, that in some patients in whom this arrangement did not yield satisfactory pacing response, probably because of localized fibrotic changes, there was immediate response to pacing after the electrodes were transferred into the left ventricular myocardium. After the position and the integrity of the myocardial wires has been examined and found in order, the tightness of the connections between the electrode wires and the extension cable, as well as those between the latter and the pulse generator, should be confirmed. If they are found in order and the patient still fails to respond to high amplitude pacing, the easiest measure is to replace the entire pacing system, especially if appropriate pacing "spikes" are not visible on the monitoring EKG. Transvenous pacing systems, such as pacing Swan-Ganz catheters, because of their unconfirmable anatomical position, should not be relied upon if suspicion of pacemaking failure exists. Therefore, in such situations they should be exchanged for intramyocardial or epicardial electrodes.

If the above measures are ineffective and the heart remains in asystole, one should pause and carefully measure up the situation. He will usually find one of the following:

1. If the inspection of the heart reveals that despite the fact that it is in flaccid asystole, its color is good and there are no localized infarcted areas, the subepicardium is neither edematous nor hemorrhagic, then one may assume that the prognosis is relatively good. In such a situation, it is preferable to convert flaccid nonresponsive asystole into coarse ventricular fibrillation by using inotropic drugs, preferably calcium chloride or epinephrine.

Ionized calcium exerts a strong influence upon cardiac contractility. Therefore, it is customary to give a bolus of 1 gm of calcium chloride intravenously, or preferably directly into the arterial return line when the completion of CPB approaches. Calcium is also useful to counteract the possible hypocalcemic effects of hemodilution, citrated blood or sodium bicarbonate which may have been used to correct metabolic acidosis. It should be also noted, however, that calcium itself carries some risk of dysrhythmia, especially if given to digitalized patients or in the presence of hypokalemia. Recent research regarding the beneficial effects of calcium channel blocker drugs in myocardial infarction also raises some very pertinent questions concerning the use of calcium in cardiac resuscitation. Despite these unsettled questions, however, the usage of calcium still appears to be a valuable adjunct in restarting forceful heartbeat.

Epinephrine is also a strong inotropic agent which increases not only myocardial tone but also augments coronary flow. The latter is achieved by both its direct action of stimulating adrenergic receptors and indirectly by raising the perfusion pressure. Epinephrine too has significant side-effects, especially that it predisposes for different dysrhythmias, particularly ventricular tachycardia. In the effort to restore effective heartbeat, epinephrine can be used most effectively in repeated small boluses of 0.1 to 0.3 mg injected directly into the arterial return line. In cases of asystole, sometimes this initiates spontaneous cardiac action. More often, however, it converts flaccid standstill into coarse fibrillation which, in turn, could be converted into heartbeat electrically. Epinephrine may be also useful in driving small air bubbles out of the coronary circulation by raising the perfusion pressure.

2. Another, more ominous type of cardiac standstill one may encounter during heart surgery is what properly may be called "terminal asystole"—a heart severely damaged by either anoxia or by other biochemical or biological insults. Such hearts are usually dilated but not necessarily overdistended, they are cyanotic, often show extensive ecchymosis and subepicardial edema, and respond extremely poorly to drugs. One seldom sees the full-blown picture of terminal asystole soon after restoration of coronary flow because these hearts usually resume initial contraction. As time passes, however, heart action becomes more and more feeble and finally end in standstill.

The prognosis of such a situation is poor. If the syndrome is recognized as such, it is advisable to delay immediate steps of resuscitation and "send the heart on a holiday," i.e., continue on a well-vented CPB to allow time to recover. During this period, atrial and ventricular electrodes should be attached if the surgeon has not already done so, and an intra-aortic balloon should be inserted. After a reasonable period of continued CPB, attempts should be made again to pace the heart or to convert asystole into fibrillation and to try to defibrillate thereafter. If heartbeat is restored, partial bypass should be continued with the heart still decompressed and the balloon pump functioning. The weaning process is usually tedious and needs to be assisted by judicious administration of different pharmacological agents. The cooperation of a well-trained anesthesiologist is essential.

SUSTAINED VENTRICULAR CONTRACTION

Nonresponsive systolic standstill is a seemingly enigmatic condition in which the heart remains in a nonbeating, systolic state, despite the fact that according to classic biological postulates heart muscle cannot be tetanized. This situation occurred relatively frequently in the mid-1960s when hypertrophied hearts were routinely operated upon without adequate measures of myocardial protection in simple normothermic ischemic arrest. The condition was at that time termed "the stone heart" by Denton Cooley. Nowadays stone hearts are seldom seen, but occasionally they still occur, and the prognosis is very poor.

The management of the stone heart should center around the principle that for someone to make a heart contract, he has to bring it first into a state of relaxation. Small doses (1 to 2 mg) of propranolol injected intravenously has been tried to achieve this goal with very limited success. In our hands, perfusion of the coronary arteries with 500 to 600 cc of 37°C potassium-cardioplegic solution proved to be somewhat more effective. After adequate relaxation of the heart muscle has been achieved, heartbeat is restored with pacing.

VENTRICULAR FIBRILLATION RESISTANT TO ELECTROSHOCK

Ventricular fibrillation resistant to electroshock may be caused by several conditions, ischemic myocardial injury the most common among them. In the management of this syndrome, patience is the key word again. Before one resorts to a large number of electroshocks with increasing amplitude as the ultimate remedy, it should be remembered that the thermal effect of these shocks themselves could further aggravate the already damaged myocardium. As a rule, therefore, electroshocks should not be repeated more than two to three times unless "something" has been done to alter the existing biological situation which provoked and/or sustained the fibrillation. This something may be based upon the underlying cause, such as uncorrected hypothermia, electrolyte imbalance, etc., but more often than not, it must be carried out on a trial and error basis and by surgical intuition.

It is certainly proper to deliver one or two electroshocks to the fibrillating heart as an initial trial. If the desired effect, however, is not achieved, there should be pause during which the surgeon and the anesthesiologist may go through the principal points of the checklist already discussed. If no significant abnormalities are detected, the next logical step is to suppose that the difficulty may be caused by coronary air embolism. This complication occurs in our view more often than generally suspected; however, most of the times it does not manifest itself clinically. To force the air out of the coronary arterial tree, the perfusion pressure should be raised by increasing the blood flow and, if necessary, by injecting minute amounts of epinephrine in the arterial return line. This effort could be enhanced by massaging the heart gently and concentrically from the apex toward the base. The high-pressure perfusion should be continued for 5 to 8 minutes after which another electroshock may be tried. Elevating the perfusion pressure is often effective even when other measures fail, because it not only drives air out of the coronary vessels but it also directly improves myocardial blood flow impaired for other reasons.

If ventricular fibrillation does not respond to the measures above, the surgeon may choose either to administer different antiarrhythmic drugs or to induce biochemical standstill.

Antiarrhythmic drugs should be given as adjuvants to defibrillatory efforts only if the heart has a good color, a good tone, and coarse fibrillatory waves. If this is not the case, the situation should be improved by waiting, by improving the conditions of the perfusion, and with inotropic agents before antiarrhythmic drugs are administered. Among the antiarrhythmic drugs, lidocaine is probably the one which is used more frequently. It is usually administered in a bolus of 1 to 1.5 mg/kg or in a continuous infusion of 2 to 4 mg/minute in an adult patient. Another substance we found effective as an adjuvant to defibrillation is prostigmine sulphate injected in a 1-mg dose into the arterial return line. One of the newer drugs used in the treatment of intraoperative dysrhythmias is bretylium, a quaternary ammonium compound found highly effective in cases refractory to other phar-

macological substances. Because the pharmacokinetics of bretylium is not well understood and it has conclusively proven to reverse ventricular fibrillation only in animal models, bretylium should be given only if more conventional antiarrhythmic agents, such as lidocaine, fail. In such cases of continued ventricular fibrillation, it should be applied in a loading dose of 5 to 10 mg/kg through a 5- to 10-minute interval.

An alternate method of antiarrhythmic drug treatment to treat ventricular fibrillation resistant to electroshocks is what we call "biochemically induced standstill," which has already been mentioned briefly in connection with the stone-heart syndrome. It is carried out in the following manner:

It is ascertained again that the heart is well perfused and adequately oxygenated and the pacing system is functional. The ascending aorta is crossclamped and 500 cc of body-temperature potassium-cardioplegic solution is infused rapidly into the aortic root. When the fibrillation ceases, the aortic crossclamp is gradually removed and the heart paced. Initially, we used this method only as a last resort when all other means of defibrillation failed. After seeing that with this gentle technique one may cope with already desperate situations, we use it at very early stages in cases where there is difficulty in terminating ventricular fibrillation electrically.

RECURRING VENTRICULAR FIBRILLATION

This syndrome occurs when ventricular fibrillation recurs repeatedly after electrical defibrillation. As in the previous conditions, the first step in handling such a situation is to eliminate the initiating cause, such as hypothermia, graft occlusion, etc., if it can be identified. It should be remembered that hyperirritability of the heart may also result from different drugs, such as epinephrine, which may have been used in the course of resuscitation. In such cases, the surgeon has to wait for 5 to 10 minutes until the effect of the drug "wears out."

Recurrent ventricular fibrillation may also

be instigated by mechanical causes, such as a "stuck" mechanical aortic valve against which the unvented left ventricle contracts. If the heartbeat can be restarted, the valve can usually be "unstuck" by enhancing the ventricular contractility with minute amounts of epinephrine and at the same time temporarily lowering the perfusion pressure (the force of which keeps the valve shut) until systolic peaks appear on the pressure monitoring screen indicating valve opening. If the heart is in asystole, the maneuver of perfusion pressure drop can still be used, but it should be supported by manual compression of the left ventricle to push the aortic valve open. Naturally, if these attempts do not result easily in prosthetic function, the aortic orifice should be reexplored without delay and the possible fault should be corrected. Another mechanical irritant which may invoke recurring ventricular fibrillation is the venting catheter itself, if it is inserted too far and its tip is lying against the ventricular endocardium. A "hint" of this possibility is the development of ectopic heartbeats at the time of the catheter's insertion. This problem can be readily solved by withdrawing the catheter away from the wall but not out of the ventricular chamber. Another way venting catheters may instigate recurrent ventricular fibrillation is by their exertion of excessive suction upon the ventricle.

If no particular cause can be identified as triggering the syndrome of recurrent ventricular fibrillation, the surgeon has no other choice but to continue to maintain the patient on a well-controlled CPB and to apply nonspecific measures, such as antiarrhythmic drugs already enumerated in the previous chapter. While this is being done, there should be a "hands off" policy until the danger of refibrillation passes with reasonable certainty. During this period, the surgeon and assistants should keep their hands away from the hyperirritable heart because any manipulation may trigger refibrillation. "Lifting out" or retracting the heart should be particularly avoided.

In the treatment of refibrillating hearts, it is very important to realize the significance of bradycardia which often acts as a precur-sor; therefore, it should not be tolerated, but should be eliminated by appropriate pacing.

It is of note that refibrillating hearts may be dismissed by the nonastute observer as hearts with continuing fibrillation. Closer inspection, however, may reveal that there is indeed a prompt response to the initial electroshock. The heart goes into standstill, but this lasts for only a few seconds after which ventricular fibrillation recurs. In such cases when the just defibrillated heart during this very short period of standstill seems to hesitate and then return to fibrillation, we found timely and immediate pacing most effective. This needs to be done in close cooperation with the anesthesiologist who should be ready to institute ventricular pacing promptly after the electroshock when the heart goes into standstill. Most hearts will respond adequately to such treatment, ventricular fibrillation will not recur, and heartbeat will remain continuous.

Another method effective in handling the refibrillating heart syndrome is application of paired electroshocks. This is done by leaving the paddles of the defibrillator adjacent to the heart just defibrillated, recharge the device immediately, and deliver a second electroshock as soon as possible. The interim period between the two electroshocks could be shortened further by using two defibrillators instead of one, thus eliminating the time necessary to recharge the capacitor.

CONCLUSIONS AND SUMMARY

This chapter deals exclusively with the management difficulties that may arise in restarting forceful heartbeat at the completion of CPB. We have discussed neither the prevention of these difficulties, nor the measures designed to support the already beating heart that fails to maintain an adequate output.

In difficult cardiac resuscitation, the following few basic situations are recognized: (1) cardiac asystole refractory to pacing; (2) sustained ventricular contraction; (3) ventricular fibrillation resistant to electroshocks; and (4) defibrillating heart syndrome.

General recommendations for the management of the above conditions include the assurance that the heart is not overdistended; the myocardium is well oxygenated; there is no metabolic or electrolyte imbalance; the parameters of perfusion hemodynamics are acceptable; and there are no mechanical causes preventing the return of forceful heartbeat.

In handling the different problem situations of the nonbeating heart, specific measures, such as the application of inotropic and antiarrhythmic agents, short-term high-pressure coronary perfusion, biochemical termination of ventricular fibrillation, as well as specific techniques of pacing and delivering electroshocks are discussed in detail.

CHAPTER 11

PERIOPERATIVE CORONARY SPASM

DONALD C. FINLAYSON, M.D.

"It is now well established that a subset of patients, with and without fixed obstruction in the coronary vasculature, exhibits disorders of vascular smooth muscle function, manifesting clinically as coronary spasm. This makes it all the more important to obtain a better understanding of vascular smooth muscle function, . . ."
D. E. L. Wilken[1]

Spasm was proposed as part of the spectrum of coronary artery disease as early as 1910,[2] but was largely ignored. The coronary arteries were thought of as passive and unresponsive conduits delivering blood to the myocardium affected only by the stenotic lesions of coronary artery disease. This view persisted until the era of angiography and the descripton of variant angina by Prinzmetal et al. in 1959.[3] Since then the differences in morphology and behavior of the more proximal and distal arteries and their respective resistive and capacitive functions have been investigated intensively and a number of reviews are available.[4–6] As a consequence, our understanding of the contributions of spasm to the development of coronary artery disease, to angina, myocardial dysfunction, and death[7] has markedly increased and is paralleled by an increase in our capacity for diagnosis and therapy that is relevant to the patient in the perioperative period.

NORMAL PHYSIOLOGY

In the normal coronary arterial system the delivery of blood to the myocardium on the input side is a function of heart rate and the coronary perfusion pressure, i.e., the result of mean aortic root pressure, chamber pressure, coronary compression during systole, and the diastolic time interval. Downstream flow is governed by a complex series of interactions between the effects of distal metabolic demand and factors acting on the vessels. The distal intramyocardial coronary arteries have little autonomic innervation, less well-developed smooth muscle, and do not constrict markedly, but do dilate in response to metabolic demand. In contrast, the more proximal epicardial vessels are richly innervated by sympathetic alpha and beta fibers. Their receptors are predominantly alpha proximally with beta-receptors more apparent distally.[8] They have well-developed smooth muscle in their media and demonstrate the phasic changes in tone fundamental to alterations of vascular resistance, to autoregulation, and to the development of spasm. In vivo, autoregulation involves a complex interaction of the autonomic nervous system, factors acting locally at the vessel wall and downstream metabolic demands of the myocardium. Normally, coronary blood flow reflects the balance of factors noted in Table 11.1.

The significance of these factors taken individually is unclear since local metabolic demands for oxygen, carbon dioxide, and nutrient homeostasis in the myocardium distally normally override physiological vasoconstrictor effects. The vasodilation which occurs in response to such demands appear to be the result of cellular production of multiple factors which may act singly and together. These may include hypoxia,[16] changes in CO_2,[17, 18] adenosine,[19] prostaglandins,[20, 21] increased cyclic adenosine monophosphate, kinins and other peptides,[22] and potassium and calcium levels.[23] Adenosine and prostaglandins may be central to the effects of these other multiple factors and central to the complex final common pathway leading to vasodilation in response to metabolic demand.[19]

Normally metabolic vasodilation readily overrides vasoconstrictor activity except in patients with variant angina, strongly sug-

Table 11.1
Factors in Coronary Spasm

Autonomic activity and circulation catecholamines:
  Proximal vasoconstriction is possible but variant angina is not always related to autonomic activity, however;
  Attacks may occur during REM sleep[9];
  Epinephrine after beta blockade may give angina[10];
  Sympathetic activity or catechols usually not found increased in variant angina[11]
Local factors intrinsic to vessel wall:
  Prostaglandins: prostacyclin (PGI₂) dilates, TxB-platelet aggregation-constriction[12, 13]
Diseases of the vessel wall—enhance constriction[14, 15]
  Elastin and atheroma—interact giving constriction with platelets, TxB, histamine, bradykinin

gesting the predominance of factors intrinsic to the vessel wall in the etiology of spasm. In addition, this appears to be a mainly calcium-calmodulin-dependent process which can be potentiated in vitro by cholesterol[14] when its effect is unopposed by the prostacyclin that is now not being secreted due to intimal disease and by thromboxane (TxB) secreted by platelets activated by such disease. This may account for the fact that spasm is more common, and more significant, in association with the obstructive lesions of coronary artery disease. Its significance stems from the fact that only a moderate amount of spasm is required to convert a partial to a complete obstruction. Since a well-developed muscular layer is a feature of the proximal epicardial rather than the distal intramyocardial segments, the picture of major and proximal ischemia in the distribution of a major vessel is usually seen.

DIAGNOSIS

Spasm is characterized by its abrupt onset, often occurring at rest or during sleep and occasionally improving with exercise. Generally, but not invariably, spasm is present at only one site,[24, 25] and affects more proximal epicardial portions. Spasm rarely affects the circumflex artery (4%), but affects the right coronary and left anterior descending arteries almost equally.[5] It may affect more distal epicardial arteries or produce only incomplete obstruction, giving ST depression rather than elevation, i.e., subendocardial ischemia. Spasm may affect vessels diseased with variant angina (70 to 85%) or angiographically normal vessels (15 to 30%).

Increased risk of spasm is associated with unstable angina,[26] introduction of beta-blockade,[27] withdrawal of calcium blocker therapy,[28] withdrawal of nitrate therapy,[29] myocardial infarction,[30] incidental ergot use, e.g., migraine,[31] vessel manipulation such as catheterization or operation, and incidental aspirin use.[32] Attacks of spasm may be provoked by parenteral ergot in over 90% with variant angina,[33] metacholine,[34] pilocarpine,[35] cold pressor test (approximately 80%),[36, 37] hyperventilation and Tris buffer,[38] and epinephrine after beta-blockade.[10] The effects of spasm occur in the following sequence: coronary sinus venous oxygen desaturation; almost immediate myocardial dysfunction with reduced DP/DT, and regional wall motion abnormalities, with possible mitral prolapse[41]; hemodynamic depression, elevation of left ventricular end-diastolic pressure or pulmonary capillary wedge pressure; ST elevation (occasionally depression) and continued hemodynamic deterioration; dysrhythmias often with block; and finally, angina, which is absent in 8 to 10% of patients[39, 40] (Table 11.2).

ANGIOGRAPHY

With angiography, increasing diagnostic capability had led to increasing recognition. Spasm was initially thought to be due to mechanical irritation at catheterization. With further study, the scope of the problem has become clearer. Spasm at coronary angiography occurred in 2.9% of 274 patients[42] and could be provoked in 134 (12%) of 1089 patients in another study.[43] Normal coronary angiograms have been frequently noted[44-47] and may be found in as many as one-third of patients. Provocation appears to confer behavior like that of the group as a whole. Patients with variant angina may have a relatively long and stable history,[47] others may be unstable and go on

Table 11.2
Diagnosis

History
    Variant or unstable angina
    Spasm after starting beta-blockers
    Recent myocardial infarction
    Provokable spasm at catheterization
    Discontinued calcium blocker therapy
    Onset without increased cardiac work
Findings
    Myocardial dysfunction—acute onset, recurrent
    Hypotension, failure, increasing resistance to Rx
    EKG
    ST depression occasionally, most often see
    ST elevation, dysrythmias, heart block
    Particularly in unoperated/normal vessels

to develop myocardial infarction.[48] However, it should be noted that unstable angina, a subset presumably including patients with variant angina, has been shown to be associated with the rapid worsening of coronary artery lesions.[49]

ELECTROCARDIOGRAM FINDINGS

ST segments may reflect subendocardial ischemia and show ST depression or complete transmural ischemia and show ST elevation. The degree of ischemia depends on the site of the spasm, the degree of obstruction to flow that is produced, and the compensating effect of the collateral circulation to the affected area. However it should be emphasized that more proximal areas are usually the site, and the obstruction is usually complete or nearly so. The picture is therefore one of dysfunction and EKG findings marked by ST elevation clearly in the vicinity of a single vessel. The provocability of spasm appears to correlate well with the clinical picture and has some implications for patient management. Dysrhythmias occurred in about 20% of attacks in half of one group of patients studied. These were predominantly ventricular in origin and occurred with equal frequency with both onset and with resolution of ST changes, i.e., reperfusion dysrhythmias with a grave prognosis could be seen.[50, 51] Six of ten such patients who developed reperfusion dysrhythmias demonstrated either ventricular tachycardia or fibrillation. Further, coronary spasm has been suggested as a possible cause of myocardial infarction without thrombosis. The provocability of spasm, and the area in which it could be demonstrated, appears to correlate well with the clinical picture and has some implications for patient management.

TREATMENT

Long-term treatment of patients with variant angina is now largely based on the use of nitrates and calcium antagonists.[52-58] The use of beta-blockers is often associated with the worsening of symptoms; although labetolol, with both α- and β-blocking capabilities has been used with success. In stable patients, particularly those with minimal coronary artery disease, conservative medical therapy may be successful.[53, 54] However, patients who are unstable or who have significant stenoses may require aortocoronary bypass—or indeed, other surgery. In such instances these drugs should be included with the premedication. Their omission may lead to exacerbation of spasm.

ANESTHESIA AND OPERATION

Perioperative incidence of spasm is unknown but may well be higher than 0.8% reported by Buxton et al.[59] after cardiopulmonary bypass—particularly since bypass is now often carried out in patients who have shown acute coronary insufficiency, unstable angina, or recent subendocardial infarctions—situations in which variant angina is common. Spasm has been documented before, at, and in most reports shortly after the end of bypass.[59-64] This period of greatest risk coincides with and may be related to the major alterations in complement, prostaglandins, and leukotrines seen during this period. It has even been reported as a late postoperative event in vein grafts.[65] The diagnosis should be considered when the previously described situations are noted perioperatively; with the sudden onset of ST elevation, or occasionally depression; hemodynamic deterioration and dysrhythmias—particularly with changes occurring in the distribution of an unoperated vessel; in patients with a high risk history; and particularly in those without evidence of antecedent increasing cardiac work (Table 11.3).

Anesthesia management objectives include adequate prophylactic vasodilator drug levels, nitrates, and calcium antagonists; monitoring for early diagnosis and therapy effects, EKG II, V_5, arterial line, and pulmonary artery catheter; respiration, normoxia, and normocarbia; and control of autonomic hyperactivity, depth of anesthesia, adequate narcotics/hypnotics, and specific vasodilators.

Prophylaxis may require starting calcium blockers, and certainly requires their continuance and inclusion with nitrates in pre-

Table 11.3
Treatment

Primary
  Nitroglycerin intravenous
  Nifedipine S.L., verapamil intravenous, brady-
    cardia
  Alpha-blocker—phentolamine
Secondary: intracoronary injection
  Nitroglycerin
  Phentolamine
  Papaverine
  Calcium blocker, verapamil, nifedipine for dila-
    tion and reperfusion protection
Tertiary: circulatory support
  Alpha- and beta-agonist, e.g., epinephrine,
    dopamine, dobutamine
  Alpha-agonist, e.g., neosynephrine may be
    contraindicated

medication. Active treatment (Table 11.3) should begin with intravenous nitroglycerin and sublingual nifedipine and may include intravenous phentolamine or verapamil. Further perioperative treatment of spasm may require escalation of therapy and should be planned. The use of sublingual nifedipine has been shown to act rapidly to give therapeutic blood levels.[66] An aggressive approach is necessary to minimize the risk of reperfusion dysfunction and arrythmias. In severe cases, where the response to initial therapy is inadequate, intracoronary injections of nitroglycerin, calcium blockers, papaverine, and phentolamine may be necessary and have been successful. Hypotension may accompany aggressive vasodilator therapy and mandate the use of an inotrope, preferably not a pure α-adrenergic agonist, for circulatory support and the maintenance of coronary artery perfusion pressure.

Isuprel as a pure beta-agonist may also prove useful even though not usually considered suitable for the patient with coronary artery disease. In any case, it must be emphasized that during antagonism of spasm a suitable coronary perfusion pressure must be maintained.

Perioperative plexectomy has also been advocated for the therapy of these patients.[67, 68] However, the technical difficulty, risk, and uncertain outcome have mitigated against widespread acceptance.

Spasm has been seen in a number of patients undergoing aortocoronary bypass and the degree of difficulty in its therapy has been reported.[69-71] All of these techniques are illustrated in our management of a patient who presented for bypass with unstable angina and several episodes of nocturnal pain immediately preceding operation (Fig. 11.1). Prior to induction, with stable vital signs, and with the patient sedated and sleeping, ST depression in lead II was noted. There were no accompanying signs or symptoms and the change disappeared promptly after infusion of nitroglycerin. The next episode (Fig. 1B), again without antecedent change in cardiac work, but with a mild respiratory alkalosis (Pa_{CO_2} 27 torr), occurred after induction of anesthesia as the patient was being draped. Seen were marked ST elevations in lead II and depression in lead V accompanied by severe hypotension. This was treated with phenylephrine then intravenous nitroglycerin, epinephrine, and sublingual nifedipine, with a return to normal within several minutes. Multiple, progressively more severe and protracted episodes recurred during operation. Reperfusion arrhythmias which included trigeminy and ventricular fibrillation were seen. Finally, unchanging ST and hemodynamic changes consistent with infarction appeared. This occurred despite large doses of intravenous and intracoronary nitroglycerin and sublingual nifedipine; intracoronary phentolamine, verapamil, and papaverine; and support of coronary perfusion pressure using dobutamine and intra-aortic balloon counterpulsation.

Interestingly, a number of cases of late spasm in a saphenous vein graft have been

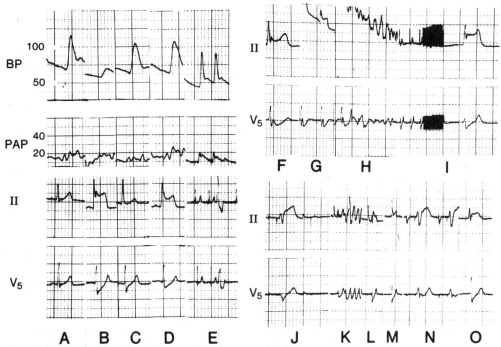

Figure 11.1. Coronary spasm is graphed *A*, before induction; *B*, after induction, draping; *C*, treatment of *B*; *D*, spasm during cannulation; *E*, reperfusion arrhythmias after treatment; *F*, beginning bypass; *GH*, spasm and fibrillation with rewarming; *IJ*, reappearance spasm with failure to pace; *K*, subsequent fibrillation; *LM*, further spasm and treatment; *NO*, end surgery-paced and nonpaced EKG. Abbreviations are: BP, blood pressure; PAP, pulmonary artery pressure; II, EKG lead II; V₅, lead V₅.

reported after operation.[65] However, perioperative risk appears to be only a short-term problem.[64] In five of six patients who demonstrated perioperative spasm, provocation of spasm could not be repeated at follow-up catheterization. It would therefore appear that the earlier skepticism about the value of revascularization in coronary spasm may be unjustified. Bypass may be more valuable and the risk of spasm less significant than at first believed. The diagnosis should be considered in all patients with perioperative circulatory collapse. In consequence, aggressive and persistent therapy with the better drugs available today, combined with heparinization and hemodilution should in most cases avert catastrophe and minimize the risk of myocardial infarction.

References

1. Wilken D: Coronary spasm. In Kalsner S (ed): *The Coronary Artery*. New York, Oxford University Press, 1982.
2. Osler W: Lumleian lectures on angina pectoris. *Lancet* 1:699, 1910.
3. Prinzmetal M, Kennamer R, Merliss R, et al: Angina pectoris I. The variant form of angina pectoris. *Am J Med* 27:375, 1959.
4. Kalsner S: *The Coronary Artery*. New York, Oxford University Press, 1982.
5. Oliva PB: Coronary arterial spasm and vasomotion (Part I), Current concepts regarding the role in ischemic heart disease. *Chest* 81:740, 1982, Part II, 82:105, 1982.
6. Hills LD, Braunwald E: Coronary artery spasm. *N Engl J Med* 229:695, 1978.
7. Maseri A, L'Abbate A, Chiercia S, et al: Coronary vasopasm as a possible cause of myocardial infarction. *N Engl J Med* 299:271, 1978.
8. Ross G: Adrenergic responses of the coronary vessels. *Circ Res* 39:461, 1976.
9. King MJ, Zir LM, Kaltman AJ, et al: Variant angina associated with angiographically demonstrated coronary artery spasm and REM sleep. *Am J Med Sci* 265:419, 1973.
10. Yasue H, Touyama M, Kato H, et al: Prinzmetal's variant form of angina as a manifestation of alpha-adrenergic receptor-mediated coronary artery spasm: Documentation by coronary angiography. *Am Heart J* 91:148, 1976.
11. Robertson RM, Bernard Y, Robertson D: Arterial and coronary sinus catecholamines in the course of spontaneous coronary artery spasm. *Am Heart J* 105:901, 1983.
12. Needleman P, Kaley G: Cardiac and coronary prostaglandin synthesis and function. *N Engl J Med* 298:1122, 1978.
13. Lewyrr I, Smith JB, Soverm J, et al: Detection of thromboxane B-2 in peripheral blood of patients with Prinzmetal's angina. *Prost Med* 5:243, 1979.
14. Yokoyama M, Henry PD: Sensitization of isolated canine coronary arteries to calcium ions after exposure to cholesterol. *Circ Res* 45:479, 1979.
15. Mudge GH, Grossman W, Mills RM, et al: Reflex increases in coronary vascular resistance in patients with ischemic heart disease. *N Engl J Med* 295:1333, 1976.
16. Gellai M, Norton JM, Detar R: Evidence for direct control of coronary vascular tone by oxygen. *Circ Res* 32:279, 1973.
17. Case RB, Greenberg H: The response of canine coronary vascular resistance to local alteration in coronary arterial pCO_2. *Circ Res* 39:558, 1976.
18. Vance JP, Smith G, Brown DM, et al: Response of mean and phasic coronary arterial blood flow to graded hypercapnia in dogs. *Br J Anaesth* 51:523, 1979.
19. Berne RM: The role of adenosine in the regulation of coronary blood flow. *Circ Res* 47:807, 1980.
20. Berger HJ, Zaret BL, Sperodd I, et al: Regional cardiac prostaglandin release during myocardial ischemia in anesthetized dogs. *Circ Res* 38:566, 1976.
21. Coker SJ, Ledingham IMCA, Parratt JR, et al: Thromboxina B2 and 6-Keto PGF1 release introcoronary venous blood: Effect of coronary artery occlusion. *J Physiol* (London) 316: 12, 1981.
22. Schror Metz U, Krebs R: The Bradykinin-induced coronary vasodilitation. Evidence of an additional prostaglandin-independent mechanism. 307:213, 1979.
23. Driscoll TM, Berne RM: Role of potassium in the regulation of coronary blood flow. *Proc Soc Exp Biol Med* 96:505, 1957.
24. El-Maraghi NR, Sealey BJ: Recurrent myocardial infarction in a young man due to coronary artery spasm demonstrated at autopsy. *Circulation* 61:199, 1980.
25. Curry RC, Pepine CJ, Sabom MB, et al: Similarities of Ergonovine-induced and spontaneous attacks of variant angina. *Circulation* 59:307, 1979.
26. Maseri A, L'Abbate A, Barolid G, et al: Coronary vasospasm is a possible cause of myocardial infarction. *N Engl J Med* 299:1271, 1978.
27. Heupler FA, Proudfit WL: Nifedipine therapy for refractory coronary arterial spasm. *Am J Cardiol* 44:798, 1979.
28. Schick EC, Liang C-S, Heupler FA, et al: Randomized withdrawal from nifedipine: placebo-control study in patients with coronary artery spasm. *Am Heart J* 104:690, 1982.
29. Lange RL, Reid MS, Tresch DD, et al: Non-atheromatous ischemic heart disease following withdrawal from industrial nitroglycerin exposure. *Circulation* 46:666, 1972.
30. Moran TJ, French WJ, Abrams HF, et al: Postmyocardial infarction angina and coronary spasm. *Am J Cardiol* 50:197, 1982.
31. Benedict CR, Robertson D: Angina pectoris and sudden death in the absence of atherosclerosis following ergotamine therapy for migraine. *Am J Med* 67:177, 1979.

32. Miwa K, Kambara H, Kawai C: Exercise-induced angina provoked by aspirin administration in patients with variant angina. *Am J Cardiol* 47:1210, 1981.

33. Heupler FA, Proudfit SL, et al: Ergonovine maleate provocation test for coronary arterial spasm. *Am J Cardiol* 41:631, 1978.

34. Endo M, Hirosana K, Kaneko N, et al: Variant angina: Coronary arteriogram and left ventriculogram during angina attack induced by methacholine. *N Engl J Med* 294:252, 1976.

35. Yasue H, Touyama M, Shimamato M, et al: Role of autonomic nervous system in the pathogenesis of Prinzmetal's variant angina. *Circulation* 50:534, 1979.

36. Raizner A, Ishimori T, Chahine R, et al: Coronary artery spasm induced by the cold pressor test. *Am J Cardiol* 41:358, 1978.

37. Shea DJ, Ockene IS, Greene HL: Acute myocardial infarction provoked by a cold pressor test. *Chest* 80:649, 1981.

38. Yasue H, Nagao M, Omote S, et al: Coronary arterial spasm and Prinzmetal's variant form of angina induced by hyperventilation and Trisbuffer infusion. *Circulation* 58:56, 1978.

39. Figueras J, Singh BN, Ganz W, et al: Mechanisms of rest nocturnal angina: Observations during continuous hemodynamic and electrocardiographic monitoring. *Circulation* 59:955, 1979.

40. Chiercia S, Brunelli C, Simonetti I, et al: Sequence of events in angina at rest: Primary reduction in coronary blood flow. *Circulation* 61:759, 1980.

41. Buda AJ, Levine DL, Myers MG, et al: Coronary artery spasm and mitral valve prolapse. *Am Heart J* 95:457, 1978.

42. Chahine RA, Raizner AE, Ishimori T, et al: The incidence and clinical significance of coronary artery spasm. *Circulation* 52:972, 1975.

43. Bertrand ME, Lablanche JM, Tilmant PY: Frequency of provoked coronary artery spasm in 273 patients with chest pain. *Am J Cardiol* 45:390, 1980.

44. Cheng TO, Bashour T, Kesler GAJ, et al: Variant angina of Prinzmetal with normal coronary arteriograms a varian of the variant. *Circulation* 47:476, 1973.

45. Benacerraf A, School JM, Achard F, et al: Coronary spasm and thrombosis associated with myocardial infarction in a patient with nearly normal coronary arteries. *Circulation* 67:1147, 1983.

46. Hart NJ, Silverman ME, King SB: Variant angina pectoris caused by coronary artery spasm. *Am J Med* 56:269, 1974.

47. Selzer A, Langston M, Ruggeroli C, et al: Clinical syndrome of variant angina with normal coronary arteriogram. *N Engl J Med* 295:1343, 1976.

48. Vincent JM, Anderson JL, Marshall HW: Coronary spasm producing coronary thrombosis and myocardial infarction. *N Engl J Med* 309:220, 228, 1983.

49. Moise A, Theroux P, Teymans Y, et al: Unstable angina and the progression of coronary atherosclerosis. *N Engl J Med* 309:685, 1983.

50. Previtali M, Clersy C, Salerno JA, et al: Ventricular tachyarrhythmias in Prinzmetal's variant angina: Clinical significance and relation to the degree in time course of S-T segment elevation. *Am J Cardiol* 52:19, 1983.

51. Tzivoni D, Keren A, Granot H, et al: Ventricular fibrillation caused by myocardial reperfusion in Prinzmetal's angina. *Am Heart J* 105:323, 1983.

52. Johnson SM, Mauritson DR, Willerson JT, et al: A controlled trial of verapamil for Prinzmetal's variant angina. *N Engl J Med* 304:862, 1981.

53. Hill JA, Feldman RL, Conti CR, et al: Longterm responses to Nifedipine in patients with coronary spasm who have an initial favorable response. *Am J Cardiol* 52:26, 1983.

54. Severi S, Davies G, Maseri A, et al: Longterm prognosis of "variant" angina with medical treatment. *Am J Cardiol* 46:226, 1980.

55. Antman E, Muller J, Goldberg S, et al: Nifedipine therapy for coronary spasm. *N Engl J Med* 302:1269, 1980.

56. Schroeder JS, Lamb IH, Gunsburger R, et al: Diltiazem for long-term therapy of coronary arterial spasm. *Am J Cardiol* 49:533, 1982.

57. Hauesler G, Holck M: Drugs which dilate the coronary arteries. cited in Kalsner, 644–666.

58. Berne RM, Belardinelli L, Harder DR, et al: Response of large and small coronary arteries to adenosine, nitroglycerin, cardiac glycosides and calcium antagonists. In Fleckstein A, Roskamm H (eds): *Calcium Antagonisms*. Spring, Berlin Heidelberg. New York, 1980, pp. 208–220.

59. Buxton AE, Goldberg S, Harken A, et al: Coronary-artery spasm immediately after myocardial revascularization. *N Engl J Med* 304:1249, 1981.

60. Kopf GS, Riba A, Zito R: Intraoperative use of nifedipine for hemodynamic collapse due to coronary artery spasm following myocardial revascularization. *Ann Thorac Surg* 34:457, 1982.

61. Zeff RH, Iannone LA, Kongtah Worn C, et al: Coronary artery spasm following coronary artery revascularization. *Ann Thorac Surg* 34:196, 1982.

62. Pichard AD, Ambrose J, Mindlich B, et al: Coronary artery spasm and perioperative cardiac arrest. *J Thorac Cardiovasc Surg* 80:249, 1980.

63. Combs DT, Wilkin JH, Blewett C, et al: Spasm of the left coronary artery with aortocoronary bypass. *Chest* 66:737, 1974.

64. Buxton AE, Hirshfeld JW, Untereker WJ, et al: Perioperative coronary arterial spasm: Long-term follow-up. *Am J Cardiol* 50:444, 1982.

65. Heljman J, Elgamal M, Michels R: Catheter-induced spasm in aorto-coronary vein grafts. *Br Heart J* 49:30, 1983.

66. Nussmeier NA, Curling PE, Murphy DA, et al: Nifedipine: Cardiovascular effects after sublingual administration during fentanyl pancuronium anesthesia in man. *Anesthesiology* 59:A-34, 1983.

67. Clark DA, Quint RA, Mitchell RL, et al: Coronary artery spasm, medical management, surgical denervation and autotransplantation. *J Thorac Cardiovasc Surg* 73:332, 1977.

68. Bertrand ME, Lablanche JM Tilmant PY: Treatment of Prinzmetal's variant angina. Role of medical treatment with nifedipine and surgical coronary revascularization combined with plexectomy. *Am J*

Cardiol 47:174, 1981.

69. Gausch WH, Lufschanowski R, Leachman RD, et al: Surgical management of Prinzmetal's variant angina. *Chest* 66:614, 1974.

70. Johnson AD, Stroud HA, Vieweg WVR, et al: Variant angina pectoris. Clinical presentations coronary angiographic patterns, and the results of medical and surgical management in 42 consecutive patients. *Chest* 73:786, 1978.

71. Wiener L, Kasparian H, Duca P, et al: Spectrum of coronary arterial spasm. Clinical, angiographic and myocardial metabolic experience in 29 cases. *Am J Cardiol* 38:945, 1976.

CHAPTER 12

DETERMINANTS OF MYOCARDIAL PERFORMANCE AND THE ADEQUACY OF SUBENDOCARDIAL BLOOD FLOW

GERALD D. BUCKBERG, M.D., F.A.C.S.
JOHN M. ROBERTSON, M.D.
DOUGLAS H. McCONNELL, M.D.
JOHN R. BRAZIER, M.D.

Inadequate cardiac output after an open heart operation is the most frequent cause of death after technically successful repair of cardiac lesions. Furthermore, impaired cardiac performance may occur in other surgical settings, so that an understanding of the factors governing myocardial performance are essential to allow one to provide appropriate perioperative care. Cardiac output is the product of heart rate and stroke volume, and its adequacy is defined by how well the heart provides oxygen supply to meet tissue oxygen demands. The three most common causes of inadequate postoperative cardiac output are: (a) hypovolemia, in which blood volume is not sufficient to fill the heart; (b) cardiac tamponade, in which venous filling of the heart is impeded; and (c) myocardial failure (where the heart's ability to empty is impaired). Currently, the most frequent cause of inadequate cardiac output is myocardial failure. This failure is most often due to ischemic injury to the heart during cardiac surgery.

The diagnosis and treatment of inadequate postoperative output are based upon an understanding of (a) the clinical and physiological consequences of inadequate tissue blood supply; (b) the physiological determinants of the bedside blood pressure measurements used to assess cardiac performance; (c) the clinical assessment of the determinants of cardiac output (preload, afterload, and contractility); and (d) the factors determining the adequacy of myocardial oxygen supply relative to cardiac oxygen demands.

Tissue oxygen supply is determined by the blood flow (cardiac output), blood oxygen content, and oxygen extraction. These factors are the components of the Fick equation, which states:

Oxygen consumption = cardiac output × (arterial-venous oxygen content difference)

It is extremely useful to know the cardiac output, but this measurement may not be accurate when output is low, and does not define how well the output provides oxygenated blood to meet metabolic demands. We believe the interpretation of the adequacy of cardiac output is more important than the measurement of its numerical value. For example, cardiac output must be higher than "normal" to provide adequately for tissue oxygen needs in the anemic or hypoxic patient whose O_2 content is reduced.

CLINICAL EVALUATION AND INTERPRETATION OF THE ADEQUACY OF CARDIAC OUTPUT

The patient with inadequate cardiac output usually shows signs of inadequate tissue perfusion. Reduced renal blood flow results in a low urinary tract output with high specific gravity (>1.020). An altered sensorium provides evidence of diminished cerebral perfusion. Inadequate coronary blood flow is associated with arrhythmias, gallop rhythms, and electrocardiographic signs of ischemia. To maintain arterial blood pressure and ensure perfusion of vital organs, peripheral resistance increases and blood flow to the skin is reduced. The extremities are cool, peripheral pulses are weak, and nail beds and lips are cyanotic. Arterial blood is usually completely saturated so that peripheral cyanosis reflects oxygen extraction by tissues in response to reduced blood flow. Oftentimes blood pressure is either normal or high.

Under the aforementioned circumstances, direct measurement of cardiac output should and can be made by placing a thermodilution floatation catheter into the pulmonary artery at the bedside. An added benefit of this measuring device is direct measurement of mixed venous (pulmonary artery) blood oxygen saturation and content. An arterial-mixed venous saturation difference greater than 30% indicates the tissue oxygen delivery (cardiac output × arterial O_2 content) is inadequate.

INTERPRETATION OF BEDSIDE BLOOD PRESSURE AND CARDIAC OUTPUT MEASUREMENTS

All vascular pressures are determined by the distensibility of the system (compliance or pressure-volume characteristics) and their contained volume. The volume is, in turn, determined by the size of the vascular bed (capacitance) and rate of entry and exit of blood (Fig. 12.1).

Arterial Blood Pressure

When arterial blood pressure is low, cardiac output is usually reduced, though depression of cardiac output may also occur with normal or high blood pressure. Systolic blood pressure is related to the stroke volume, compliance of the major arteries, and peripheral resistance (runoff of blood out of the arterial system) (Fig. 12.1). Reduction of arterial compliance (e.g., aging or atherosclerosis) results in an increased peripheral resistance and a higher systolic pressure for

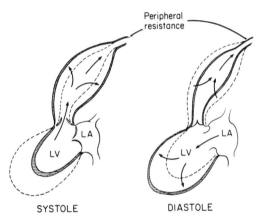

Figure 12.1. Systolic blood pressure (*left panel*) is determined by (a) the volume of blood ejected from the left ventricle (stroke volume), (b) compliance of the walls of the arterial system, and (c) rate of runoff (peripheral resistance). Diastolic blood pressure is determined by (a) volume of blood remaining in the arterial system, (b) compliance of the arterial wall, and (c) peripheral resistance (regulating the rate of runoff of blood). Left ventricular diastolic pressure, which equilibrates with left atrial pressure, is determined by compliance of the left ventricular wall and left ventricular volume. This volume is determined by (a) rate of entry of blood from the left atrium (venous return) and (b) completeness of emptying the ventricle during the last systole (ejection fraction).

any given stroke volume. If peripheral resistance is increased, which occurs when cardiac output is reduced, then arterial blood pressure maintained as runoff from the arterial bed becomes impaired. Blood pressure falls only after cardiac output is reduced markedly. Consequently a normal arterial blood pressure in a vasoconstricted patient should raise the suspicion that cardiac output is low.

Diastolic blood pressure is related principally to the compliance of the arteries, their elastic recoil, and peripheral resistance. Though systolic blood pressure is commonly the primary focus of attention, it must be remembered that the left ventricle, especially the subendocardium, is nourished during diastole, so that a low diastolic blood pressure may be detrimental to coronary perfusion.

Such lowering of diastolic blood pressure may occur under conditions of low peripheral resistance (i.e., anemia, arterial venous fistula, patent ductus arteriosus, surgical systemic pulmonary shunt, fever, etc.) or when vasodilator drugs are given. These conditions may be associated with a normal or high cardiac output, but myocardial failure may occur due to inadequate maintenance of perfusion to subendocardial muscle.

Venous Pressure

Venous pressure is determined by the volume of blood in the venous system, the pressure-volume characteristics of the venous bed (compliance) (Fig. 12.2A); the size of the venous bed (capacitance), and the ability of the heart to eject its venous return. When the circulation is intact, two pumps are in series with competent valves interposed between them. Therefore, though the principles determining pulmonary and systemic venous pressures are similar, different volumes of blood are contained within the venous system on either side of the heart. The compliance of the receiving chambers (left and right ventricles) are different, and the ability of each ventricle to eject its volume may differ depending upon the pre-existent lesions and injury incurred during operation.

CENTRAL VENOUS PRESSURE

Central venous pressure provides a guide to systemic blood volume and right ventricular performance. Approximately 60% of the blood volume resides in the peripheral venous system (large capacitance). Veins are compliant structures so that when venous pressure is low, large increments of blood volume may be necessary before venous pressure rises (Fig. 12.2B). When venous pressure is high (15 mm Hg), however, the steep part of the venous pressure-volume curve is reached, so that small increments in blood volume are associated with a large rise in venous pressure. This physiological factor is useful in deciding how much volume may be required when central venous pressure is low.

PULMONARY VENOUS PRESSURE

Pulmonary venous pressure provides a guide to pulmonary blood volume and left ventricular performance. Pulmonary venous pressure can be estimated from left atrial pressure or pulmonary arterial wedge pressure. Although isolated segments of pulmonary veins may have the same pressure volume characteristics as isolated segment as systemic veins (Fig. 12.2A), the capacitance of the pulmonary venous system (5% of total blood volume) is significantly less than that of the peripheral venous system (60% of total blood volume) as seen in Figure 12.2B. Assuming a 70-kg person has a blood volume of approximately 5000 ml (i.e., 7% body weight), a sudden shift of only 2% of total blood volume (100 cc) into the pulmonary venous system, as would occur with acute left ventricular failure would increase pulmonary blood volume by 40%. If the rise in pulmonary blood volume occurs while the pulmonary venous system is close to the steep part of the pressure-volume curve, pulmonary venous pressure may rise precipitously and cause pulmonary edema even though systemic venous pressure does not change appreciably. (Systemic venous volume would have decreased only 3.3%).

Under these circumstances, a test transfusion of 5% of the blood volume (250 cc of saline) would lead to pulmonary edema. Conversely, such a test transfusion would

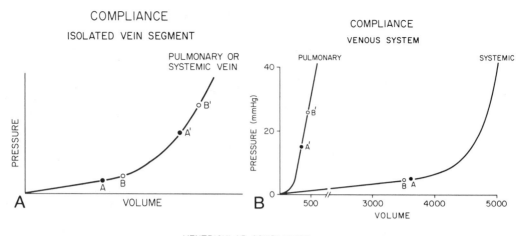

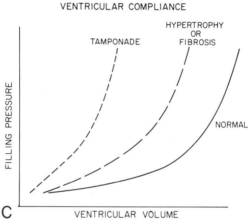

Figure 12.2. *A*. Pressure-volume characteristics (compliance) of isolated segments of pulmonary or systemic veins are shown. Note: When the vessel is empty, it accommodates a large volume before pressure rises (A to B). When the vessel becomes full, small changes in volume causes large changes in pressure (A¹ to B¹). This change in the slope of the compliance curve of these venous segments has important physiological implications (see text). *B*. Compliance of the entire pulmonary and systemic venous systems is shown. Although compliance of isolated pulmonary and systemic veins is similar, the venous systems differ in their capacitance. The pulmonary system (*left curve*) has less capacitance (accommodates less volume)—normal pulmonary venous volume is approximately 350 cc. In contrast, the systemic venous system has large capacitance (normal systemic venous volume is approximately 3500 cc). The results of translocation of small volumes of fluid (100 cc) are seen when these two systems are operating on different points on their pressure-volume curve. Loss of 100 cc from the systemic venous system causes only a negligible change in systemic venous pressure (moving from point A to B). However, addition of 100 cc of blood to the pulmonary venous system (A¹ to B¹) causes a large increase in pulmonary venous pressure. This relationship explains why small shifts of blood from the systemic to pulmonary venous system may cause pulmonary edema; pulmonary venous and systemic venous pressures must be monitored separately. *C*. The pressure-volume relationship (compliance) of the left ventricle is shown. The normal left ventricle is compliant (*far right*). When either the ventricle is hypertrophied or fibrotic (center curve) or prevented from distending by a taut pericardium or surrounding mediastinum (*center* and *left* curves); compliance becomes reduced. These changes in compliance result in the need for higher filling pressures in order to achieve the same diastolic ventricular volume (fiber stretch) in order to augment contractility (Starling effect) (Fig. 12.3*A*).

not be considered if the decision was made after the knowledge of both central venous and pulmonary artery wedge pressures.

The venous pressures on both sides of the heart also provide an estimate of the ventricular end-diastolic pressure. This pressure reflects the volume of blood contained within the ventricular cavity, the distensibility and capacitance of the combined heart and pericardial sac, and the ability of each side of the heart to eject their venous return.

INTERPRETATION OF BLOOD PRESSURE AND HEART RATE RESPONSE

While arterial blood pressure does not accurately reflect stroke volume, directional changes in blood pressure after volume replacement are useful in assessing cardiac performance. The basis of this relationship is the Frank-Starling mechanism of cardiac function. Isolated muscle fibers (Fig. 12.3A) develop more contractile tensions as their length is increased. Increased contractile tension in the intact heart (Fig. 12.3B) results in an increased stroke volume which, in turn, is reflected by an augmented blood pressure (Fig. 12.3C).

Venous pressure (central venous or left atrial) is used to characterize the changes in fiber stretch of the ventricular muscle. As indicated previously, the pressure developed for any given volume is also a reflection of the compliance of the ventricle. The left ventricle is usually less compliant than the right, and ventricular compliance is reduced when the normal ventricle becomes either hypertrophied, fibrotic, or ischemic, or when a taut pericardium does not allow the muscle fibers to stretch. Consequently, different filling pressures are required in order to achieve the same end-diastolic volume (fiber stretch) under these different conditions (Fig. 12.2C).

Small changes in fiber length of normal muscle fiber are accompanied by large increases in contractile tension. The clinical correlate of this is that stroke volume and blood pressure are augmented markedly with small changes in filling pressure (fiber length). Conversely, the ischemic muscle develops less tension and contractile force than the normal muscle when it is stretched to the same fiber length. Consequently, a greater end diastolic volume (filling pressure) will be necessary to achieve the same stroke volume in the ischemic heart (Fig. 12.3A–C).

The principal determinants of stroke volume (fiber shortening) are preload (stretch of the muscle fiber), afterload (the force resisting fiber shortening) and the contractile state of the myocardium (properties of heart muscle which characterize the force of contraction independent of preload and afterload). For any level of contractile state, the extent of fiber shortening will vary directly with the preload and inversely with the afterload. Heart rate is the remaining determinant of cardiac output because the total extent of muscular shortening per minute depends on the frequency of contractions. These four determinants of cardiac output are interdependent so that a change in one will affect the others. For example, when peripheral resistance (afterload) is high, left ventricular emptying is more difficult and the systolic ejection period is prolonged. End-diastolic volume must increase in order to stretch the muscle fiber (increase preload) and ensure adequate stroke volume. The compensatory mechanism of increased preload has been used to compensate for increased afterload. The resultant increase in left ventricular end diastolic volume raises ventricular diastolic pressure and the prolongation of systole shortens diastole. The consequences of these changes in terms of the adequacy of coronary flow will be discussed later.

CLINICAL ASSESSMENT

Cardiac output is heart rate multiplied by stroke volume. Abnormalities of heart rate and rhythm are obvious by looking at the EKG recorded continually at the bedside in all monitored patients. In the patient with clinically inadequate cardiac output, consideration must be given to both the appropriateness of heart rate and the normality of conduction before the determinants of the stroke volume are manipulated. Whereas the normal heart rate varies between 70 and 90 beat/minute, heart rate should rise as

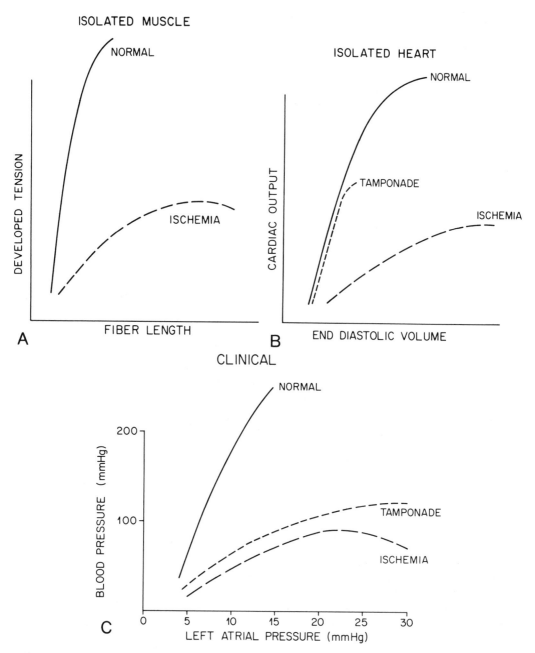

Figure 12.3. *A*. Developed tension of an isolated muscle segment is plotted against its fiber length. As fiber length (preload) is increased in the normal muscle, developed tension increases markedly. Ischemic muscle, however, cannot develop as much tension as normal muscle, and requires increased fiber length to achieve comparable levels of tension. *B*. The isolated heart performs much in the same way as the isolated muscle strip; a small increase in preload by raising end-diastolic volume (fiber length) results in a marked augmentation of stroke volume (cardiac output)—a normal ventricular function curve. Impairment of myocardial contractile properties by ischemia reduces the stroke volume achieved for any given change in diastolic volume (fiber length)—a depressed ventricular function curve.

stroke volume is impaired (i.e., hemorrhage, cardiac failure, etc). For example, the hypovolemic patient should develop tachycardia and peripheral vasoconstriction as a normal response. This normal tachycardia response may be impaired pharmacologically (i.e., propranolol) or pathologically (intrinsic atrial ventricular conduction defects). Under these circumstances, atropine or isoproterenol (pharmacological intervention) or atrial pacing (mechanical intervention) can improve cardiac output markedly. Cardiac output decreases markedly in patients with heart disease who develop interruption of normal atrial ventricular conduction as occurs with the development of nodal rhythm or atrial-fibrillation. Both conduction abnormalities interfere with the presystolic accentuation of ventricular filling. Use of atrial pacing to overcome nodal rhythm or drugs to slow the ventricular response to atrial fibrillation (i.e., digitalis) or direct countershock to convert fibrillation may produce marked improvement in cardiac output.

The preload (fiber stretch) of the left and right ventricle is assessed from central venous and left atrial pressures, and knowledge of the structural characteristics of each ventricle (i.e., the presence of fibrosis or hypertrophy will require a higher filling pressure to acheive the same end-diastolic volume).

The afterload (impedance to left ventricular emptying) is determined by the peripheral resistance, structural characteristics of the arteries (compliance), and the volume of blood contained within the arterial system. If the extremities are cool, nail beds and lips are cyanotic, and peripheral pulses are weak, it is safe to assume that peripheral resistance is high. Conversely, a full peripheral pulse with warm, pink extremities will usually reflect a normal or decreased peripheral resistance and help assure the adequacy of cardiac emptying.

Myocardial performance, or the contractility of the heart, can be assessed from ventricular response to a volume challenge and from the characteristics of the arterial pulse contour in addition to the measured cardiac output. The normal ventricle generates an arterial pressure curve characterized by a brisk upstroke at the beginning of systole and relatively short systolic ejection period (Fig. 12.4A). Conversely, the poorly contracting ventricle generates a systolic pressure wave with a sluggish upstroke and the systolic ejection period is prolonged for any given heart rate (Fig. 12.4B). At the bedside, we often inscribe a clinical ventricular function curve by observing the response of arterial and venous blood pressures to an increased preload (transfusion) in patients with and without thermodilution floatation catheters in place.

The measured cardiac output must be normalized for patients' size and interpreted in relation to tissue metabolic needs. In the normal resting patients, cardiac output is 70 to 90 ml/kg or 2.5 to 3.5 liter/m^2. The term cardiac index applies to this normalization. It is apparent that a healthy 50-kg patient with a cardiac output of 4.0 liter/min (i.e., 80 ml/kg) has a normal cardiac output whereas a similar output in another 50-kg patient must be evaluated in terms of tissue needs. For example, if the patient was anemic, a higher cardiac output would be

With tamponade, the ventricle has normal contractility, but, due to the mechanical restriction of ventricular filling, it cannot achieve the end-diastolic volume required to augment cardiac output. C. By observing the effects of transfusion (increased preload) on blood pressure and left atrial or central venous pressure, a clinical ventricular function curve is inscribed. Blood pressure is used to indicate stroke volume and left atrial or central venous pressure to indicate end-diastolic ventricular volume. With transfusion the normal ventricle increases its output and blood pressure rises markedly while left atrial pressure increases only slightly. The ischemic ventricle does not increase its output in response to transfusion; blood pressure falls or does not change and left atrial pressure rises markedly. An intermediate response is seen with tamponade; blood pressure increases (as contractility may be normal) but left atrial pressure also rises as small changes in preload cause large changes in left ventricular pressure due to decreased compliance (Fig. 12.2C).

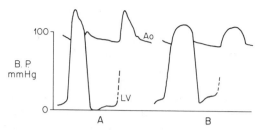

Figure 12.4. *A.* Normal left ventricular pressure recordings; systolic ejection is brisk and the duration of systole is short. *B.* Left ventricular failure; note the sluggish upstroke of aortic systolic pressure, prolonged systole, and narrow aortic pulse pressure.

needed until blood oxygen content could be adjusted (transfusion) so that a normal cardiac output under these circumstances, is, in reality low.

The availability of measurements of intravascular pressures (arterial, central venous, left atrial), cardiac indices, and arterial and mixed venous blood gases improves our ability to detect and manage inadequate cardiac output clinically. However, the clinical signs of organ hypoperfusion (i.e., reduced urine output, peripheral vasoconstriction, and altered mental state) can exist in a patient whose cardiac output is either normal or high and when arterial mixed venous oxygen differences are normal or narrow. Such clinical conditions include septic shock, hepatic disease with multiple arterial fistula, myocardial infarction with ventricular septal defect and congenital heart disease with too large a pulmonary systemic shunt or breakdown of intraventricular repair. Under these circumstances, the determinants of cardiac output must be manipulated to make cardiac output meet tissue demands, rather than accepting these normal values of cardiac index and arterial venous oxygen difference.

Hypovolemia

The two most common causes of hypovolemia (decreased preload) are (a) inadequate blood volume replacement, and (b) pharmacological venodilatation so that blood volume pools in the venous capaci-

tance bed. Both forms of hypovolemia are clinically similar, but they may be differentiated by their response to volume replacement. Noncompliant ventricles (hypertrophied and fibrotic) may require higher filling pressure to achieve a fiber length sufficient to provide an optimum stroke volume.

In the presence of hemorrhagic or hypovolemic hypotension, both left atrial and central venous pressure are low. If the ventricle has not experienced an ischemic insult during surgery, then a blood transfusion is usually accompanied by a prompt rise in arterial blood pressure with only a small increment in left atrial and central venous pressure—a normal ventricular function curve. In the normal heart, it is extremely difficult, short of massive hypervolemia, to raise left atrial pressure above 15 mm Hg. Consequently, failure to achieve a high central venous and left atrial pressure with volume replacement while blood pressure continues to rise, should not be interpreted as a sign of continued bleeding. The concept of citrate toxicity must be considered when rapid transfusions are given. Clinical and experimental studies have shown that ionic calcium is chelated by the excess citrate contained as the principle anticoagulant in most "banked" blood. This lowering of the circulating ionic calcium results in an impaired myocardial contractility during massive transfusion. When blood is replaced more rapidly than one unit each 5 to 10 minutes, calcium chloride (100 mg/100 cc of blood/min) should be administered simultaneously into a separate central intravenous site.[1, 2]

If hypotension is due to pharmacological venodilatation (morphine), the administration of blood or other fluids is not usually associated with an increase in either venous or arterial blood pressure. The failure to raise venous pressure with volume replacement indicates either that the rate of bleeding exceeds the rate of transfusion or that the added volume has not been returned to the heart, i.e., transfusion into an infinite capacitance bed. This syndrome can be diagnosed by the administration of a narcotic antagonist, which will have little or no effect if hypotension is not caused by excessive narcosis.

Tamponade

Inadequate cardiac output during cardiac tamponade and hypovolemia has a similar principal cause. Although blood volume is sufficient, myocardial compression is an impedance to cardiac filling. In contrast to hypovolemia, where filling pressure are low on both sides of the heart, left- and right-sided pressures are high during tamponade. In the early phase of tamponade, the high filling pressures reflect the diminished compliance of both ventricles due to external compression rather than cardiac failure (Figs. 12.2C and 12.3C)

Volume replacement usually augments blood pressure, but in contrast to the response in hypovolemia, filling pressures are also increased. Increased filling pressure is required to obtain the stretch of the muscle fibers required to augment cardiac performance; the filling pressures represent the combined compliance of the muscle and the pericardium and overlying mediastinum (Fig. 12.2C).

The postcardiac surgical patient with cardiac tamponade usually has had moderate chest tube drainage (200 to 300 cc/hour) with previously low filling pressures. Drainage may gradually or suddenly decrease as blood pressure falls and filling pressure rises. Such changes in vital signs and drainage should alert the clinician to the possibility of tamponade. The chest tube should be evacuated promptly and plans should be made for mediastinal exploration. Because reduced stroke volume from impaired filling is the major problem, four physiological mechanisms may be used for the treatment of tamponade or preparations are made to return the patient to the operating room for decompression. (a) Volume replacement will increase preload, which provides greater stretch on the muscle fibers and increases myocardial contraction. (b) Increased heart rate is essential because stroke volume is usually fixed, and increased heart rate will raise cardiac output (atropine may be useful). (c) Decreasing afterload may allow ventricular emptying to occur more easily and increase stroke volume. This may be dangerous because blood pressure is usually maintained by intense peripheral constriction. (d) Increasing contractility with inotropic drugs will usually ensure a greater ejection fraction and augment output. We find isoproterenol most useful because it augments contractility, reduces peripheral resistance (decreases afterload), and increases heart rate.

If tamponade is allowed to persist, ischemic myocardial failure may supervene because arterial hypotension (reduced diastolic blood pressure), tachycardia (shortened diastole), and high left ventricular diastolic pressures are detrimental to coronary perfusion.

Myocardial Failure

Reduced myocardial contractility is the most frequent cause of inadequate postoperative cardiac output. Patients who develop myocardial failure will frequently show impaired cardiac performance within the first 24 hours after operation. Arterial blood pressure is usually low, but may be normal or increased. If the right ventricle is failing, central venous pressure will be high and left atrial pressure low. This may occur after correction of congenital defects (tetralogy of Fallot, pulmonary stenosis), and after mitral replacement in patients who have pulmonary hypertension. When left ventricular failure develops, left atrial pressure is high (greater than 25 mm Hg) and central venous pressure is normal or increased (its level determined by the blood volume).

In contrast to the blood pressure response to volume replacement in patients with tamponade, blood transfusion in patients with myocardial failure usually results in markedly increased cardiac filling pressure, while arterial pressure does not change or falls—a depressed ventricular function curve (Fig. 12.3C).

In our experience, myocardial failure due to ischemic cardiac injury during operation is the most common cause of inadequate postoperative cardiac output. The region of the heart affected most severely is the left ventricular subendocardium. Subendocardial necrosis is shown on autopsy either grossly, microscopically, or histochemically in over 90% of patients who die after open heart operations. Necrosis occurs despite the absence of anatomically obstruction to the coronary arteries.[3-5]

Subendocardial ischemia with patient coronaries can be predicted, prevented, and treated. To avoid successfully this potentially fatal complication, one must understand the determinants of subendocardial oxygen supply and demand, which hearts are vulnerable to this injury, how the heart can be preserved optimally during operation, and how to detect postoperative subendocardial ischemia so that the supply/demand relationship may be used to avoid ischemic injury.

SUPPLY/DEMAND RELATIONSHIP

Supply

Oxygen supply to the heart, as to other organs, is determined by the coronary blood flow, blood oxygen content, and oxygen extraction. Blood flow and oxygen content are the principal determinants, since almost all the oxygen received by the heart is extracted under resting conditions. Therefore, coronary blood flow must increase if raised oxygen requirements are to be met adequately.

Myocardial flow depends upon the driving pressure and vascular resistance. Coronary vascular resistance is determined not only by the vasomotor tone in the coronary arteries, but also by how these vessels are compressed as the heart contracts. Intramyocardial systolic compressive forces are greatest in the subendocardial region (Fig. 12.5) so that the inner shell of the left ventricle must receive most or all of its blood supply during diastole. Conversely, the outer shell of the left ventricle and the entire right ventricle can receive blood supply throughout the cardiac cycle. The left ventricular subendocardium is therefore the part of the heart most vulnerable to ischemic damage because it receives its blood supply only during diastole. The same considerations apply to the right ventricle if pulmonary hypertension is present.

If perfusion pressure falls, flow may at first be maintained by autoregulation (coronary artery dilation). When the coronary vessels become maximally dilated, flow is determined by the coronary driving pres-

RIGHT AND LEFT VENTRICULAR BLOOD SUPPLY

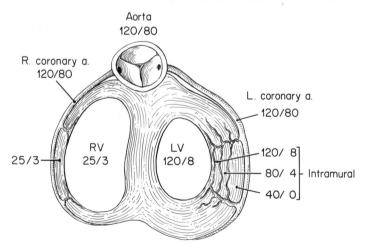

Figure 12.5. Diagrammatic cross-section of the heart indicates intramyocardial compressive forces in different parts of the myocardium. Pressures are systolic and end-diastolic. Note that intramyocardial compressive forces during systole are similar to intracavitary and intravascular pressures. Consequently, the left ventricular subendocardium must receive its blood supply during diastole.

sure and duration of diastole. In the absence of coronary artery obstruction, subendocardial driving pressure is equal to the aortic diastolic pressure minus the opposition force to flow offered by either left ventricular diastolic pressure or coronary sinus pressure, whichever is greater. These factors are represented by the area between the superimposed aortic and left ventricular pressure curves in diastole, which we have referred to as the diastolic pressure time index (DPTI)[6] (Fig. 12.6).

To assess DPTI at the bedside, one can monitor the arterial pressure and left atrial pressure (or pulmonary artery wedge pressure which are similar to left ventricular diastolic pressure) and the coronary sinus pressure, which equal right atrial of central venous pressure (Fig. 12.7A). The area of potential subendocardial blood supply can become compromised if aortic diastolic pressure is lowered (fever, arteriovenous fistula, aortic insufficiency, vasodilator drugs, anemia), left ventricular diastolic pressure is raised (cardiac failure, overtransfusion, poorly compliant left ventricular wall, pericardial tamponade), or diastole is shortened

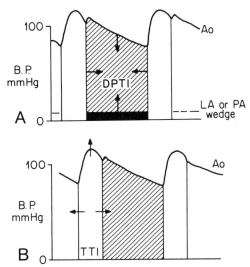

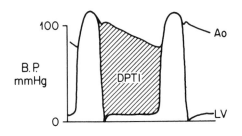

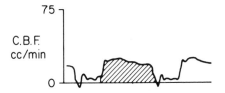

Figure 12.6. Area for potential blood supply to left ventricular subendocardium— DPTI is shown as the *cross-hatched area* between the left ventricular and aortic pressure curves. Note that phasic coronary flow to the left ventricle is predominantly diastolic.

Figure 12.7. *A.* The DPTI can be estimated at the bedside by using arterial and left atrial pressure recordings. Diastole extends from the dicrotic notch to the beginning of the next systole. Left atrial or pulmonary wedge pressure is subtracted from the total area beneath the diastolic pressure tracing. This area can be compromised by (a) reducing diastolic blood pressure, (b) tachycardia (shortening diastolic time interval), (c) increased left atrial pressure, or (d) prolongation of systole (reducing diastolic perfusion time). *B.* TTI is used to estimate myocardial oxygen demands of the left ventricle and is represented by the area beneath aortic pressure tracing from the beginning of systole to the dicrotic notch. This area can be increased by (a) raising systolic blood pressure, (b) increasing the duration of systole, and (c) tachycardia (more frequent systole).

by tachycardia or prolonged ventricular ejection (aortic stenosis, systemic hypertension, ischemic myocardium).

Although DPTI reflects potential subendocardial blood supply, oxygen supply to the subendocardium is determined by both blood flow and the arterial oxygen content. We have shown that DPTI × O_2 content provides an estimate of subendocardial oxygen supply. Oxygen content can be assessed readily at the bedside by measuring hemoglobin, blood oxygen saturation, and P_{O_2}.[7]

Oxygen Demands

The four principal determinants of myocardial oxygen requirements are (a) the external work or the product of mean blood pressure and cardiac output; (b) the developed tension or the product of pressure multiplied by the radius from the LaPlace relationship; the dilated heart must develop more tension to the same systolic pressure as the nondilated heart (i.e., cardiac failure versus normal heart); (c) heart rate, the ventricle must develop tension more frequently each minute as its rate increases; (d) contractile state of the myocardium, the heart requires more oxygen to perform the same amount of external work during inotropic stimulation (calcium, digitalis, catecholamines).

Sarnoff et al.[8] have shown that the oxygen demands of the heart can be estimated from the area beneath the left ventricular pressure curve in systole which he called the tension time index (TTI) (Fig. 12.7B). The TTI increases if left ventricular systolic pressure rises, or the duration of systole is prolonged (longer systolic ejection or tachycardia). Although myocardial oxygen needs during inotropic stimulation may be underestimated 25 to 30% using TTI, it is a method of assessing oxygen requirements under clinical circumstances.

We have proposed that the ratio DPTI × O_2 content/TTI provides an estimate of the supply/demand relationship of the subendocardium.[7] When hemoglobin exceeds 12 g%, and the blood is more than 95% saturated, DPTI/TTI ratios of more than 0.7 are usually sufficient to ensure satisfactory subendocardial perfusion. When hemoglobin is less than 12 g%, or the arterial blood is desaturated, the oxygen content of arterial blood is a critical factor in determining the supply/demand relationship.

VULNERABILITY TO ISCHEMIC INJURY

Ventricles that are hypertrophied or ischemic before surgery are more vulnerable to develop hypoxic damage and resultant myocardial failure from an intraoperative ischemic insult than are normal hearts. The mechanism of ischemia with coronary disease is readily understood because there is an anatomical obstruction to coronary blood flow (Fig. 12.8). In coronary disease there is a reduced oxygen supply (decreased driving pressure beyond the obstruction) with normal oxygen demand. Avoidance of (a) presurgical hypotension (which reduces supply still further), (b) hypertension (which increases oxygen requirements and raises left ventricular diastolic pressure impairing subendocardial flow), and (c) tachycardia (which shortens the diastolic filling of the coronary arteries and increases oxygen requirement) will minimize the ischemic damage which is added to that sustained during the surgical procedure. While pre-existing ischemia is readily accepted with coronary artery disease most patients with aortic valvular disease (stenosis or insufficiency) and mitral insufficiency also have ischemic left ventricles before operation, and their vulnerability to ischemic damage is enhanced because of coexistent ventricular hypertrophy. Preoperative EKGs almost always show evidence of this subendocardial ischemia. Figure 12.8 shows the basis for the unfavorable supply-demand relationship in these conditions.

Aortic Stenosis

Myocardial oxygen requirements (TTI) are high because of ventricular systolic hypertension and prolongation of systole. At the same time, DPTI is reduced and diastole shortened due to prolonged ventricular ejection, and left ventricular diastolic pressure is raised due to poor ventricular compliance (hypertrophy and fibrosis) as well as myocardial failure. The diastolic blood pressure may be normal but is decreased if associated aortic insufficiency is present. Tachycardia must be avoided in these patients as diastole is always shortened due to prolonged emptying across a fixed valvular obstruction.

Aortic Insufficiency

Although the increased volume work performed by patients with aortic insufficiency

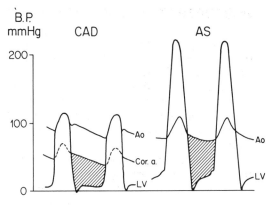

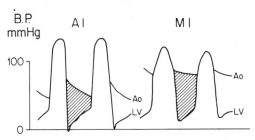

Figure 12.8. Mechanisms of ischemia are produced by altered supply/demand relationship (DPTI/TTI). *Top*. Coronary artery disease (CAD); note reduced coronary perfusion pressure beyond obstruction resulting in lowered DPTI (*stippled area*); TTI is normal. Aortic stenosis (AS); note increased myocardial oxygen requirements due to systolic hypertension and prolonged systole. DPTI is reduced because (a) diastole is shortened by systole, (b) left ventricular diastolic pressure is raised (myocardial failure and reduced compliance). *Bottom*. Aortic insufficiency (AI); note DPTI is reduced because (a) aortic diastolic pressure is low, and (b) left ventricular diastolic pressure is high. Mitral insufficiency (MI); DPTI is reduced because (a) left ventricular diastolic pressure is high (myocardial failure and increased volume) and (b) diastole is shortened by prolonged systole (which simultaneously increases TTI).

is not excessively costly in terms of oxygen requirements, these ventricles are dilated so that wall tension is high despite normal or slightly increased systolic blood pressure.

Regurgitation across the aortic valve reduces DPTI by (a) lowering diastolic blood pressure and (b) raising left ventricular diastolic pressure. In contrast to aortic stenosis where coronary flow becomes impaired with increased heart rate, coronary perfusion is impaired when patients with aortic insufficiency develop bradycardia. Slow heart rates are associated with more time for regurgitation (lower diastolic pressure and higher left ventricular diastolic pressure) and should be avoided during the surgical procedure.

Mitral Insufficiency

These patients have dilated hearts and left ventricular wall tension is high despite normal or low systolic blood pressures. When myocardial failure develops, DPTI is lowered further and left ventricular rate raises and impedes diastolic coronary flow. If hypotension develops, either during the period of induction or during the surgical procedure, it should be treated with inotropic drugs rather than peripheral constrictors. Increasing only peripheral resistance raises systemic blood pressure at the expense of increased regurgitation across the insufficient valve. This results in (a) decreased systemic blood flow, (b) increased ventricular wall tension, (c) raised left ventricular diastolic pressure (decreased DPTI).

PREOPERATIVE CONSIDERATIONS

In all patients who are either suspected of having or known to have either coronary artery disease or valvular heart disease, ischemia can be minimized by monitoring the arterial blood pressure and pulmonary arterial wedge pressure and optimizing supply and demand balance (DPTI:TTI).

Hypotension should be avoided because subendocardial blood supply will fall and ischemia will occur in all hearts that have lost autoregulatory capacity. Ischemia may worsen, however, if appropriate decisions are not based on wedge pressure recordings. Myocardial depression (anesthetic drugs) will reduce DPTI by lowering the arterial blood pressure and raising left ventricular diastolic pressure. Treating this cause of hypotension with alpha-adrenergic drugs (e. g., vasoxyl, neosynephrine) may accentuate ischemia by increasing afterload, which raises left ventricular oxygen needs (TTI). The rise in arterial blood pressure may be transient and followed by a return of hypotension.

Hypertension (e.g., insufficient anesthesia), however, may provide a false sense of security about the adequacy of subendocardial perfusion. High peripheral resistance (increased afterload) raises left ventricular oxygen requirements (TTI) markedly; left ventricular emptying becomes impaired, left ventricular diastolic pressures increases, DPTI falls, and subendocardial flow is impeded. Pharmacological vasodilators, such as nitroprusside or phentolamine may cause a marked improvement in the myocardial supply and demand balance despite lowering diastolic blood pressure.[9]

The effects of heart rate on the various disease states must also be recognized and optimized. Tachycardia, for example, shortens the diastolic filling period of the coronary arteries and causes ischemia in patients who have coronary artery disease. Rapid heart rate should also be avoided in patients who have aortic stenosis because the diastolic interval is compromised, even at slow heart rates, due to prolonged systolic ejection across the stenotic valve. Conversely very slow heart rates are deleterious to subendocardial perfusion in patients with aortic insufficiency, because more time is available for regurgitation. This increased regurgitant volume leads to a marked decreased in DPTI by lowering aortic diastolic pressure while increasing left ventricular diastolic pressure. Atrial pacing can substantially improve the adequacy of subendocardial perfusion in this condition.

Patients suffering from anemia must also be recognized and treated appropriately. Anemia produces tachycardia and raises myocardial oxygen requirements (TTI); and coronary blood flow may be incapable of increasing so as to maintain adequate oxygen delivery when blood oxygen content is reduced only mildly in patients with severe coronary artery disease or left ventricular hypertrophy.

POSTOPERATIVE CONSIDERATIONS

In the postoperative period, the major objectives should be to identify any myocardial ischemic injury that may have occurred and/or to limit its progression. The successful accomplishment of this goal is based upon ensuring an optimal supply/demand relationship (DPTI $\times$ O$_2$ content/TTI).

We have produced subendocardial ischemia in beating working normal hearts by reducing coronary diastolic blood pressure, raising left ventricular diastolic pressure (impeding left ventricular subendocardial flow), shortening diastole, or raising oxygen demands by causing left ventricular hypertension. Consequently, postoperative hypotension (reduced aortic diastolic blood pressure), myocardial failure or volume overload (increased left ventricular diastolic pressure), tachycardia (shortened diastole), or systolic hypertension (raised oxygen requirements) would accentuate ischemic injury present before operation or caused during surgery.

Our experimental studies indicate that subendocardial ischemia will be present when the supply/demand ratio falls below 0.7 provided hemoglobin is greater than 12 g% and and the blood more than 95% saturated. Clinical studies suggest that similar ratio may be applicable in man.[6,10] Attention should be directed toward each component of this ratio so that the decision regarding therapeutic intervention can be made appropriately. The ratio describing the supply/demand relationship can be calculated easily since aortic, left atrial, as well as central venous pressure may be recorded at the bedside.

MANAGEMENT OF IMPAIRED MYOCARDIAL PERFORMANCE

Blood Oxygen Content

Oxygen delivery to all organs is determined by blood flow and oxygen content. Consequently, higher cardiac outputs and coronary flows are necessary to ensure adequate myocardial and systemic oxygen delivery in the patient with anemia or arterial desaturation. Hemoglobin should be raised to 10 to 12 g% to increase oxygen-carrying capacity in the patient with postoperative anemia. Arterial desaturation should be corrected by increasing inspired oxygen or adjusting the mechanics of respiration (assisted ventilation, positive end-expiratory pressure, improved pulmonary toilet).

Compensatory mechanisms (e.g., tachycardia, which increases TTI and simultaneously decreases DPTI by shortening the coronary diastolic filling period) in anemic or hypoxic patients may adversely affect supply/demand relationships and the adequacy of myocardial and tissue oxygen delivery (Fig. 12.9). High cardiac output cannot be maintained, and signs of congestive failure worsen when subendocardial ischemia is caused by anemia.[7]

Determinants of Cardiac Output

The mechanism of maximizing preload, reducing afterload, optimizing heart rate, and increasing contractility are all available to improve myocardial performance in ischemic failing hearts after operation.

PRELOAD

Diastolic fiber length should be optimized before resorting to pharmacological or mechanical support modalities. Left atrial pressure (the barometer of left ventricular fiber stretch) is usually adequate when kept between 15 and 20 mm Hg, but higher filling pressures may be necessary in ventricles with reduced compliance (hypertrophy, fibrosis, ischemia) or with tamponade. This can be tested by volume infusion. If effective, transfusion increases both left atrial pressure and DPTI by raising arterial diastolic pressure as stroke volume rises. If contractility improves, the systolic ejection period may shorten and diastolic augmentation of DPTI occurs, if heart rate falls (Fig. 12.10). If a small transfusion (200 to 300 cc) fails to increase arterial blood pressure or decreases it while raising left- and right-sided filling pressures further, then alteration of preload cannot be used to augment cardiac performance.

DETERMINANTS OF SUBENDOCARDIAL
OXYGEN SUPPLY AND DEMAND

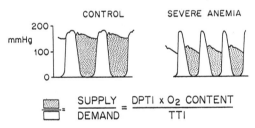

$$\frac{\text{SUPPLY}}{\text{DEMAND}} = \frac{\text{DPTI} \times O_2 \text{ CONTENT}}{\text{TTI}}$$

Figure 12.9. In the presence of anemia or arterial desaturation, compensatory mechanisms (e.g., tachycardia, which increases TTI and decreases DPTI by shortening the coronary diastolic filling period) adversely affect the supply/demand relationship and, hence, the adequacy of myocardial and tissue oxygen delivery. Note: (a) more rapid upstroke of systolic pressure recording, (b) widened pulse pressure, (c) lowered diastolic pressure (coronary perfusion pressure), and (d) tachycardia with shortened diastolic filling period of the coronary arteries.

INCREASED PRELOAD

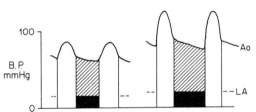

Figure 12.10. Increased preload is used to improve postoperative cardiac output. Before transfusion (*left*), note low diastolic blood pressure, prolonged systole, slow upstroke of aortic pulse pressure (which is narrowed), and left atrial pressure of 15 mm Hg: DPTI/TTI is reduced. After transfusion (*right*), DPTI/TTI improves despite increased systolic blood pressure and raised left atrial pressure. Note: (a) more rapid upstroke of systolic pressure recording, (b) higher systolic and diastolic blood pressure, (c) widened pulse pressure, (d) reduction of systolic time interval and slowing of heart rate (longer diastole).

AFTERLOAD

Cardiac output may be inadequate with normal or increased arterial blood pressure when peripheral resistance is increased markedly. Ischemic myocardium does not empty efficiently if afterload is high. DPTI may be impaired, despite diastolic hypertension, because (a) prolonged systolic ejection shortens coronary diastolic filling period and (b) raised left ventricular diastolic pressure impedes subendocardial flow. Simultaneous oxygen requirements (TTI) are high because systolic hypertension (a) increases pressure work, (b) prolongs the ejection period, and (c) raises myocardial wall tension (Fig. 12.11).

Blood volume must be adequate before vasodilator drugs are used; blood pressure is maintained by intense peripheral vasoconstriction in patients with low output syndrome. Vasodilator drugs may cause sudden profound hypotension when they lower peripheral resistance if blood volume is not adequate to fill the increased vascular bed. Vasodilator drugs (arfonad, nitroprusside, dibenzyline) improve the supply/demand relationship in several ways. Decreasing afterload in hypertensive patients reduces TTI by lowering systolic arterial pressure and duration, and reduces wall tension. The unloaded ventricle empties more easily and has a lower diastolic pressure and longer coronary diastolic filling period due to a more rapid systolic ejection. DPTI may not, therefore, be impaired significantly despite reduced arterial diastolic pressure.

Afterload reduction in normotensive or hypotensive patients with high left atrial pressures (25 to 30 mm Hg) may not alter or even increase arterial blood pressure. This occurs when cardiac output increases more than peripheral resistance falls so that more volume is present in the aorta and arterial system. It is often necessary, however, to augment preload during afterload reduction if left atrial pressure falls significantly.

HEART RATE

Atrial pacing is preferable to ventricular pacing because it provides more uniform ventricular filling and maximizes the Starling response by providing presystolic ventricular fiber stretch. Cardiac output is the product of stroke volume and heart rate, so that increasing heart rate should improve the output of failing hearts. The normal heart does not, however, change its output with tachycardia as stroke volume falls (pacing narrows pulse pressure, reduces systolic and increases diastolic blood pressures). Two questions arise in regard to pacing: (a) why isn't subendocardial flow impaired by increasing heart rate in as much as tachycardia shortens the diastolic coronary filling period and (b) how can optimum heart rate be determined?

Increasing heart rate improves cardiac performance most effectively in patients with wide pulse pressures. Their coronary arteries are usually dilated maximally. DPTI/minute increases despite shortened diastole, because the time for peripheral runoff is reduced and mean aortic diastolic

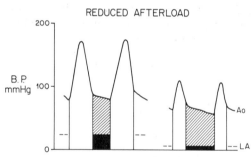

Figure 12.11. Postoperative hypertension causes myocardial ischemia (*left*). TTI is high due to (a) systolic hypertension and (b) prolonged systolic ejection time; DPTI is low (despite diastolic hypertension) because diastole is shortened by prolonged systole and left atrial pressure is high due to impaired cardiac emptying and myocardial ischemia. Afterload reduction by nitroprusside (*right*) results in reduced TTI (systolic pressure falls and systole shortens as the ventricle empties more easily), DPTI increases as left atrial pressure is lowered and systole is shortened so that the diastolic filling period of the coronary arteries is prolonged. Note: DPTI/TTI increases despite reduction of diastolic blood pressure.

pressure rises more than diastole is shortened.[3] Although pulse pressure narrows, both systolic and diastolic pressure increases when cardiac output rises (Fig. 12.12). The systolic ejection period shortens if contractility increases, so that diastolic filling period is not compromised as severely as expected. Cardiac size also decreases as the heart empties more completely due to inotropic effects of tachycardia, and subendocardial perfusion improves. The ideal heart rate is one which provides a maximum increase in the supply/demand (DPTI/TTI) ratio.[3]

If stroke volume is increased by pacing, arterial blood pressure rises and left atrial pressure falls; DPTI/TTI improves. If stroke volume does not change arterial pressure remains constant but cardiac output increases. Any reduction of systolic blood pressure suggests stroke volume has decreased and heart rate is excessive (Fig. 12.12).

INCREASING HEART RATE

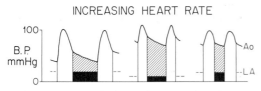

Figure 12.12. Increased heart rate is used to improve postoperative myocardial function and subendocardial perfusion. *Left.* Note wide aortic pulse pressure and prolonged systole. DPTI is low as diastolic pressure continues to fall as diastole is prolonged (slow heart rate). *Center.* Increasing rate (atrial pacing) raises DPTI as (a) aortic diastolic pressure is raised more than diastole is shortened, (b) systolic ejection period is reduced (more time for diastole), (c) left atrial pressure falls as the heart empties more complete (improved contractility resulting from increased subendocardial perfusion); cardiac output improves. *Right.* When heart rate is too rapid there is (a) failure of systolic pressure to rise, (b) excessive shortening of diastole, (c) increased left atrial pressure (reflecting accentuation of myocardial failure); DPTI/TTI falls.

CONTRACTILITY

Catecholamines, commonly used to raise myocardial contractility, can produce subendocardial necrosis.[11] These drugs cause necrosis by reducing available oxygen supply relative to simultaneous cardiac oxygen demands rather than by direct toxicity.

ISOPROTERENOL

The maximal benefit achieved with isoproterenol (Isuprel) relates to its effect on the supply/demand relationship, rather than to its absolute infusion rate.[12] Ischemia develops at higher supply/demand ratios (~1.0) with inotropic drugs because TTI underestimates oxygen requirements by approximately 30% during catecholamine stimulation.[13]

Isoproterenol increases oxygen requirements by (a) increasing contractility, (b) increasing heart rate (raised TTI/minute), and (c) increasing volume work by raising output. As it dilates coronary arteries, it simultaneously reduces the DPTI by (a) lowering aortic diastolic pressure (peripheral vasodilation) and (b) shortening coronary diastolic filling period by tachycardia. Isoproterenol can augment or impair cardiac performance (Fig. 12.13). If contractility is increased, both systolic and diastolic pressures rise, and, despite tachycardia systolic ejection period shortens and limits the reduction in diastolic time for any given heart rate. Patients show increased peripheral perfusion (warmer extremities) indicating lowered peripheral resistance. The association of increased blood pressure and reduced resistance indicates that cardiac output rose more than peripheral resistance fell. Isoproterenol can also cause tachycardia and diastolic hypotension sufficient to reduce available subendocardial blood supply relative to demands. When this occurs, DPTI/TTI falls below 1.0, arrhythmias are encountered frequently, and blood pressure cannot be maintained despite increased infusion rates.

NOREPINEPHRINE

The tachycardia and diastolic hypotension seen with isoproterenol do not occur when norepinephrine is used. However, norepinephrine increases oxygen demands

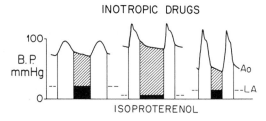

Figure 12.13. Inotropic drugs are used to improve cardiac function. *Left*. Pressure tracing when cardiac output is inadequate; arterial pressure is low, pulse pressure is narrow, left atrial pressure is high and DPTI/TTI is reduced. *Center*. With isoproterenol infusion, systolic and diastolic blood pressures rise, systole is shortened, systolic ejection is brisk, left atrial pressure falls, and DPTI/TTI is raised. When too much isoproterenol is given (*right*), peripheral vasodilation causes a reduction in diastolic blood pressure and tachycardia shortens diastole; DPTI/TTI falls and ischemia results. Systole now becomes more prolonged and left atrial pressure increases. In this instance, isoproterenol may augment any myocardial ischemia present as shown in the *left* panel.

by raising contractility and increasing peripheral vascular resistance. Consequently afterload is increased and ventricular emptying may become impaired. The increase in blood pressure associated with norepinephrine may not necessarily reflect an improved cardiac output, but indicates the retention of more blood in the arterial system due to reduced runoff. If both arterial pressure and left atrial pressure rise, DPTI/TTI is reduced and subendocardial ischemia may worsen.

EPINEPHRINE

Although epinephrine causes vasoconstriction, peripheral resistance does not rise as much as with norepinephrine. As with isoproterenol, there is a tendency for tachycardia, arrhythmia, and increased contractility. The combined effects may reduce DPTI/TTI and worsen subendocardial ischemia.

DOPAMINE

This drug is a naturally-occurring precursor of norepinephrine and has both alpha- and beta-receptor stimulating properties. It differs from the previously mentioned catecholamines in that it can specifically cause dilation of the renal and mesenteric blood vessels in doses that may not increase the heart rate or blood pressure (1 to 5 μg/kg/minute). At higher doses (5 to 10 μg/kg/minute) this drug has general beta-receptor stimulating properties on the heart which results in increased cardiac output. At dosages greater than 10 μg/kg/minute, dopamine stimulates alpha-adrenergic receptors and results in peripheral vasoconstriction with subsequent afterloading of the ventricle and increasing left atrial pressure.

DOBUTAMINE

This new synthetic catecholamine produces myocardial beta-adrenergic stimulation and hence increases myocardial contractility. Unlike the previously mentioned catecholamines, dobutamine rarely causes tachycardia and produces little vasoconstriction at the usual therapeutic doses (2.5 to 10 μg/kg/minute).

COUNTERPULSATION

The intra-aortic balloon is suited ideally to improve the myocardial supply/demand relationship (Fig. 12.14). Counterpulsation reduces myocardial oxygen requirements by lowering the TTI (decreasing systolic pressure and shortening systolic ejection) and increasing the DPTI by (a) augmenting aortic diastolic pressure, (b) reducing left ventricular diastolic pressure, and (c) prolonging diastole. It is effective only if cardiac rhythm is regular. In the normal heart, coronary flow is not augmented by counterpulsation because the coronary arteries autoregulate to maintain a given flow. In the ischemic heart the coronary arteries are dilated maximally. Flow is pressure dependent and increases when counterpulsation raises the DPTI. It is our view that balloon counterpulsation should be used if small doses of inotropic drugs do not produce an adequate cardiac output. Intra-aortic bal-

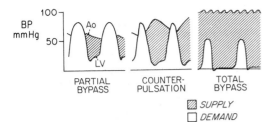

Figure 12.14. Effects of partial bypass, of diastolic aortic counterpulsation, and of total (vented) bypass on supply/demand relationship are shown. The *cross-hatched* area is the DPTI. The open area is the TTI. *Left.* With partial bypass, the supply/demand ratio remains depressed because the left ventricle does pressure and volume work (increasing demands), and high left ventricular diastolic pressure and diastolic aortic hypotension decrease supply. *Center.* While counterpulsation increases DPTI markedly by raising diastolic perfusion pressure and reduces TTI by lowering systolic pressure with ventricular unloading, some volume and isometric ventricular pressure is still necessary. Note ventricular diastolic pressure remains elevated. *Right.* With *total* bypass, adequate venting reduces oxygen demand and removes impedance to subendocardial perfusion by lowering high left ventricular diastolic pressure. Supply is optimized by raising aortic blood pressure with increased extracorporeal flow rate and/or administration of a peripheral vasoconstrictive drug.

loon counterpulsation should not be considered "an intervention of last resort" and reserved until organ failure is advanced. Conversely, arterial complications from this device do occur so that indiscriminate use is not warranted.

Philips and Bregman and their associates[10, 14] report DPTI/TTI to be useful in detecting subendocardial ischemia postoperatively and employ balloon counterpulsation when this ratio falls below 0.8. If counterpulsation increases the ratio above this level cardiac output increases, left atrial falls, an electrocardiographic evidence of

ischemia improves. They report survival only in those patients who maintain supply and demand ratios above 0.8 when counterpulsation is discontinued.

EXTRACORPOREAL CIRCULATION

Extracorporeal circulation is another form of mechanical circulatory support which can be instituted, using local anesthesia, via the femoral artery and vein of the patient who does not respond to the aforementioned attempts to improve the adequacy of cardiac output. In the cardiac surgical patient, whose output is inadequate when extracorporeal circulation is discontinued intraoperatively, the unique opportunity exists to reduce left ventricular oxygen requirements markedly by venting the ventricle and placing the heart in the beating empty state. Simultaneously, subendocardial blood (oxygen) supply can be raised by increasing aortic blood pressure and increasing the extracorporeal flow rate and red cell mass (transfusion) expecially if extreme hemodilution has been used.

The effectiveness of cardiopulmonary bypass in reducing ischemia and relieving the heart of its work load is achieved best when the left ventricle vented completely.[15] The partially bypassed heart must perform both pressure and volume work; because of impaired function it frequently has a high left ventricular diastolic pressure, which may reduce coronary driving pressure and impede subendocardial blood supply. Partial bypass can be continued postoperatively without the need of an oxygenator, if necessary, by using the left atrial aortic method described by Litwak et al.[16] Perhaps the most efficient use of partial bypass (with an oxygenator) is in the patient suffering from right ventricular failure (coronary embolism, right ventricular infarction). Unfortunately, the need for anticoagulation may lead to coagulopathies which are difficult to manage so that partial bypass is usually reserved for extreme circumstances.

References

1. Bunker JP: Metabolic effects of blood transfusion. *Anesthesiology* 27:466, 1967.

2. Cooper N, Brazier J, Hottenrott C, et al: Myocardial depression following citrated blood transfusion—an avoidable complication. *Arch Surg* 107:756, 1973.

3. Buckberg GD, Fixler DE, Archie JP, et al: Variable effects of heart rate on phasic and regional left ventricular muscle blood flow in anesthetized dogs. *Cardiovasc Res* 9:1, 1975.

4. Najafi H, Henson D, Dye WS, et al: Left ventricular hemorrhagic necrosis. *Ann Thorac Surg* 7:550, 1969.

5. Taber RC, Morales AR, Fine G: Myocardial necrosis and the postoperative low cardiac output syndrome. *Ann Thorac Surg* 4:12, 1967.

6. Buckberg GD, Towers B, Paglia DE, et al: Subendocardial ischemia after cardiopulmonary bypass. *J Thorac Cardiovasc Surg* 64:669, 1972.

7. Brazier J, Cooper N, Buckberg G: The adequacy of subendocardial oxygen delivery: The interaction of determinants of flow, arterial oxgyen content, and myocardial oxygen need. *Circulation* 49:968, 1974.

8. Sarnoff SJ, Braunwald E, Welch GH: Hemodynamic determinants of oxygen consumption of the heart with special reference to the tension time index. *Am J Physiol* 192:148, 1958.

9. Hoar PF, Hickey RF, Ullyot DJ: Systemic hypertension following myocardial revascularization. *J Thorac Cardiovasc Surg* 71:859, 1976.

10. Philips P, Mary A, Miyanoto A: A clinical method for detecting subendocardial ischemia following cardiopulmonary bypass. *J Thorac Cardiovasc Surg* 69:30, 1975.

11. Ferrans VJ, Hibbs RG, Black WC, et al: Isoproterenol induced myocardial necrosis. A histochemical and electron microscopic study. *Am Heart J* 68:71, 1964.

12. Buckberg GD, Kattus AA: Factors determining the distribution and adequacy of left ventricular myocardial blood flow. In Bloor, Olsson, (eds): *Current Topics in Coronary Research*. Plenum Press, New York, 1973, pp. 95–113.

13. Krasnow N, Rolett EL, Yurchak PM, et al: Isoproterenol and cardiovascular performance. *Am J Med* 37:514, 1964.

14. Bregman D, Parodi EN, Edie RN, et al: Intraoperative unidirectional intraaortic balloon pumping (IABP) in the management of left ventricular power failure. *J Thorac Cardiovasc Surg* 70:1010, 1975.

15. Pennock JL, Pierce WS, Waldhausen JA: Quantitative evaluation of left ventricular bypass in reducing myocardial ischemia. *Surgery* 79:523, 1976.

16. Litwak RS, Koffsky RM, Jurado RA, et al: Use of a left heart assist device after intracardiac surgery: technique and clinical experience. *Ann Thorac Surg* 21:191, 1976.

CHAPTER 13

AFTERLOAD MISMATCH IN THE PERIOPERATIVE PERIOD

JOHN J. ROSS, JR., M.D.

The concept of afterload mismatch carries certain implications for the preoperative selection and postoperative management of cardiac patients. However, before developing these applications, it will be necessary first to consider some basic physiological principles that lead to a relatively simple framework for considering left ventricular (LV) function, LV pressure-volume or wall stress-volume (SV) loops, and the linear relation at end-systole between LV pressure and volume or wall stress and volume. This framework will then be used to consider briefly the effects of acute cardiac overload, as in sudden valvular regurgitation; the immediate effects of operation on the left ventricle in selected valvular lesions; and postoperative myocardial failure with correction of afterload mismatch by vasodilators. The importance of the venous return will also be discussed.

AFTERLOAD MISMATCH

Afterload mismatch may be described as the inability of the ventricle to deliver a normal SV against a given level of systolic load at any level of myocardial contractility (inotropic state).[1] A number of examples of such a mechanism can be developed, but three will serve to illustrate the concept under conditions when left ventricular contractility is normal or near normal:

1. In the normal heart, when the preload is artificially maintained at a fixed level and the afterload is progressively increased, the SV progressively falls[2,3]; under these conditions, Frank-Starling reserve is absent because the preload is held fixed and afterload mismatch develops with *any* increase in systolic load.

2. Afterload mismatch can be induced in the normal heart by marked volume and pressure overloading to reach the limit of preload reserve; in this setting, with further loading the SV also falls due to afterload mismatch, even if myocardial contractility is normal, because the preload reserve is exhausted.[2]

Such mismatch can occur when the preload is fully utilized in the presence of acute valvular lesions such as aortic or mitral regurgitation or ventricular septal defect, or acute malignant hypertension[4]; in these settings, since myocardial contractility is basically intact, it may be anticipated that relief of the excessive mechanical loading conditions will result in normal LV function.[3] If the venous return is limited by peripheral factors, afterload mismatch can occur in the normal heart, even when the preload reserve is not fully utilized.

Afterload mismatch can also occur in several situations when myocardial contractility is decreased:

1. In chronic pressure overload due to aortic stenosis, inadequate use of the Frank-Starling reserve could occur because of excessive diastolic wall stiffness, or because the afterload is excessive relative to the

levels of myocardial contractility and hypertrophy in the late phase of this disorder; correction of aortic stenosis by valve replacement in the latter setting would be expected to result in immediate improvement of LV function.[5]

2. In chronic mitral regurgitation with depressed myocardial contractility, afterload mismatch may occur in the immediate postoperative period when the low impedance leak into the left atrium is corrected by mitral valve replacement.[5]

3. In chronic myocardial disease with moderate depression of LV contractility, compensatory mechanisms including use of the Frank-Starling reserve may prevent afterload mismatch at rest, but it can be induced by an acute pressor stress such as infusion of angiotensin or phenylephrine; in this setting the ventricle behaves *as if* the preload were held fixed. This can also occur in some patients with aortic regurgitation in whom the preload reserve is fully utilized.[6]

4. Afterload mismatch can exist in the *basal state*, even when there is a normal level of systolic pressure. In chronic severe heart failure or acute postoperative heart failure, as in some patients with preoperative LV dysfunction, correction of afterload mismatch can be accomplished by pharmacological interventions.[7]

Changes in the afterload are usually associated with changes in the LV and aortic systolic pressures, although it should be recognized that afterload is better represented by the *wall stress* on the myocardial fibers. In simplest terms: wall stress = pressure · radius/2 · wall thickness. The impedance to ejection has also been employed to represent the afterload, although we have recently shown that the wall stress effectively represents the systolic load, and encompasses impedance effects.[8]

The preload reserve can be analyzed at the sarcomere level. Experiments in hearts fixed at end-diastole at a normal filling pressure have shown midwall sarcomere lengths of approximately 2.0 μ,[9] and after acute volume overloading to filling pressures in excess of 20 mm Hg, sarcomeres are recruited from the inner and outer wall to yield sarcomere lengths in excess of 2.2

across the wall (the maximum sarcomere lengths obtainable in the normal heart experimentally).[10] Indeed, even at extremely high filling pressures (over 50 mm Hg) the sarcomeres do not extend beyond 2.2 to 2.3 μ because of the inherent stiffness of the ventricular myocardium at elevated filling pressures and high volumes.[11] Thus, the limit of preload reserve in the normal heart in the open chest animal is approximately 25 mm Hg (Fig. 13.1). Even in the chronically dilated heart, it has been shown that the sarcomeres do not extend beyond 2.2 μ in animals (Fig. 13.1), a marked increase in LV end-diastolic volume occurring while more sarcomeres are added in series.[12] This suggests that in the chronically-dilated and failing heart the preload reserve is maximally utilized under resting conditions when the filling pressures are substantially elevated.

A FRAMEWORK USING END-SYSTOLIC RELATIONS

In isolated cardiac muscle it has been shown that regardless of the preload or afterload the muscle when it shortens tends to reach the isometric length-tension curve; that is, the isometric length-active tension relation provides the limit for shortening.[13] If the length-active tension relation is shifted by a positive or negative inotropic influence a new limit of shortening is established. In the intact left ventricle a nearly linear relation between calculated peak systolic wall stress and end-diastolic volume in isovolumetric beats was shown, and in ejecting beats the relationship between LV volume and wall tension at the end of ejection appeared to fall on this relation.[14] Similar relations were demonstrated in the isolated heart ejecting under isovolumetric and isotonic conditions.[15] In detailed experiments in the isolated heart by Suga, Sagawa, and associates,[16, 17] the end-systolic pressure-volume relation was shown to be linear and to provide the limit of end-systolic volume for the pressure-volume loop, and this relation could also be shifted by a positive inotropic intervention.

As shown diagrammatically in Figure

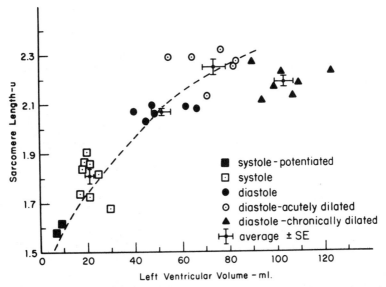

Figure 13.1. Relations between LV volume and sarcomere length at the midwall in the dog are shown. The hypothetical curve for an ellipse is shown by the *dashed line* and the volume-sarcomere length relations at various ventricular volumes are shown (for further discussion, see text). The *solid triangles* indicate the diastolic sarcomere length volume relations in the chronically-dilated ventricle due to chronic volume overload. Reproduced by permission of John Ross, Jr. and the American Heart Association, Inc. From Ross et al.[6]

13.2, in the ventricle operating from a normal end-diastolic volume if the afterload (peak systolic pressure in this instance) is increased while the end-diastolic volume is held constant, a drop in the SV will occur as the ventricle shortens to the linear end-systolic relation (Beat 1 to Beat 2, Fig. 13.2). Ordinarily under these circumstances in the ensuing beats the ventricle will compensate by increasing its end-diastolic volume, and through the Frank-Starling reserve the SV may be restored to normal (Beat 3). However, if the limit of preload reserve is reached at this point (LV end-diastolic pressure of 20 mm Hg or more) little further increase in ventricular volume will occur as the end-diastolic pressure rises, and if the systolic pressure is then further elevated the SV will drop (Beat 4, Fig. 13.2). Both Beats 2 and 4 represent examples of afterload mismatch, the first with the preload held fixed, the second with an increase in systolic pressure when limit of Frank-Starling reserve is fully utilized. Of course, if a positive

inotropic agent were given to shift the linear end-systolic relation upward and to the left with a steepened slope, a larger SV could ensue from any given level of preload and systolic pressure.

Afterload mismatch can result in an apparent descending limb of a Starling Curve relating LV end-diastolic volume or pressure to the SV, as shown experimentally[2] in open chest animals subjected to acute pressure and volume overloading in which mitral regurgitation did not occur. The relationship between end-diastolic pressure and SV became flat as filling pressures were elevated by transfusion above 20 mm Hg, and at about 35 mm Hg further infusion resulted in a drop in the SV while calculated wall stress rose further.[2] It has been proposed that the descending limb of function under these circumstances is not due to a descending limb of the Frank-Starling curve (sarcomere overstretch) but rather to effects of afterload mismatch when the preload reserve is fully utilized.[1,2]

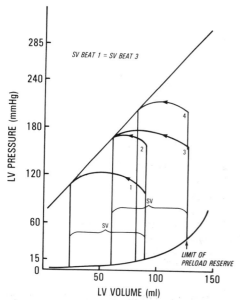

Figure 13.2. The diagram shows response to changes in afterload of the normal left ventricle. Pressure-volume loops are shown, the *arrows* indicating the direction of volume change during LV ejection and at end-ejection these loops reach the linear relation between LV end-systolic pressure and end-systolic volume. SV Beats 1 and 2 show the effect of elevating LV systolic pressure when the LV end-diastolic volume is held fixed; a sharp reduction in the SV ensues. Beat 3 shows the compensation for increased afterload by use of the Frank-Starling reserve (increased preload) with restoration of the SV to normal (SV1 = SV3). If the ventricle has reached the limit of its preload reserve at that end-diastolic volume, with any further increase in LV systolic pressure the ventricle will behave as if the preload were fixed, and the SV will fall (Beat 4).

Thus, the concept of afterload mismatch with limited preload reserve is conveniently described by the pressure-volume loop and by end-systolic pressure-volume relations or wall SV relations, although other frameworks such as the force-velocity-length relation and the ventricular function curve can also be utilized.[1,18] This is not to suggest it is necessary to determine end-systolic relations at the bedside in the acute care setting; rather, this theoretical framework is useful for understanding and predicting hemodynamic responses that may occur in this setting.

ACUTE VALVULAR REGURGITATION OR SEVERE HYPERTENSION

With marked pressure volume and/or pressure overloading, it would be expected that the ventricle could reach the limit of preload reserve; thus, when faced with a very high systolic pressure due to uncontrolled hypertension, severe acute aortic regurgitation, or acute mitral regurgitation due to infective endocarditis or chordal rupture, afterload mismatch may develop. As indicated in Figure 13.2, a sharp drop in the SV may occur under such circumstances, without depression of the intrinsic inotropic state of the ventricles, and acute severe heart failure may ensue. Use of a vasodilator to treat the acute, severe hypertension usually restores the SV and cardiac output to normal, even if there is some intrinsic depression of the hypertrophied ventricle in patients with malignant hypertension. Likewise, in the presence of acute valvular regurgitation, a vasodilator such as nitroprusside will both decrease the degree of valvular regurgitation, and also will lower the afterload (wall stress) on the ventricle during ejection, thereby improving the forward cardiac output, lowering the filling pressures, and allowing time to prepare for corrective operation. Immediately after operation, it may be predicted that ventricular function will return to normal or near normal, since the deterioration of LV performance was due primarily to afterload mismatch rather than to intrinsic depression of myocardial contractility.

AFTERLOAD MISMATCH AND CHRONIC MITRAL REGURGITATION

It is recognized that a fraction of patients with chronic severe mitral regurgitation respond poorly to mitral valve replacement and exhibit continuing LV failure. Recent studies have identified preoperatively two groups of patients in whom the response to operation differs.[19] In one group there is only a moderate increase in LV end-diastolic dimension (by echocardiography) and the ejection fraction (EF) is in the high normal range, and in the other group there is a much larger end-diastolic dimension with the LV EF in the low normal range (Fig. 13.3). Postoperatively, the EF fell in both groups, but in the first group the fall was only slight and it remained within the normal range, whereas in the second group there was a marked drop in the EF (Fig. 13.3).[19] None of these patients showed evidence of intraoperative myocardial damage, and therefore the latter response can be attributed to the presence of depressed LV function preoperatively.

Such responses are diagrammed in Figure 13.4. The usual response to volume overload is a shift to the right of the diastolic pressure-volume relation, and the mean systolic wall stress is maintained at a relatively normal level[20] by the large regurgitant leak early and late during ventricular ejection into the low impedance left atrium (Fig. 13.4, *top*). Therefore, in compensated initial regurgitation the EF is maintained at a high normal range, with the enlarged ventricle delivering an enhanced SV with normal shortening of each unit of the enlarged circumference. Postoperatively, the end-diastolic volume may return to nearly normal and the ejection function is well maintained (Fig. 13.4, *top*). In patients with preoperative depression of myocardial contractility, the linear end-systolic wall SV relation is shifted downward and to the right. Nevertheless, because of the low-impedance leak into the left atrium the ventricle may be able to maintain a nearly normal EF due to the lowered instantaneous afterload early and late during ejection, even if the peak wall stress is elevated to some degree (Fig. 13.5). Under these conditions, when the mitral valve is replaced the left ventricle must now deliver all of its SV into the high impedance of the aorta. The wall stress throughout systole therefore rises, and the SV may drop markedly with a severe reduction of the EF postoperatively (Fig. 13.5, Panel B).[5] Under these conditions, the left ventricle is unloaded preoperatively, and afterload mismatch develops in the immediate postoperative period. Here, knowledge of the nature of the lesion and the preoperative cardiac status could allow prediction of how surgical treatment will alter LV dynamics. It may also be anticipated that such patients will exhibit LV failure in the postoperative period, with low cardiac output, and early institution of vasodilator and/or inotropic therapy should be planned. It seems clear that we are waiting too long to recommend operation in such patients. Therefore, new

MITRAL REGURGITATION SUBGROUPS

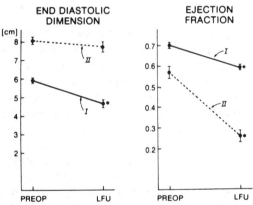

Figure 13.3. Average echocardiographic measurements are shown in patients with mitral regurgitation before (*PREOP*) and at late follow-up (*LFU*, average 15 months) after mitral valve replacement. Group II (*dashed lines*) indicates a subgroup with large left ventricles (end-diastolic diameter over 70 mm and end-systolic diameter over 50 mm). Notice that in Group I there is a fall of heart size postoperatively and only a small drop in ejection fraction. In contrast, in Group II heart size fails to decrease significantly and there is a marked drop in the ejection fraction. Modified from Schuler et al.[39]

MITRAL REGURGITATION

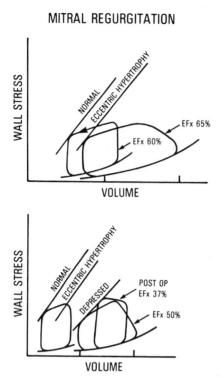

AORTIC STENOSIS

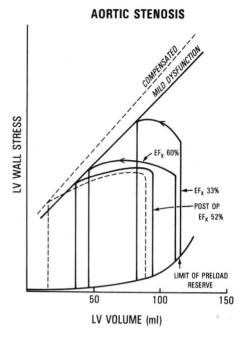

Figure 13.4. A diagram of wall SV loops and end-systolic volume-wall stress relations in severe mitral regurgitation is shown. *Top.* The shift to the right of the diastolic and end-systolic relations allows the volume overloaded left ventricle to maintain a high SV. Mean wall stress during ejection is somewhat reduced, and in mitral regurgitation the EF is high normal when contractility is normal. *Bottom.* With the development of depressed contractility, the end-systolic wall SV relation is shifted to the right before operation. Despite severely depressed contractility, the ventricle is able to deliver a nearly normal EF because of the very large ventricular volume and the relatively low mean wall stress during ejection (EF = 50%). Contractility remains depressed after mitral valve replacement, and with correction of the low impedance leak the ventricle must now deliver the total SV into the aorta against a higher wall stress; the EF therefore falls to 37% (Beat 1). Reproduced by permission from J. Ross Jr.[29]

Figure 13.5. Loops showing the relationship between LV volume and wall stress throughout contraction under various conditions in the presence of aortic stenosis. With fully compensated aortic stenosis (*dashed lines*), the linear end-systolic relation between wall stress and volume is normal, and the volume-wall stress loop shows a normal level of wall stress (afterload) during ejection. With the development of mild depression of the inotropic state, the linear end-systolic relation is shifted somewhat to the right. The end-diastolic volume of the ventricle increases to some degree, but LV function is well maintained (loop showing EF) [EF_x] of 60%). With further progression of the degree of aortic stenosis, the left ventricle may reach the limit of its preload reserve (*arrow*) and high LV systolic pressure and volume result in a higher LV wall stress during ejection leading to afterload mismatch; the ejection fraction in this case drops to 33%. Following aortic valve replacement (postop) since there is only mild myocardial dysfunction, relief of the obstruction results in a normal wall stress and a return of the EF to near normal (52%).

methods, such as use of the end-systolic wall SV index,[21] must be developed to identify such patients prior to the development of irreversible myocardial changes.[5]

AFTERLOAD MISMATCH AND AORTIC STENOSIS

The response to operation in this lesion in patients who have LV dysfunction is opposite to that in mitral regurgitation, in that afterload mismatch is usually corrected by aortic valve replacement. Studies have now shown that even if the LV ejection fraction is severely depressed preoperatively (as low as 18 to 20%), in many such patients a striking improvement in the EF occurs postoperatively.[22] Recent patient studies suggest that this response may occur very early in the postoperative period, as might be expected from correction of afterload mismatch by valve replacement.[23] The LV ejection fraction was severely depressed preoperatively (approximately 25%) when studied by left ventriculography at cardiac catheterization. However, only 5 days postoperatively a radionuclide EF revealed that the LV EF had returned entirely to normal (65%).[23] Under conditions of chronic concentric LV hypertrophy due to pressure overload, experimental studies have shown that as the concentric hypertrophy develops the chamber size remains normal, and the enhanced wall thickening is able to counterbalance the elevated systolic pressure. Therefore, the LV wall stress remains normal in the compensated state, and the SV and EF are normal.[24] As diagrammed in Figure 13.5, in many patients with severe aortic stenosis who develop heart failure depression of myocardial contractility may be relatively mild; however, as the stenosis progresses the ventricle reaches the limit of its preload reserve and afterload mismatch ensues with a drop in the EF. Under these conditions, replacement of the aortic valve with a prosthesis will relieve the mismatch and allow the EF to return to normal in the immediate postoperative period. Therefore, it may be predicted that such patients will ordinarily not require intensive cardiac therapy in the postoperative period.

In the selection of patients for operation, such findings imply that operation should not be denied patients with hemodynamically severe aortic stenosis, even if there is severe preoperative depression of LV function.[5]

AFTERLOAD MISMATCH AND HEART FAILURE

In chronic heart failure with LV dilation it has been shown that the left ventricle responds to a pressor stress, such as angiotensin infusion, by an increase in the end-diastolic pressure and a sharp drop in the SV.[25] It has been suggested that this type of response indicates that the failing heart is operating at the limit of its preload reserve in the resting state, and under these conditions *any* increase in the systolic LV pressure will result in a further drop in SV, since the ventricle behaves *as if* the preload were fixed (the preload reserve is exhausted).[1] Indeed, when the SV is low at rest, the ventricle may exhibit afterload mismatch under basal conditions due to depressed inotropic state and elevated wall stress, even when the systolic pressure is normal.

A number of investigators have shown that infusion of a vasodilator in patients with heart failure results in a fall in LV filling pressure and a rise in SV, provided that the LV filling pressure or mean pulmonary artery wedge pressure is elevated above approximately 15 mm Hg. In contrast, if the filling pressure is below 15 mm Hg, a fall in the LV filling pressure is usually accompanied by a drop in the SV and cardiac output.[26]

Venous Return

Differences in the cardiac output response to vasodilator may be explained by recent studies concerned with venous return and cardiac output curves, using the framework defined by Guyton et al.[27] In brief, the venous return curve may be plotted as an inverse relation between the mean right atrial pressure and the level of venous return (increases in right atrial pressure with the heart excluded from the circulation decreasing the gradient for venous return);

increases in intravascular volume, shift the venous return curve upward in a parallel manner, whereas depletion of intravascular volume shifts the relationship downward.[27] Other peripheral factors (the tone, resistance, and compliance) of the systemic circulation also can importantly affect the venous return and hence the cardiac output, independently of cardiac function.[27] The cardiac output curve can be plotted on the same diagram (mean right atrial pressure against cardiac output), and in the Guyton framework the cardiac output curve can be shifted upward by influences in addition to an increase in inotropic state, including decreased afterload, whereas the curve may be shifted downward by negative inotropic influences and increased afterload. The intersection between the venous return curve and the cardiac output curve identifies a given steady-state equilibrium.[27]

THE ROLE OF VENOUS RETURN IN AFTERLOAD REDUCTION THERAPY

The importance of venous return in the cardiac output response to vasodilators has been emphasized by recent experiments from our laboratory in dogs with normal hearts and those in which acute cardiac failure was induced by multiple coronary artery ligations.[28] These studies indicate that vasodilator therapy with nitroprusside is effective in increasing cardiac output only if peripheral factors allow an increase in venous return to occur.

When nitroprusside was administered intravenously in the relatively normal circulation, a fall in the cardiac output resulted, despite lowered systemic vascular resistance (and therefore more favorable loading conditions on the normal left ventricle). This response occurred because nitroprusside-induced concomitant dilation of the venous bed, which was only partially compensated for by a small shift of blood volume from the central to the peripheral circulation (2.4 ± 0.4 SEM ml/kg).[28] Therefore, the venous return curve was displaced downward and to the left due to a reduction of the effective systemic blood volume (Fig. 13.6). The consequent reduction of venous return to the right heart was responsible for a reduction in right ventricular output and hence in LV

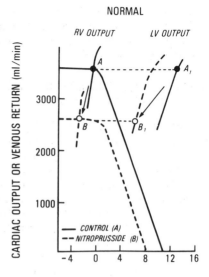

Figure 13.6. The relation between cardiac output and venous return in acute heart failure is shown. Under control conditions (*solid lines*), the intersect between right ventricular output and venous return (*Point A*) is on the ascending portion of the venous return curve, cardiac output being limited by the failing left ventricle which is operating on a flat and depressed cardiac output curve (*Point A₁*). Following nitroprusside infusion (*dashed lines*) there is no shift of the venous return curve, a downward shift being prevented by a redistribution of the central blood volume to the periphery (see text). There is now a marked shift upward of the function curve of the left ventricle due to reduced afterload with correction of afterload mismatch, and a marked drop in the LV filling pressure occurs. The shift upward of the LV and right ventricular (RV) output curves is now accompanied by an increase in the cardiac output (*Point B*), and at equilibrium the left ventricle (*Point B₁*) is now operating at a lower filling pressure with an improved cardiac output. Modified from Pouleur et al.[28]

output, despite reduction of the afterload on the left ventricle (Fig. 13.6).[28]

In the presence of acute experimental LV failure (produced by multiple coronary artery ligations) in which the LV end-diastolic pressure was elevated to more than 20 mm Hg, an opposite effect occurred marked by an increase in the cardiac output during nitroprusside infusion. Again, nitroprusside produced venodilation in the peripheral circulation; however, under conditions of failure there was a large shift of blood volume from the distended central circulation to the peripheral circulation during infusion of the vasodilator (7.4 ± 1.3 ml/kg), presumably because the failing left ventricle was now able to unload more effectively and thereby release blood stored behind it in the lungs. Under these circumstances, the venous return curve was *not* shifted downward by nitroprusside (Fig. 13.7), indicating that the blood volume shift from the central circulation counterbalanced the tendency for nitroprusside to reduce the effective systemic blood volume. Consequently, the marked shift upward of the cardiac output curve due to correction of the afterload mismatch on the failing ventricle could now be expressed as an increase in the cardiac output because the left ventricle, not the venous return, was the limiting factor (Fig. 13.7).[28] (In the Guyton framework, such shifts need not indicate a change in inotropic state.[27]

Thus, it is clear that the effects of vasodilator drugs on the peripheral circulation, as well as on the heart, are important in determining overall circulatory responses.

CORRECTION OF AFTERLOAD MISMATCH IN HEART FAILURE

As shown in Fig. 13.8, when venous return is able to increase, the response to correction of afterload mismatch can be diagrammed within the wall SV framework. In Beat 2 the ventricle is operating in a steady state of afterload mismatch, with a reduced SV; lowering the afterload on the left ventricle by administration of a vasodilator allows the end-diastolic pressure and volume to fall to some degree while at the same time the SV is considerably enhanced (Fig. 13.8, Beat 1). Even when the heart size changes little and the peak systolic pressure is maintained during vasodilator therapy, the cardiac output can still rise appreciably, since lowering of the impedance to ejection

HEART FAILURE

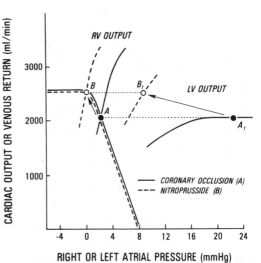

Figure 13.7. The relation between cardiac output and venous return in the normal heart (open chest, anesthetized dog) is shown. The inverse relation between right atrial pressure and venous return is shown under control conditions (*solid lines*) and during nitroprusside infusion (*dashed lines*). Segments of cardiac ouput curves relating right ventricular output (*RV output*) to right atrial pressure and *LV output* to left atrial pressure are also shown in these two circumstances. Under control conditions, the cardiac output is limited by the venous return, and the equilibrium point (*Point A*) where the venous return and cardiac output curves intersect is on the plateau of the venous return curve. In the steady-state, the RV and LV outputs are in equilibrium (*dashed horizontal line* and *Point A₁*). During nitroprusside infusion, venodilation produces a drop in mean systemic pressure and shift downward of the venous return curve, the right ventricle reaching a new equilibrium point at a lower cardiac ouput (*Point B*) which, in turn, is in equilibrium with a lower left ventricular output at a lower mean left atrial pressure (*Point B₁*). Thus, despite upward shifts of the RV and LV function curves due to lowered impedance to ejection, with reduced afterload, the cardiac output falls with nitroprusside. Modified from Pouleur et al.[28]

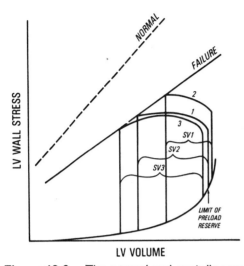

LV VOLUME

Figure 13.8. The normal end-systolic pressure-wall stress relation is shown by the *dashed lines*, and in severe heart failure this relation is shifted downward and to the right. In Beat 1, the left ventricle is shown operating on a steep portion of the passive pressure-volume curve and at the limit of its preload reserve (sarcomeres maximally elongated). With acute pressure loading (as with angiotensin infusion) there is a rise in end-diastolic pressure but little further change in end-diastolic volume, and since the ventricle behaves as if the preload were fixed, the SV (SV2) drops (Beat 2). Note also that in Beat 2 there is a further rise of end-systolic wall stress compared with wall stress at the onset of ejection. Beat 3 indicates the hypothetical response to vasodilator treatment of the failing ventricle and illustrates how there could be a substantial increase in the SV (SV3) compared with that of Beat 1 (SV1). The impedance reduction in Beat 3 is produced primarily by a fall of the instantaneous afterload early and late during ejection, with only a small reduction in end-diastolic volume. Under these circumstances there is only a minor change in peak LV wall stress in Beat 3 compared to Beat 1, and systolic pressure need not change appreciably. Reproduced by permission from J. Ross Jr.[4]

in the aorta early and late during systole by the vasodilator can lower the instantaneous wall stress and substantially augment the SV (Fig. 13.8, Beat 3).

From these considerations, it is evident that the use of a vasodilator alone may be ineffective in increasing the cardiac output, or may even cause a fall in the cardiac output, if the filling pressure in the central circulation is not sufficiently high. Of course, the use of concomitant volume expansion, as is often done in the postoperative setting with careful monitoring of the pulmonary artery wedge and right heart pressures, may allow proper compensation for venodilation. Also, drugs such as hydralazine that have little venodilator effect may be effective in patients with somewhat lower filling pressures, even without volume loading. The inotropic reserve of the failing ventricle also can be enhanced if necessary by adding drugs such as dopamine or dobutamine, as well as digitalis. In any case, for correction of afterload mismatch to be effective in the therapy of heart failure, regardless of the combination of drugs employed, it is critical that the important interactions between the peripheral circulation and the heart be considered.

CONCLUSION

An understanding of how loading conditions affect heart function, and how various forms of therapy affect both the heart and the peripheral circulation, have become basic to patient management. It would appear that by proper preoperative patient selection and by careful postoperative management, we should now have reached the point where lethal postoperative cardiac dysfunction is rare.

References

1. Ross J Jr: Afterload mismatch and preload reserve: A conceptual framework for the analysis of ventricular function. *Prog Cardiovasc Dis* 18:255, 1976.
2. MacGregor DC, Covell JW, Mahler F, et al: Relations between afterload, stroke volume, and descending limb of Starling's curve. *Am J Physiol* 227:884, 1974.
3. Ross J Jr, Covell JW, Sonnenblick EH, et al: Contractile state of the heart characterized by force-velocity relations in variably afterloaded and isovolumic beats. *Circ Res* 18:149, 1966.

4. Ross J Jr: Mechanisms of cardiac contraction: what roles for preload, afterload and inotropic state in heart failure? *Eur Heart J* 4(A):19, 1983.

5. Ross J Jr: Left ventricular function and the timing of surgical treatment in valvular heart disease. *Ann Intern Med* 94:498, 1981.

6. Ricci DR: Afterload mismatch and preload reserve in chronic aortic regurgitation. *Circulation* 66:826, 1982.

7. Ross J Jr: Role of vasodilator therapy. In Karliner J, Gregoratos G (eds) *Coronary Care*. Churchill Livingstone Publishers, New York, 1980.

8. Pouleur H, Covell JW, Ross J Jr: Effects of alterations in aortic input impedance on the force-velocity-length relationship in the intact canine heart. *Circ Res* 45:126, 1979.

9. Sonnenblick EH, Ross J Jr, Covell JW, et al: Alterations in resting length-tension relations of cardiac muscle induced by changes in contractile force. *Circ Res* 19:980, 1966.

10. Yoran C, Covell JW, Ross J Jr: Structural basis for the ascending limb of left ventricular function. *Circ Res* 32:297, 1973.

11. Monroe RG, Gamble WJ, LaFarge CG, et al: Left ventricular performance at high end-diastolic pressures in isolated, perfused dog hearts. *Circ Res* 26:85, 1970.

12. Ross J Jr, Sonnenblick EH, Taylor RR, et al: Diastolic geometry and sarcomere lengths in the chronically dilated canine left ventricle. *Circ Res* 28:49, 1971.

13. Braunwald E, Ross J Jr, Sonnenblick EH: *Mechanisms of Contraction of the Normal and Failing Heart*. Little, Brown & Co., Boston, 1968.

14. Taylor RR, Covell JW, Ross J Jr: Volume-tension diagrams of ejecting and isovolumic contractions in the left ventricle. *Am J Physiol* 216:1097, 1969.

15. Burns JW, Covell JW, Ross J Jr: Mechanics of isotonic left ventricular contractions. *Am J Physiol* 224:725, 1973.

16. Suga H, Sagawa K, Shjoukas AA: Load independence of the instantaneous pressure-volume ratio of the canine left ventricle and effects of epinephrine and heart rate on the ratio. *Circ Res* 32:314, 1973.

17. Sagawa K: The ventricular pressure-volume diagram revisited. *Circ Res* 43:677, 1978.

18. Ross J Jr: Assessment of cardiac function and myocardial contractility. In Hurst JW (ed): *The Heart*, 5th Ed. McGraw Hill Book Co., New York, 1982.

19. Schuler G, Peterson KL, Johnson A, et al: Temporal response of left ventricular performance to mitral valve surgery. *Circulation* 59:1218, 1979.

20. Grossman W, Jones D, McLaurin LP: Wall stress and patterns of hypertrophy in the human left ventricle. *J Clin Invest* 56:56, 1975.

21. Carabello BA, Nolan ST, McGuire LB: Assessment of preoperative left ventricular function in patients with mitral regurgitation: Value of the end-systolic wall stress-end-systolic volume ratio. *Circulation* 64:1212, 1981.

22. Smith N, McAnulty JH, Rahimtoola SH: Severe aortic stenosis with impaired left ventricular function and clinical heart failure: Results of valve replacement. *Circulation* 58:255, 1978.

23. Ross J Jr, Stein JB: Diagnosis and treatment of valvular aortic stenosis. *Cardiol Consult* 3:9, 1982.

24. Sasayama S, Ross J Jr, Franklin D, et al: Adaptations of the left ventricle to chronic pressure overload. *Circ Res* 38:172, 1976.

25. Ross J Jr, Braunwald E: The study of left ventricular function in man by increasing resistance to ventricular ejection with angiotensin. *Circulation* 29:739, 1964.

26. Chatterjee K, Parmley WW: The role of vasodilator therapy in heart failure. *Prog Cardiovasc Dis* 19:301, 1977.

27. Guyton AS, Jones CE, Coleman TG: *Circulatory Physiology: Cardiac Output and its Regulation*, 2nd Ed. W. B. Saunders Co., Philadelphia, 1973.

28. Pouleur H, Covell JW, Ross J Jr: Effects of nitroprusside on venous return and central blood volume in the absence and presence of acute heart failure. *Circulation* 61:328, 1980.

29. Ross J Jr: Pathophysiology of the human heart. In Krayenbuehl RC, Kubler BJ (eds): *Kardiologie in Klinik und Praxis*. George Thieme Verlag, Stuttgart, 1981.

CHAPTER 14

CORONARY BYPASS SOON AFTER ACUTE MYOCARDIAL INFARCTION

ELIS L. JONES, M.D.
RICHARD MICHALIK, M.D.

Between January, 1976 and April, 1982, 131 patients had urgent myocardial revascularization for clinical instability after acute myocardial infarction (AMI). Group 1 (21 patients) had coronary bypass grafting within 24 hours of AMI; Group 2 (29 patients) had coronary bypass grafting within 2 to 7 days after MI; and Group 3 (81 patients) had coronary bypass grafting 8 to 30 days after infarction. Indications for operation were persistent or recurrent pain (81%), pain plus ventricular arrhythmias (12%), and pain plus compelling anatomy (7%).

The incidence of single-vessel, triple-vessel, and left main coronary artery disease was 26%, 31%, and 8%, respectively. There were no hospital deaths in this series. The incidence of inotropic requirements, postoperative intra-aortic balloon pumping (IABP), ventricular arrythmias, and perioperative infarction was higher in patients operated in within 7 days of AMI than for patients having coronary bypass grafting after this time. This was especially true for patients who were operated upon within the first 24 hours. There have been six late deaths during a mean follow-up of 19 months. Actuarial survival was 97% at 30 months. Sixty-eight percent of patients are presently pain free. Graft patency was 84% in 17 patients catheterized after coronary

bypass grafting and in 14 patients, grafts placed into the area of infarction were patent. This study suggests that the frequency of perioperative complications will be increased in patients operated on within 1 week of AMI, but after this period coronary bypass grafting can be accomplished with the same morbidity as that of elective operations.

The unstable clinical course of some patients following AMI has been documented in recent reports.[1–8] At the Massachusetts General Hospital, early mortality of patients with transmural MI was 29% and of those with subendocardial infarction, 14%.[7] Although immediate prognosis after subendocardial infarction appears fairly good, Madigan and co-workers[9] found the incidence of unstable angina or later transmural infarction to be 46% and 21%, respectively. If left ventricular (LV) power failure and cardiogenic shock occur as a complication of acute infarction, mortality has been exceptionally high with medical therapy, approaching 80 to 90% in most series.[10–14]

Recently there has been renewed interest in applying the coronary bypass operation to selected patients early after AMI in order to prevent extension of infarction and preserve myocardial muscle mass and LV function.[7, 8, 15–18] The following report deals with 131 consecutive patients undergoing urgent myocardial revascularization for persistent pain within 30 days of AMI. The clinical profile of the patient population, criteria for operation, and methods of reducing early surgical mortality form the basis of this report.

CLINICAL PROFILE

Between January, 1976 and April, 1982, 131 patients had urgent myocardial revascularization for clinical instability within 30 days of AMI. Seventy-seven percent of this series (101 of 131) were male and the mean age of the patient population was 55.5 years. Infarction was defined as prolonged ischemic pain accompanied by EKG evidence of new 0.04-second Q waves (70% of patients) or acute S-T depression or T-wave inversion or both of these (30% of patients) associated with elevation of creatinine phosphokinase (CK) to twice normal levels for our laboratory (290 μmole/ml). Although in the early years of the study CK MB analysis was not performed in all patients, for the past 2 years all patients entered into the series had a positive CK MB fraction. No patient in this study underwent emergency operation secondary to a complication of cardiac catheterization.

Patients were arbitrarily divided into three groups defined by the interval between infarction and revascularization. Group 1 (21 patients) underwent operation within 24 hours of AMI; Group 2 (29 patients) had revascularization 2 to 7 days (mean 4.5 days) following infarction; and Group 3 (81 patients) had revascularization 8 to 30 days (mean 18 days) after infarction. Clinical instability was defined as persistent pain despite maximal therapy with vasodilator drugs, narcotics (Group 1) and propranolol; recurrent or persistent pain following infarction (Groups 2 and 3); or persistent or recurrent pain associated with ventricular arrhythmias (premature ventricular contractions, ventricular tachycardia, or ventricular fibrillation).

CRITERIA FOR OPERATION

Indications for operation were medically uncontrollable pain or recurrent pain following infarction in 81% of the 131 patients.

The indication for operation in 12% was pain with ventricular arrhythmias, and in 7% the indication for operation was the young age of the patient or compelling anatomy, such as high grade left main obstruction. There was no important difference in the indications for operation among the three groups.

There was a higher incidence of transmural than subendocardial infarction in the entire series. Seventy percent had transmural infarction and 30% subendocardial infarction. If a transmural infarction occurred it was more likely to be inferior or posterior (41%) than anterior (29%), except in Group 1 patients who had a very high incidence (71%) of anterior wall transmural infarction. This finding was statistically significant ($p < .01$).

CARDIAC CATHETERIZATION

Left Ventricular Function

Mean ejection fraction (EF) for the entire series was 0.55 with no significant difference among the three groups. Mean EF was equal to or less than 0.40 in 17% (19 of 111) of patients and equal to or less than 0.35 in 11% of patients. No patient operated on within 24 hours of infarction had EF equal to or less than 0.35 (Table 14.1). LV wall motion was normal in 38% of patients (44 of 117) and hypokinetic or akinetic in 18% and 41% of patients, respectively. Resting LV end-diastolic pressure was normal in 73% (23 of 79) and abnormal in 27% of

Table 14.1
Preoperative LV Function in Patients with Recent Acute MI

Patient Group	Ejection Fraction*		
	Mean	≤0.40 (%)	≤0.35 (%)
Series (N = 111)	.55	17	11
Group 1 (N = 17)	.58	6	0
Group 2 (N = 22)	.54	18	9
Group 3 (N = 22)	.54	19	14

* p = not significant between groups.

patients. It was equal to or greater than 20 mm Hg in 9% (10 of 108) of patients.

Coronary Artery Disease

At least 75% of the lumenal area of the left main coronary artery was obstructed in 8% of the patients in this series (Table 14.2). A higher percentage of patients in Group 1 and Group 2 had left main coronary disease than patients in Group 3 (12% and 13% versus 5%, respectively), but this difference was not statistically significant. The incidence of triple-vessel disease was 31% (37 of 118). The incidence of single-vessel disease was 26% for the series (31 of 118). There was at least one totally occluded artery in 55% of the entire series (65 of 118). The left anterior descending coronary artery was greatly obstructed in 89% of patients (105 of 118). This artery was the only artery involved with a hemodynamically significant lesion in 14% of the series (17 of 118).

OPERATION

Precise monitoring of rate pressure product, inferior and lead V_5 precordial EKG changes, pulmonary capillary wedge pressure, and cardiac output was performed in most patients before bypass. Swan-Ganz catheters were not routinely employed in those patients who had ventricular arrhythmias in the preoperative period. Anesthesia was maintained primarily by frequent doses of morphine sulphate, with diazepam, and nitrous oxide, as indicated to control blood pressure or heart rate. For most patients

(except those with evidence of reduced cardiac output) propranolol therapy was continued until 12 hours prior to anesthetic induction. However, if either tachycardia or hypertension occurred before bypass, it was managed promptly with small doses of intravenously administered propranolol or trinitroglycerin drip, respectively.

Adverse changes in the variables monitored were treated quickly to avoid acute deterioration in ventricular function prior to cardiopulmonary bypass. Otherwise, the operative technique in these patients was no different from that used in others having coronary artery bypass.[19] Moderate systemic hypothermia was employed and LV depressive factors such as ventricular distention and fibrillation were minimized. However, LV venting was not used in the latter part of the series. No patient in this series had endardarectomy, infarctectomy, or aneurysmectomy combined with coronary bypass grafting. Myocardial preservation was accomplished with either a cold (4°C) hyperkalemic or hyperkalemic hyperosmolar solution injected into the aorta at the time of aortic crossclamping. A single aortic crossclamp was used for all distal anastomoses, regardless of the degree of ventricular dysfunction or the number of bypass grafts to be performed. Single coronary bypass grafting was performed in 14% of patients (19 of 131), and three or more coronary bypasses were performed in 58% of patients (76 of 131). The incidence of multiple grafting was approximately the same for all groups. The average number of grafts for patients in the entire series was 2.7.

HOSPITAL MORTALITY AND MORBIDITY

There were no hospital deaths in this series of patients. Inotropic drugs were required postoperatively in 6% of patients. Although requirement for inotropic drugs was only 5% for patients operated on within 24 hours of infarction it must be noted that IABP was required in 10% of cases. Inotropic requirements for patients operated 2 to 7 days after infarction were quite high (14%) and this was significantly higher than

Table 14.2
Distribution of Coronary Artery Disease in Patients with Coronary Bypass and Recent Infarction

Patient Group	Single-Vessel Disease* (%)	Triple-Vessel Disease* (%)	Left Main Coronary Artery Disease* (%)
Series	26 (31/118)	31 (37/118)	8 (0/118)
Group 1	29 (5/17)	29 (5/17)	12 (2/17)
Group 2	17 (4/23)	39 (9/23)	13 (3/23)
Group 3	28 (22/78)	30 (23/78)	5 (4/78)

* No statistically significant difference between groups.

for patients operated on after the first week of infarction. This contrasted markedly to the 5% incidence of inotropic usage in 3466 consecutive isolated coronary bypass patients serving as a control (Fig. 14.1). Inotropic requirement for patients having elective bypass was approximately the same as for patients having revascularization more than 1 week after infarction.

Postoperative pharmacological treatment of ventricular arrhythmias consisting of multifocal premature ventricular contractions, ventricular tachycardia, or fibrillation was required in 2% of the patients (3 of 131). The incidence of arrhythmias requiring treatment was 10% in patients operated on within 24 hours of infarction, and was significantly greater than the 1% incidence of ventricular arrhythmias in the control population (Fig. 14.1). IABP to wean the patient from cardiopulmonary bypass was used in 8% of patients in this series. Postoperative use of IABP for elective bypass over a comparable period of time was less than 1%. Postoperative use of IABP was much more frequent for patients in Group 1 and Group 2 than in Group 3 (Fig. 14.1). Perioperative infarction (new Q wave) oc-

curred in 5% of the 93 patients in whom it could be evaluated by serial EKG. This compared to 3% of control patients having elective operation during this same period. The incidence of perioperative infarction was significantly higher for patients operated on within 24 hours of infarction (Fig. 14.1).

Figures 14.2 and 14.3 depict perioperative complications in five different clinical conditions. In 78 patients with unstable angina pectoris (rest pain > 20 minutes plus transient ST-T wave changes) inotropes were required in 12% versus 5% of control patients. The incidence of new Q wave in the unstable angina group was 4% versus 3% for the elective bypass group. The incidence of ventricular arrhythmias was 1.3% versus 1% for this control group. Hospital mortality for the 78 patients with unstable angina was 1.2% versus 0.8% for the 3466 control elective bypass patients.

The incidence of perioperative complications in patients having revascularization within 24 hours of infarction was quite different from either the control or the unstable angina patients. In patients with revascularization within 24 hours of infarction, inotropic usage was only 5% and not dissimilar

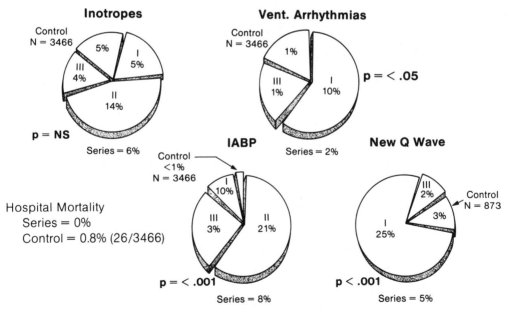

Figure 14.1. Perioperative complications may follow coronary bypass within 30 days of infarction.

Perioperative Complications During Acute Cardiac Ischemia

A Comparative Analysis of 5 Clinical States

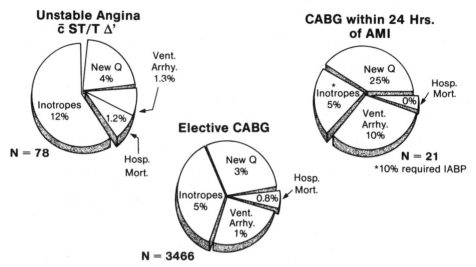

Figure 14.2. Comparison of perioperative complications for patients with unstable angina, coronary bypass within 24 hours of infarction and elective surgery is shown. CABG = coronary bypass grafting.

Perioperative Complications During Acute Cardiac Ischemia

A Comparative Analysis of 5 Clinical States

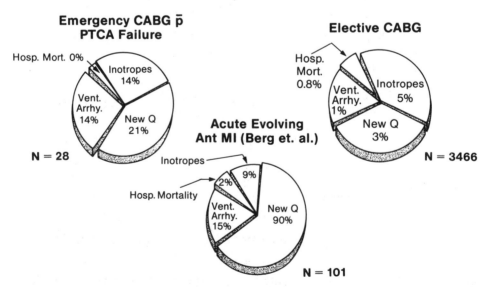

Figure 14.3. Comparison of perioperative complications in patients with coronary bypass for angioplasty failure, acute evolving anterior infarction, and for elective surgery is shown.

from the control group. However, it must be noted that 10% of patients in this group required IABP and thus demonstrated significant LV dysfunction. The incidence of ventricular arrhythmias requiring pharmacological treatment was 10% in Group 1 patients and was significantly greater than the incidence in both the controls and patients with unstable angina (Fig. 14.2). Likewise, the incidence of perioperative infarction was 25% in patients having revascularization shortly after infarction (24 hours) compared to 4% in the unstable angina patients and 3% in elective bypass patients.

Figure 14.3 depicts perioperative complications in two additional acute clinical states, namely, emergency bypass after failure of percutaneous coronary angioplasty and emergency revascularization for acute evolving anterior myocardial infarction.[6] Complications occurring after emergency bypass for percutaneous transluminal coronary angioplasty failure and acute evolving anterior MI were as follows: new Q wave, 21% and 90%, ventricular arrhythmias 14% and 15% and inotropic requirement 14% and 9%, respectively. The frequency of perioperative complications for these two clinical entities were quite dissimilar to those of patients having elective bypass (Fig. 14.3).

In order to elucidate some of the factors responsible for preservation of myocardial function and influencing occurrence of perioperative complications, a more extensive examination of the 28 patients having coronary artery bypass early after angioplasty failure (within 24 hours) was performed. The mean interval from angioplasty failure to complete revascularization in these patients was 5 hours. In 11 patients revascularization was completed within 2 hours of angioplasty failure. The angioplasty-revascularization interval was 124 minutes in six patients who developed new postoperative Q waves but was 190 minutes in 21 patients in whom no new Q wave appeared after coronary bypass grafting for percutaneous transluminal coronary angioplasty failure. In four of these 21 patients this interval could not be determined.

LATE FOLLOW-UP

There have been six late deaths during a short follow-up (mean = 19 months). There was no significant difference in the death rate among patients in the three groups. Of the five patients who died, only one had an EF less than 0.40. Sixty-eight percent of patients (77 of 113) are presently pain free, and 30% although improved do complain of some residual chest discomfort, thought to represent angina pectoris. Only 2% of patients are worse or unchanged following revascularization (Table 14.3).

Repeat cardiac catheterization was performed 1 to 19 months following operation in 17 patients. Graft patency was 84% (36 of 43) for the series and in 76% of patients (13 of 17) all grafts were patent. In 14 of the 17 patients, grafts placed into the area of MI were patent at the time of restudy. Mean EF following revascularization increased slightly in those restudied. Normal wall motion by angiography was present in 47% of patients (8 of 17) after operation, compared with 23% of patients (8 of 35) at the time of original catheterization. Most patients demonstrated either an improvement in ejection fraction when this value had been depressed preoperatively or very little deterioration when EF had been high preoperatively. Only one patient exhibited severe deterioration in ejection fraction and this patient had an MI after catheterization and just prior to operation. Improvement in segmental wall motion following revascularization occurred in seven patients; there was no change in six patients and deterioration in movement occurred in two patients. Actuarial survival was 97% at 30 months (Fig. 14.4).

PRINCIPLES OF MANAGEMENT

The annual incidence of AMI in the United States is approximately 1.5 million

Table 14.3
Functional Status of Patients Having CABG Soon after Infarction (mean interval = 19 months)

Patient Group	Late Cardiac Deaths (%)	Anginal Status (%)		
		No Pain	Rest Pain	Improved
Series	4.6	68	17	98
Group 1	5	82	12	100
Group 2	7	78	4	100
Group 3	4	62	22	97

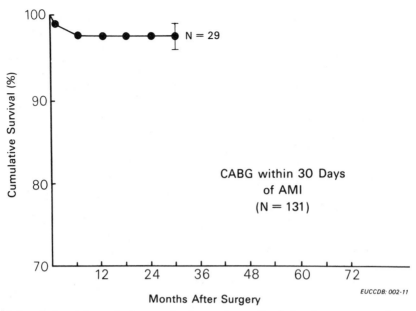

Figure 14.4. Actuarial survival curve is shown for patients having coronary bypass within 30 days of MI.

individuals per year. The morbidity and loss of life following these infarctions represents a staggering national health problem. Studies published by the *American Journal of Public Health* in 1968 revealed that 23% of patients die before reaching a hospital, another 15% die after reaching the hospital and there is an additional 5% mortality the first 6 months following discharge. Total 6-month mortality is approximately 43%.[20]

The unstable clinical course of some patients following AMI has been well documented.[1,2,7] Overall hospital mortality has been reported as 10% to 15% during the first year and 20% to 30% by the third year after infarction. Over one-half of these deaths are sudden.[8] Stenson and associates[21] identified a group of patients with persistent or recurrent pain and S-T segment elevation after infarction in whom mortality was very high on medical therapy and observation alone. Infarct extension soon after the initial infarction accounts for a large number of these deaths. The true incidence of this phenomenon is unknown but has been reported to be between 33% and 86%.[4,5] In 1979, Fraker and co-workers[3] retrospectively analyzed 458 patients admitted to their coronary care unit and found the incidence of infarct extension to be less than reported previously, but still around 13%. Extension of the infarction occurred an average of 3.4 days after admission to the hospital. Hospital mortality in these patients was 36% versus 9% for patients without infarct extension. One-year survival for patients with extension was 76% and 91% for matched patients without extension.

Persistent or recurrent pain following acute infarction in our patients was interpreted as incomplete infarction distal to an obstructed artery (borderzone ischemia) or loss of collateral blood supply to a myocardial region away from the original infarction but supplied by another greatly obstructed artery. Schuster and Bulkley[6] corroborated this clinical supposition by describing two morphological classifications of infarction thought to be important in the production of postinfarction angina. They identified 20 patients in whom angina occurred in association with transient ischemic EKG changes after infarction. In 12 of these patients, the angina was associated with EKG changes in the EKG area of the original infarct. In the remaining patients, there was EKG evidence of ischemia developing at a site distant from the area of initial infarction which they interpreted as infarction-induced interruption of collaterals to a distant site supplied by a second chronically narrowed coronary vessel. In the majority of these patients, rest pain developed within the first 36 hours after infarction. Death was due not to cardiogenic shock but ventricular arrhythmias. This led the authors to conclude that patients in whom ischemia distant from the site of infarction develops following AMI may be especially suited for therapeutic interventions directed at limiting ischemia, ischemia-related arrhythmias, and necrosis. In contrast, patients with ischemia in the infarct zone at postmortem examination appeared more likely to have AMI with a large mass of irreversible necrotic myocardium, a setting in which any intervention would be of limited value.

In recent years there has been much interest in the surgical treatment of patients during or shortly after AMI.[6,7,9,15,17,18,22–25] Since the early reports of Keon,[26] Hill,[27] Dawson,[28] Johnson,[29] Loop,[30] and their associates, interest in the clinical management of these patients has continued.[7,8,17,18] Careful selection is important in assuring a successful outcome in patients undergoing coronary bypass shortly after AMI. Continued or recurrent pain after infarction implies the event is not yet complete and suggests improved patient salvage may be attained by surgical intervention. Our data indicate this is particularly true if residual LV function is adequate, suitable distal vessels are visualized on arteriograms, and medical therapy after catheterization is not pursued to such a point that infarction occurs again and irreparable LV damage is done.

The low morbidity and mortality seen in our patients are probably a reflection of the aggressiveness of our medical and surgical staff in treating patients with persistent or recurrent pain after infarction in addition to selection of good candidates for surgical therapy. Our incidence of single-vessel disease was higher than that reported by Levine, Brundage, and their co-workers[7,18] in which hospital mortality after revascularization was 8.8% and 9%, respectively. In

the study of Levine and colleagues,[7] preoperative IABP was used in 72% of patients. Brundage and associates[18] reported a series of 22 patients having revascularization an average of 15.8 days after AMI in which triple-vessel disease was present in 82%, the mean age of the patient population was 61.4 years, and there was a high incidence of left main coronary artery stenosis. Whereas IABP was used by Levine and colleagues[7] for relief of angina and hemodynamic instability and for hemodynamic instability in the report of Brundage and associates,[18] our use of this device before operation has been very limited, confined primarily to a few patients with intractable pain until the patient could undergo myocardial revascularization. IABP has been used in some patients prior to cardiopulmonary bypass to reduce or terminate refractory ventricular arrhythmias, minimize ischemic trauma associated with anesthetic induction, and reduce LV work associated with return of cardiac function at the conclusion of the operative procedure. Although intra-aortic balloon support may be advantageous in stabilizing the patient's condition before cardiac catheterization, it was not used in any of our patients. We agree with others[25,31,32] that cardiac catheterization can be performed safely in patients soon after MI.

The three groups of patients in this study were arbitrarily defined according to the infarction-revascularization interval to discern if hospital morbidity or mortality could be correlated with the temporal relationship between infarction and operation. In our initial series of 35 patients reported in 1978,[15] it appeared that difficulty in the perioperative period was unrelated to this interval. As the series was extended, however, it was found that the incidence of postoperative inotropic requirements, IABP, ventricular arrhythmias, and perioperative infarction was found to be more frequent in those patients having myocardial revascularization in the first week and especially in the first 24 hours after infarction. Although difficulty in the postoperative period appears to be increased in patients operated on within a week of infarction, hospital mortality and long-term survival do not appear to be affected adversely. Use of inotropic drugs or IABP in the postoperative period could not be predicted prior to operation by preoperative descriptors such as extent of vessel disease, EF, or angiographically documented wall-motion abnormalities.

Although the follow-up period is short and many of the patients had operation recently, we believe our major objectives of therapy have been realized: There have been no hospital deaths and only five late deaths with an 18-month actuarial survival of 97%. Although all but one patient dying late had preoperative angiographic LV wall-motion abnormality, preoperative descriptors such as multivessel disease and depressed EF were not predictive of poor late survival. Only a small percentage of patients had an unfavorable result, and the patency rate for most patients was gratifying. Our findings of a high patency rate in grafts performed to the area of infarction agree with the clinical studies of others.[16,17,32] LV function was preserved and frequently improved as demonstrated by postoperative changes in the EF and LV segmental wall motion.[15] However, this study is not proof that myocardial revascularization following infarction improves LV function and regional wall motion. It is well known that during an acute ischemic event, with or without infarction, myocardial wall motion and EF can be markedly depressed but can be improved considerably once the initial insult has passed. This finding is true regardless of whether patients are treated medically or surgically. The effect on LV function for early revascularization soon after MI is a major concern and must be resolved before any large scale implementation of coronary artery bypass graft for acute evolving infarction.

Although conclusive data regarding the best mode of therapy in this particular patient population would best be obtained by a medical and surgical randomized study, we attempted to show that adequate revascularization can be accomplished safely and effectively in a group of patients previously deemed at very high operative risk. Improvement in anginal status in this series was practically identical to that of patients having elective operation. It might be argued that more persistent medical therapy would be effective in temporarily controlling ventricular arrhythmias, pain, or even reduced cardiac output. However, we believe that revascularization of the ischemic and injured myocardium can be accomplished effectively with low operative risk and offers the best chance of minimizing LV muscle damage and patient mortality. This study suggests that the frequency of perioperative complications will be increased in patients operated on within a week of infarction but after this period, revascularization can be accomplished with the same morbidity as that of elective operation. Patients with infarction should not be treated medically for an arbitrary period of time before operation is considered because this will only enhance the chances of irreparable ventricular damage from infarct extension. Each patient must be evaluated individually with all clinical factors known to the responsible physicians. If these recommendations are followed, we believe that myocardial revascularization can be accomplished with very low mortality, morbidity, and satisfactory long-term survival.

References

1. Madigan NP, Rutherford BD, Frye RL: The clinical course, early prognosis and coronary anatomy of subendocardial infarction. *Am J Med* 60:634, 1976.
2. Levy WK, Cannorn DS, Cohen LS: Prognosis of subendocardial myocardial infarction. *Circulation* 51, 52:Suppl 2:107, 1975.
3. Fraker RD Jr, Wagner GS, Rosati RA: Extension of myocardial infarction: Incidence and prognosis. *Circulation* 60:1126, 1979.
4. Reid RR, Taylor DR, Kelly DT, et al: Myocardial infarct extension detection by precordial ST-T segment mapping. *N Engl J Med* 290:123, 1974.
5. Kronenbery MK, Hodges M, Akiyama T, et al: S-T segment variations after acute myocardial infarction: Relationship to clinical status. *Circulation* 54:756, 1976.
6. Schuster EH, Bulkley BH: Ischemia at a distance after acute myocardial infarction: A cause of early postinfarction angina. *Circulation* 62:509, 1980.
7. Levine FH, Gold HK, Leinbach RC, et al: Safe early revascularization for continuing ischemia after acute myocardial infarction. *Circulation* 60:I-5, 1979.
8. Rogers WJ, Smith LR, Oberman A, et al: Surgical

vs. nonsurgical management of patients after myocardial infarction. *Circulation* 62:I-67, 1980.

9. Madigan NP, Rutherford BD, Barnhorst DA, et al: Early saphenous vein grafting after subendocardial infarction: Immediate surgical results and late prognosis. *Circulation* 56:Suppl 2:1, 1977.

10. Cronin RFP, Moore S, Marpole DG: Shock following myocardial infarction: A clinical survey of 140 cases. *Can Med Assoc J* 93:57, 1965.

11. Killip J, Kimball JJ: Treatment of myocardial infarction in a coronary care unit: A two-year experience with 250 patients. *Am J Cardiol* 290:457, 1967.

12. Nielsen BL, Marner IL: Shock in acute myocardial infarction. *Acta Med Scand* 175:65, 1964.

13. Scheidt S, Ascheim R, Killip T: Cardiogenic shock after acute myocardial infarction. *Am J Cardiol* 26:556, 1970.

14. Lown B, Vassaux G, Hoop SB, et al: Unresolved problems in coronary care. *Am J Cardiol* 20:494, 1967.

15. Jones EL, Douglas JS Jr, Craver JM, et al: Results of coronary revascularization in patients with recent myocardial infarction. *J Thorac Cardiovasc Surg* 76:545, 1978.

16. Berg R Jr, Kendall RW, Duvoisin GE, et al: Acute myocardial infarction: A surgical emergency. *J Thorac Cardiovasc Surg* 70:432, 1975.

17. Phillips SJ, Kongtahworn C, Zeff RH, et al: Emergency coronary artery revascularization: A possible therapy for acute myocardial infarction. *Circulation* 60:241, 1979.

18. Brundage BH, Ullyot DJ, Winokur S, et al: The role of aortic balloon pumping in postinfarction angina: A different perspective. *Circulation* 62:I-119, 1980.

19. Jones EL: Coronary artery bypass grafting: Simplification and refinement of surgical technique. *Ann Thorac Surg* 30:84, 1980.

20. Weinblatt E, Shapiro S, Frank CW, et al: Prognosis of men after first myocardial infarction: Mortality and first recurrence in relation to selected parameters. *Am J Public Health* 58:1329, 1968.

21. Stenson RE, Flamm MD Jr, Zaret BL, et al: Transient ST-segment elevation with post-myocardial infarction angina: Prognostic significance. *Am Heart J* 89:449, 1975.

22. Bardet J, Rigaud M, Kahn JC, et al: Treatment of post-myocardial infarction angina by intra-aortic balloon pumping and emergency revascularization. *J Thorac Cardiovasc Surg* 74:299, 1977.

23. Kongtahworn C, Zeff RH, Iannone L, et al: Emergency myocardial revascularization during acute evolving myocardial infarction. *Chest* 72:403, 1977.

24. Mundth ED, Buckley MJ, Leinbach RC, et al: Myocardial revascularization for the treatment of cardiogenic shock complicating acute myocardial infarction. *Surgery* 70:78, 1971.

25. Cheanvechai C, Effler DB, Loop FD, et al: Emergency myocardial revascularization. *Am J Cardiol* 32:901, 1973.

26. Keon WJ, Bedford P, Shankar KR, et al: Experience with emergency aortocoronary bypass grafts in the presence of acute myocardial infarction. *Circulation* 47, 48:Suppl 3:151, 1973.

27. Hill JD, Kerth WJ, Kelly JJ, et al: Emergency aortocoronary bypass for impending or extending myocardial infarction. *Circulation* 43, 44:Suppl 1:105, 1971.

28. Dawson JT, Hall RJ, Hallman GL, et al: Mortality in patients undergoing coronary artery bypass surgery after myocardial infarction. *Am J Cardiol* 33:483, 1974.

29. Johnson WD, Flemma RJ, Lepley D Jr: Direct coronary surgery utilizing multiple-vein bypass grafts. *Ann Thorac Surg* 9:436, 1970.

30. Loop FD, Cheanvechae C, Sheldon WC, et al: Early myocardial revascularization during acute myocardial infarction. *Chest* 66:478, 1974.

31. Cohn LH, Gorlin R, Herman MV, et al: Aortocoronary bypass for acute coronary occlusion. *J Thorac Cardiovasc Surg* 64:503, 1972.

32. Begg RF, Kooros MA, Magovern GJ, et al: The hemodynamics and coronary arteriography patterns during acute myocardial infarction. *J Thorac Cardiovasc Surg* 58:647, 1969.

CHAPTER 15

PERIOPERATIVE ARRHYTHMIAS—USE OF EPICARDIAL WIRE ELECTRODES FOR DIAGNOSIS AND TREATMENT

ALBERT L. WALDO, M.D.

Cardiac rhythm and conduction disturbances are quite common following open heart surgery. In most instances, they are transient and amenable to standard modes of therapy. However, uniquely for the post-open heart surgical patient, temporary wire electrodes can be placed on the epicardium of both the atria and the ventricles at the time of operation. These wire electrodes can then be brought out through the anterior chest wall for diagnostic and therapeutic use in the postoperative period.[1-21] At our medical center (the University of Alabama in Birmingham), one pair of atrial stainless steel wire electrodes and at least one and often a pair of ventricular stainless steel wire electrodes are routinely placed at the time of open heart surgery. These electrodes have proven invaluable in the management of arrhythmias following open heart surgery. They can be used with great effectiveness both diagnostically and therapeutically using techniques which are safe, easy to implement, reliable, and rapid.[1-21]

Temporary atrial wire electrodes can be used diagnostically in two ways. First, they can be used to record atrial electrograms, that is, electrical activity recorded directly from the atria. The ability to record atrial electrograms provides a clear record of atrial activity and is particularly valuable in the diagnosis of arrhythmias in which the nature of atrial activation and/or the relationship of atrial activation to ventricular activation is unclear from the standard EKG.[1, 2, 8, 9, 15-17, 20] Second, they can be used to pace the heart to assist in the diagnosis of an arrhythmia.[9, 15-17, 19-21] For example, atrial pacing may be required to diagnose a narrow QRS complex tachycardia with a regular R-R interval and a 1:1 atrioventricular (AV) relationship at a rate of 150 beat/minute, and it may also be used to assess AV conduction. In addition, these temporary epicardial atrial wire electrodes can be used in the effective pacing treatment of virtually all abnormalities of rhythm and conduction with the exception of artial fibrillation, Type II atrial flutter, sinus tachycardia, and ventricular fibrillation.[1, 2, 4, 7-21] Thus, atrial pacing may be used to suppress premature atrial or ventricular beats, terminate tachyarrhythmias, increase heart rate as treatment of bradyarrhythmias, or override or suppress undersirable rhythms with continuous rapid atrial pacing.

Temporary ventricular epicardial wire electrodes are of great value also. Although they are rarely of use diagnostically, they are of great use therapeutically, particularly in the treatment of various bradyarrhythmias associated with AV block, but also for the treatment of serious tachyarrhythmias such as AV junctional tachycardia or recurrent ventricular tachycardia.[12, 16–18, 20, 21]

By the very nature of a chapter such as this, it is not possible to detail all the uses of these epicardial wire electrodes. For this purpose, the reader is referred to several rather detailed articles and monographs on this subject.[1–21] However, this review will discuss and illustrate some of the more common applications of techniques which utilize the wire electrodes.

DIAGNOSIS AND TREATMENT OF POSTOPERATIVE BRADYCARDIAS

Sinus bradycardias (rates less than 60 beat/min) and relative sinus bradycardias (rates between 60 to 75 or 60 to 80 beat/min) are common postoperative arrhythmias.[16] They may be associated with a low cardiac output and rate-related supraventricular and ventricular arrhythmias. Ventricular extrasystoles that would not be present at a more rapid heart rate are the most obvious examples. By pacing the atria or ventricles at a more rapid rate than the spontaneous rate, it is possible to increase the cardiac output solely by this rate augmentation and at the same time to suppress the ventricular arrhythmias. If AV conduction is intact, this is best accomplished by overriding the spontaneous heart rate with atrial pacing at an appropriate rate, often as fast as 100 to 110 beat/minute.

If the bradycardia is the result of second- or third-degree AV block, ventricular pacing at an appropriate rate (virtually always in a demand mode) is indicated. If the cardiac output during ventricular pacing in the face of second- or third-degree AV block is less than satisfactory, it may be desirable to initiate AV sequential pacing in order to include the atrial contribution to cardiac output. This may be particularly important in treatment of complete heart block that re-

sults following surgical repair of congenital heart disease in infants.[17]

DIAGNOSIS AND TREATMENT OF SUPRAVENTRICULAR TACHYCARDIAS

Atrial Fibrillation

Although this arrhythmia usually is easily diagnosed from an EKG, the recording of an atrial electrogram for diagnostic purposes may be quite helpful and, in fact, is sometimes necessary. Bipolar atrial electrograms recorded from patients with atrial fibrillation and characterized by complexes having a myriad of sizes, shapes, polarities, and amplitudes, as well as a broad range of rates and beat-to-beat intervals.[15] In fact, based on recorded bipolar atrial electrograms, the hallmark of atrial fibrillation is the characteristic beat-to-beat variability of these parameters (Figs. 15.1 and 15.2).

As is clear from Figures 15.1 and 15.2, despite the fact that the atrial electrograms recorded during atrial fibrillation are characterized by variability in morphology, polarity, amplitude, and cycle length, not all atrial fibrillation is chaotic. Some forms of atrial fibrillation appear to be rather well ordered (Fig. 15.1*A* and *B*). Furthermore, although the atrial rates as measured from atrial electrograms recorded during atrial fibrillation range widely, surprisingly low rates, in fact, as low as 263 beat/minute, have been documented during atrial fibrillation.[15] Also, it is not unusual to find atrial rates during atrial fibrillation within the range associated with atrial flutter.[15, 19] Thus, should the rate of atrial fibrillation be relatively slow and the atrial electrogram be relatively organized, atrial fibrillation may mimic atrial flutter (Fig. 15.1*A*). In such instances, it is important to identify the rhythms properly, because classical atrial flutter can be treated effectively with rapid atrial pacing whereas atrial fibrillation cannot.[11, 13–17, 19–21] While it remains to be seen whether or not the identification of different types of atrial fibrillation on the basis of the recorded bipolar atrial electrogram has any mechanistic implications, this characteriza-

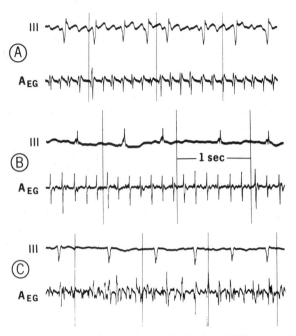

Figure 15.1. In each of the three panels in this figure, EKG lead III has been recorded stimultaneously with a bipolar atrial electrogram (A_{EG}). *Panel A* demonstrates the characteristic A_{EG} for Type I atrial fibrillation (characterized by A_{EG}s with discrete complexes of variable morphology, polarity, amplitude, and cycle length separated by an isoelectric baseline free of perturbation), *Panel B* for Type II atrial fibrillation (characterized by discrete beat-to-beat A_{EG} complexes of variable morphology, polarity, amplitude, and cycle length, but different from Type I atrial fibrillation in that the baseline is not isoelectric, having perturbations of varying degrees), and *Panel C* for Type III atrial fibrillation (characterized by A_{EG}s which are chaotic in apperance and which fail to demonstrate either discrete complexes or isoelectric intervals). Note that the EKG in *Panel A* mimics atrial flutter, but careful examination of the recorded bipolar A_{EG} clearly demonstrates that the rhythm is atrial fibrillation. Time lines are at 1-second intervals. Modified from Wells et al.[15]

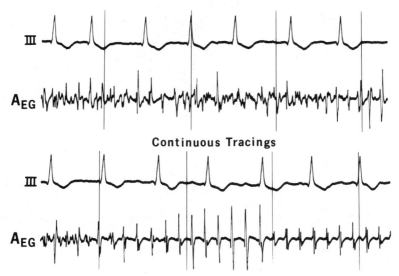

Figure 15.2. EKG lead III recorded simultaneously with a bipolar A_{EG} demonstrating the A_{EG} characteristic of Type IV atrial fibrillation (characterized by A_{EG}s consistent with Type III, alternating with periods of A_{EG}s consistent with Type I and/or Type II). Time lines are at 1-second intervals. Reproduced with permission from Wells et al.[15]

tion is clinically useful in distinguishing atrial fibrillation from atrial flutter.

Atrial Flutter

DIAGNOSIS

For rhythms with rapid ventricular rates, the differential diagnosis often includes atrial flutter. However, it may be difficult to identify atrial flutter waves in the EKG, especially if one of the flutter waves is masked with the QRS complex. In such cases, by recording a bipolar atrial electrogram, atrial activation is readily identified and the nature of the atrial rate and rhythm is usually easily established (Fig. 15.3).

Recent studies in patients following open heart surgery have identified two types of atrial flutter, labeled Type I (classical) and Type II.[19] Both types of atrial flutter resemble each other in that they are rapid, regular atrial rhythms. The bipolar atrial electrograms recorded during each type of atrial flutter characteristically are of uniform morphology, polarity, and amplitude; have a remarkably regular beat-to-beat interval; and have an isoelectric interval between the discrete electrogram complexes (Fig. 15.4).

Occassionally, the recorded bipolar atrial electrogram in each type of atrial flutter demonstrates a beat-to-beat electrical alternans, and sometimes the latter is also associated with an alternans in the beat-to-beat cycle length.[19]

The two types of atrial flutter differ from each other in that Type I atrial flutter can always be influenced by rapid atrial pacing from the high right atrium (i.e., from the usual atrial location of the temporary, epicardial atrial wire electrodes), whereas Type II atrial flutter cannot be so influenced.[14, 19] They also differ in their range of atrial rates, the range of Type I atrial flutter being about 230 to 340 beat/minute and the range of Type II atrial flutter being about 340 to 433 beat/minute, the upper and lower limits for each being somewhat variable.[19]

TREATMENT OF TYPE I (CLASSICAL) ATRIAL FLUTTER

Rapid atrial pacing from the temporary atrial epicardial wire electrodes placed high in the right atrium is the treatment of choice for patients who develop Type I atrial flutter following open heart surgery.[14, 17, 19–21] We currently recommend a ramp atrial pacing

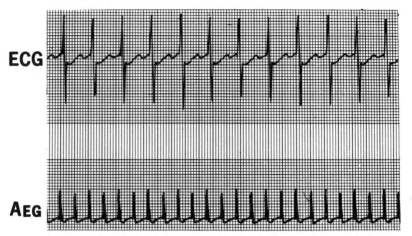

Figure 15.3. Monitor EKG lead recorded simultaneously with a bipolar A_{EG} during an episode of Type I atrial flutter. The atrial rate is 280 beat/minute and there is 2:1 AV conduction. Note that atrial complexes are not readily discerned from the EKG alone, but the bipolar A_{EG} clearly establishes the nature of atrial activation and its relationship to ventricular activation. Reproduced with permission from Waldo and MacLean.[17]

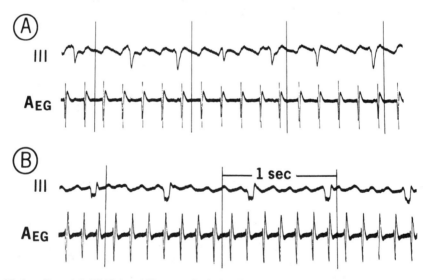

Figure 15.4. *Panel A.* EKG lead III recorded simultaneously with a bipolar A_{EG} from patient demonstrating the A_{EG} characteristic of Type I (classical) atrial flutter. *Panel B.* EKG lead III recorded simultaneously with a bipolar A_{EG} from another patient demonstrating the A_{EG} characteristic of Type II atrial flutter. Time lines are at 1-second intervals. Modified from Wells et al.[19]

technique, in which bipolar atrial pacing at a rate about 10 beats faster than the spontaneous atrial rate is begun and EKG lead II is recorded continuously. When it is demonstrated that the atrial rate has increased to the pacing rate, the atrial pacing rate is gradually increased until the atrial complexes (flutter waves) in lead II, which previously had been negative, become frankly positive. When this occurs, because it is almost always a marker of interruption of the atrial flutter, the atrial pacing may be abruptly terminated or the pacing rate may be quickly slowed. The latter permits control of the atrial rhythm until a desirable atrial rate such as 100 to 110 beat/minute is achieved. A representative example is illustrated in Figure 15.5.

In another pacing technique, the constant-rate technique, rapid atrial pacing is initiated at a rate faster than the spontaneous rate. Pacing at this rate is continued for 30 seconds and then is either abruptly terminated or rapidly slowed to a desirable atrial rate. Because we have found that the most successful rate for interruption of Type I atrial flutter is approximately 120 to 130% (range 111 to 135%) of the spontaneous

atrial rate, if using this second technique, one could start pacing at a rate within this range of the spontaneous atrial flutter rate (e.g., 125% of the spontaneous rate) and pace either for 30 seconds or until the atrial complexes in EKG lead II change from negative to positive. If pacing at the initial rate does not interrupt atrial flutter, the atrial pacing rate may be increased in increments of 5 to 10 beat/minute until successful interruption of the atrial flutter has been achieved.[14, 17, 19–21] A representative example is illustrated in Figures 15.6 to 15.8.

With either of the above two pacing techniques, the atria may be paced at rates faster than the spontaneous rate, but such pacing

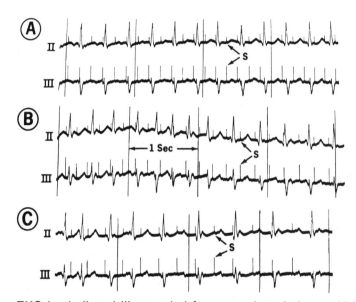

Figure 15.5. EKG leads II and III recorded from a patient during rapid high right atrial pacing to treat atrial flutter (intrinsic rate 200 beat/min). As the pacing rate was increased from 350 beat/minute to a high of 382 beat/minute, the atrial complexes became completely positive in both leads II and III. In fact, close observation of the records in *Panel A* reveals that this occurred at a pacing rate of about 370 beat/minute. When the pacing rate was slowed, atrial capture was maintained (*Panels B and C*). Note at the end of *Panel B* at a pacing rate of 270 beat/minute (i.e., a rate which is much slower than that of the spontaneous atrial flutter) the P waves remained positive, and as the pacing rate was decreased further, the atrial flutter did not recur (*Panel C*). In fact, atrial capture was maintained as the pacing rate was decreased to a rate of 110 beat/minute. Thus, in this patient, the atrial flutter was interrupted by the rapid atrial pacing when an appropriate pacing rate was achieved. The hallmark of the appropriate pacing rate was the appearance of positive atrial complexes in leads II and III. Time lines are at 1-second intervals. S = stimulus artifact. Modified from Waldo et al.[14]

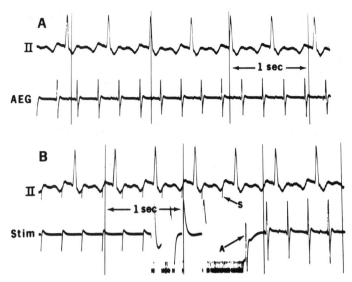

Figure 15.6. *Panel A.* EKG lead II recorded simultaneously with a bipolar A$_{EG}$ demonstrating Type I (classical) atrial flutter at a cycle length of 264 msec. *Panel B.* Recordings from the same patient at the termination of 30 seconds of rapid atrial pacing at a cycle length of 254 msec. Note that despite the fact that the atrial rate increased to the pacing rate during the rapid atrial pacing, the morphology of the atrial complexes during the rapid pacing was essentially unchanged when compared to that during the spontaneous rhythm. Time lines are at 1-second intervals. S = stimulus artifact; A = atrial electrogram. Modified from Waldo et al.[14]

may not interrupt the atrial flutter despite the fact that the atrial rate increased to the pacing rate (Figs. 15.6 and 15.7).[14,17] This phenomenon, called transient entrainment,[14,18,22] should not be considered evidence that rapid atrial pacing will be unsuccessful. Rather, it provides evidence that pacing at a more rapid rate is required to interrupt the atrial flutter.[14,17] Also, as illustrated in Figure 15.8, when using the constant-rate technique for interruption of the atrial flutter, a critical duration of pacing (average 11 sec) at the critical rate is required.[14]

Occasionally, atrial pacing rates of over 400 beat/minute may be required to interrupt Type I atrial flutter when using either the ramp or constant-rate pacing technique.[14,17] In a small percentage of patients, rapid atrial pacing produces atrial fibrillation. Atrial fibrillation precipitated by rapid atrial pacing is most often transient, lasting seconds to minutes before spontaneously converting to sinus rhythm. For those few patients in whom the atrial fibrillation persists, it is usually a more desirable rhythm than the continuation of Type I atrial flutter because atrial fibrillation is almost always associated with a slower ventricular response rate than that during atrial flutter.[13,14,16,17] Also, in almost all instances the ventricular response rate to atrial fibrillation can be quite easily controlled with digitalis or occasionally with verapamil or propranolol as well. For those patients in whom Type I atrial flutter recurs despite its interruption by rapid atrial pacing, continuous rapid atrial pacing to precipitate and sustain atrial fibrillation may be indicated.[13]

Paroxysmal Atrial Tachycardia

DIAGNOSIS

The diagnosis of paroxysmal atrial tachycardia usually should be suspected from examination of the standard EKG, particu-

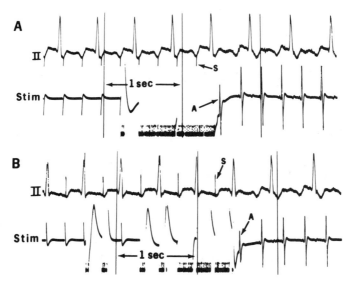

Figure 15.7. *Panels A and B* were recorded from the same patient as in Figure 15.6. *Panel A* was recorded at the termination of 30 seconds of atrial pacing and at a cycle length of 242 msec, and *Panel B* at the termination of 30 seconds of atrial pacing at a cycle length of 232 msec. Once again, note in each panel that the atrial rate increased to the atrial pacing rate during the rapid atrial pacing, yet following termination of the pacing the atrial flutter returned promptly. Furthermore, note that the morphology of the atrial complexes during the atrial pacing in *Panel A* was virtually identical to that of the spontaneous atrial flutter, and in *Panel B* it was only minimally changed from that of the spontaneous atrial flutter. Thus, during the rapid atrial pacing, the atrial rate increased to the pacing rate, but the atrial flutter was not interrupted. Time lines are at 1-second intervals. S = stimulus artifact; A = atrial electrogram. Modified from Waldo et al.[14]

larly when a 1:1 AV relationship is established during a regular rhythm with a narrow QRS complex at rates between 180 to 200 beat/minute. However, the range of rates of paroxysmal atrial tachycardia is quite broad (about 130 to 220 beat/min), and the differential diagnosis for regular rhythms with rates in this range includes several arrhythmias. In order to establish the diagnosis, the recording of a bipolar atrial electrogram is quite helpful because it clearly identifies atrial activation and its relationship to ventricular activation. For instance, during tachycardia with a regular ventricular rate of 150 beat/minute, a bipolar atrial electrogram recording which demonstrates a rate of 150 beat/minute would quickly eliminate atrial flutter as the underlying rhythm. However, the rhythm could still be a sinus tachycardia, an automatic AV junctional tachycardia, paroxysmal atrial tachycardia, a sinus node re-entrant tachycardia, and, in the presence of a wide QRS complex, a ventricular tachycardia with 1:1 retrograde conduction to the atria. If the atrial electrogram were recorded simultaneously with or just after the QRS complex, it would make a sinus node re-entrant rhythm most unlikely. The diagnosis is further assisted by the response of the arrhythmias to rapid atrial pacing. If the rhythm were successfully interrupted by rapid atrial pacing in the presence of a narrow QRS complex, the rhythm would almost certainly have to be paroxysmal atrial tachycardia. Thus, rapid atrial pacing would be both diagnostic and therapeutic, permitting the diagnosis to be established and also

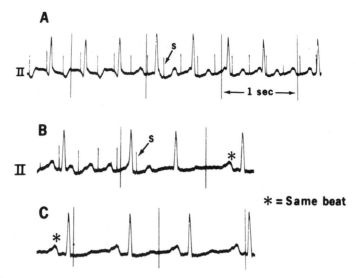

Figure 15.8. EKG and II recording from the same patient as in Figures 15.6 and 15.7 during atrial pacing at a cycle length of 224 msec. In *Panel A*, note that with the seventh atrial beat, and 22 seconds after the onset of atrial pacing at this cycle length, the morphology of the atrial complexes in the EKG suddenly changed from the negative complex characteristic of the spontaneous atrial flutter to a positive complex characteristic of pacing from the high right atrium (the site which was the location of the temporarily fixed epicardial atrial wire electrodes). *Panel B* was recorded several seconds after the tracing in *Panel A* and demonstrates that now when atrial pacing was abruptly terminated a spontaneous sinus rhythm developed. The first beat in *Panel C (asterisk)* is identical to the last beat in *Panel B (asterisk)*. Thus, this figure illustrates both the critical pacing rate and critical duration of pacing to interrupt Type I atrial flutter. Time lines are at 1-second intervals. S = stimulus artifact. Modified from Waldo et al.[14]

providing effective therapy (Figs. 15.9 and 15.10).

TREATMENT

Paroxysmal atrial tachycardia probably is the simplest tachyarrhythmia to interrupt with atrial pacing, and in patients following open heart surgery, atrial pacing is the treatment of choice. There are several acceptable methods of cardiac pacing to interrupt this arrhythmia.[17, 20–22] Paroxysmal atrial tachycardia can often be interrupted with an appropriately timed premature atrial beat. Therefore, one can initiate atrial pacing at a rate significantly slower than the paroxysmal tachycardia, for example, 100 beat/minute, and interrupt the faster rhythm because the random occurrence of a premature

atrial beat at an appropriate interval following a spontaneous atrial beat often will interrupt this re-entrant rhythm. However, since paroxysmal atrial tachycardia can always be interrupted with atrial pacing at a rate faster than the spontaneous rate, this simple and more predictable method of pacing therapy is recommended. Using this latter technique, the atria are paced at a rate about 10 to 20 beat/minute faster than the spontaneous rate of the tachycardia. After achieving atrial capture, atrial pacing may be abruptly terminated (Fig. 15.10), or the atrial pacing rate may be slowed rapidly to a predetermined pacing rate (e.g., 100 to 110 beat/min). Because paroxysmal atrial tachycardia (both the intranodal type and the AV bypass type) will be transiently en-

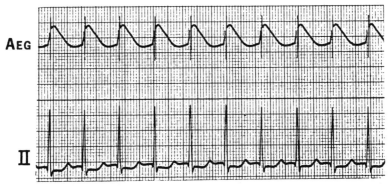

Figure 15.9. Bipolar A$_{EG}$ (*top trace*) recorded simultaneously with EKG lead II (*bottom trace*) in a patient who developed a paroxysmal tachycardia with a ventricular rate of 140 beat/minute. No P waves could be identified in any EKG leads. Vagal maneuvers neither elicited any changes in the rhythm nor provided evidence of atrial activation in the EKG. Simultaneous recording of the A$_{EG}$ with the EKG established a 1:1 relationship between atrial and ventricular activation. This clearly eliminates the possibility of atrial flutter with 2:1 AV conduction. The differential diagnosis therefore lies between sinus tachycardia with a prolonged P-R interval; AV junctional tachycardia with retrograde activation of the atria; and paroxysmal atrial tachycardia. A sinus node re-entrant tachycardia is also a remote possibility. Reproduced with permission from Waldo et al: Utilization of the cardiac catherization laboratory for the diagnosis and treatment of cardiac arrhythmias and conduction disturbances. *Alabama J Med Sci* 11:119, 1974.

Pace Atria-160 beats/min

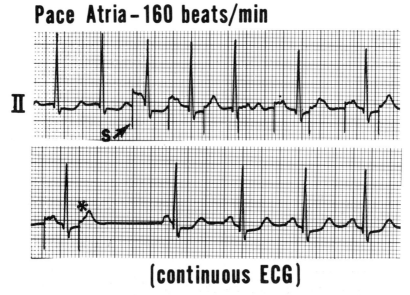

(continuous ECG)

Figure 15.10. Continuous EKG led II recorded from the patient illustrated in Figure 15.9. The first two beats in the *top trace* illustrate again the cycle length of the rapid spontaneous rhythm. Because of the likelihood of the diagnosis of paroxysmal atrial tachycardia, atrial pacing at a rate of 160 beat/minute was initiated (*top trace*). Atrial capture with second-degree AV block was obtained during the pacing. Following the 10th paced atrial beat (*asterisk*), pacing was abruptly stopped. The rhythm then returned to a spontaneous sinus rhythm. This demonstrates the ease in successfully treating paroxysmal atrial tachycardia with rapid atrial pacing. It also demonstrates that atrial pacing may not only successfully convert a re-entrant tachyarrhythmia to sinus rhythm, but also by so doing, may establish the diagnosis. S = stimulus artifact. Reproduced with permission from Waldo et al: Utilization of the caridac catherization laboratory for the diagnosis and treatment of cardiac arrhythmias and conduction disturbances. *Alabama J Med Sci* 11:119, 1974.

trained at some overdrive pacing rates, occasionally, overdrive pacing to interrupt paroxysmal atrial tachycardia may require pacing at rates 20 to 50 beat/minute faster than the spontaneous rate of the paroxysmal atrial tachycardia.[17,22] For those patients in whom paroxysmal atrial tachycardia recurs despite its successful interruption by rapid atrial pacing, continuous rapid atrial pacing techniques may be required to suppress the arrhythmia and to control ventricular rate.[13,17]

Ectopic (Nonparoxysmal) Atrial Tachycardia

DIAGNOSIS

Ectopic atrial tachycardia is a poorly understood rhythm that is generated in the atria and is characterized by an atrial rate ranging from about 130 to 240 beat/minute.[17] When the atrial rate is greater than 160 beat/minute, it is usually characterized by second degree AV block. As for virtually all the tachyarrhythmias, there are times when these arrhythmias may be difficult to diagnose because atrial activation in the EKG may not be readily apparent (Fig. 15.11). In such cases, recording an atrial electrogram is invaluable.

TREATMENT

When present, ectopic atrial tachycardia is commonly associated with 2:1 AV conduction such that, despite rapid atrial rates (e.g., 200 beat/min) the ventricular rate (e.g., 100 beat/min) is clinically quite acceptable. Thus, therapy to interrupt the ar-

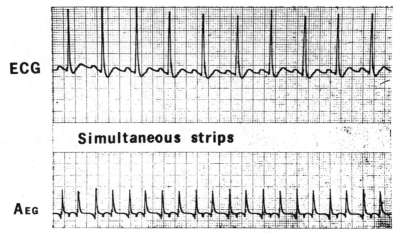

Figure 15.11.   Monitor EKG recorded simultaneously with a bipolar A$_{EG}$ demonstrating ectopic atrial tachycardia with 2:1 AV conduction. This rhythm was recorded from a patient who previously had demonstrated an ectopic atrial tachycardia with variable AV block. The rhythm then was noted to have become regular at a rate of about 100 beat/minute. The routine monitor EKG suggested that a sinus rhythm had developed, but the simultaneous recording of the bipolar A$_{EG}$ with the EKG clearly demonstrated that the ectopic atrial tachycardia was still present. Finally, note the irregularity of the beat-to-beat cycle length evident in the recorded A$_{EG}$s. This is a common, though not invariable, characteristic of this rhythm. Reproduced with permission from Waldo et al.[16]

rhythmia may not be required. Usually, the rhythm will spontaneously revert to the preoperative rhythm (e.g., sinus rhythm or atrial fibrillation) over a period of 1 or 2 days. However, because the degree of AV conduction may be variable and therefore the ventricular rate often rapid, atrial pacing may be utilized to interrupt the rhythm. The recommended pacing technique is similar to the constant pacing rate technique described for Type I atrial flutter. Utilizing the atrial wire electrodes, atrial pacing at a rate 10 beat/minute faster than the intrinsic rate of the arrhythmia should be initiated. Pacing should be continued for at least 30 seconds and then should either be abruptly terminated or quickly slowed to a desirable atrial pacing rate (e.g., 100 beat/min). Should the overdrive atrial pacing fail to interrupt the arrhythmia (because of transient entrainment), overdrive atrial pacing should be reinitiated, increasing the pacing rate in 5 to 10-beat increments, until the arrhythmia has been interrupted[17] (Fig. 15.12).

During rapid atrial pacing to interrupt ectopic atrial tachycardia, the arrhythmia commonly is transiently entrained to the pacing rate until a sufficiently rapid pacing rate is achieved to which the arrhythmias cannot be entrained (Fig. 15.12). Therefore, failure to interrupt the arrhythmia with rapid pacing at rates faster than the pacing rate should not be interpreted as indicating that this rhythm is not interruptable by pacing.[17,21] Also, for some patients, continuous rapid atrial pacing to achieve and maintain 2:1 AV conduction may be required to control the ventricular rate.[13]

Sponataneous Sinus and Atrioventricular Junctional Automatic Tachycardias

DIAGNOSIS

Generally, sinus and AV junctional automatic tachycardias in the postoperative period are transient and benign, and do not require special attention apart from seeking the etiology of the tachycardia (e.g., for sinus tachycardia—fever, anemia, cardiac tamponade, or hypovolemia) and initiating appropriate therapy.[17] Sinus and AV junctional automatic tachycardias are not readily

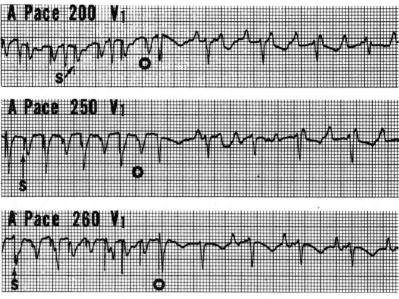

Figure 15.12. EKG lead V₁ recorded at the termination of 30 seconds of atrial pacing at rates of 200 beat/minute (*top trace*), 250 beat/minute (*middle trace*) and 260 beat/minute (*bottom trace*) in a patient who had an ectopic atrial tachycardia at a rate of 180 beat/minute with 2:1 AV conduction. In each trace, the *circle* marks the last paced atrial beat. The ectopic atrial tachycardia was not interrupted by atrial pacing at rates of 200 (*top trace*), 210, 220, 230, 240, and 250 (*middle trace*) beat/minute. However, atrial pacing at 260 beat/minute (*bottom trace*) interrupted the ectopic atrial tachycardia, with the development of a sinus rhythm following abrupt cessation of atrial pacing (*bottom trace*). S = stimulus artifact. Reproduced with permission from Waldo and MacLean.[17]

amenable to therapy with standard atrial pacing techniques.[17] Although they can be overdriven, as soon as the external pacemaker is turned off or its rate is slowed to a rate less than that of the spontaneous rate, the spontaneous automatic tachycardia again becomes the rhythm of the heart. In fact, these latter characteristics are utilized to help establish the diagnosis of the tachycardia when it is uncertain. Both these rhythms demonstrate overdrive suppression during rapid pacing of the appropriate chamber (atrium for sinus tachycardia and either atrium or ventricle for AV junctional tachycardia).[23] With abrupt cessation of the overdrive pacing, both rhythms demonstrate a warm-up period.[23] When it is not clear whether a tachyarrhythmia is a sinus tachycardia with first-degree AV block or an AV junctional tachycardia with 1:1 ret-

rograde AV conduction, the relationship of atrial to ventricular activation following abrupt termination of pacing should differentiate between these two rhythms.[17] The persistence of atrial activation preceding ventricular activation indicates a sinus mechanism, and the opposite indicates an AV junctional mechanism.

Treatment of Atrioventricular Junctional Tachycardia

Usually an AV junctional tachycardia occurring in the postoperative period will subside spontaneously over a period of several days. On occasion, it may be desirable to overdrive an AV junctional tachycardia in order to provide an atrial contribution to cardiac output.[16, 17] This usually may be accomplished simply by pacing the atria at a rate just faster than the AV junctional rate

(Fig. 15.13). On occasion, the enhanced AV junctional pacemaker responsible for the spontaneous tachycardia may be associated with a significant degree of anterograde AV block, such that an atrial impulse produced by pacing the atria at a rate faster than that of the AV junctional pacemaker will block proximal to the focus of the AV junctional pacemaker and thus will not overdrive the AV junctional rhythm. In such circumstances, it may be desirable to initiate AV sequential pacing at a rate appropriately faster than the AV junctional rate. Whenever an automatic AV junctional tachycardia becomes life-threatening, generally because of marked hypotension and low cardiac output, ventricular paired-pacing may be required and should be effective.[12,17,24–26]

Pacing to Produce a Desirable Supraventricular Tachyarrhythmia

CONTINUOUS RAPID ATRIAL PACING TO PRECIPITATE AND SUSTAIN ATRIAL FIBRILLATION

On occasion, some arrhythmias which have been successfully interrupted with rapid atrial pacing techniques may recur despite their successful interruption. In these instances, particularly when these arrhythmias are associated with rapid ventricular rates, it may be desirable to precipitate and sustain atrial fibrillation by pacing the atria continuously at 450 beat/minute.[13,17] The ventricular response rate may be clinically acceptable without need for additional drug therapy, but if it is too rapid, it can virtually always be easily controlled with digoxin, verapamil, and/or propranolol.[17] The most common indication for the use of this technique is recurrent Type I atrial flutter (Fig. 15.14).[13,17] When using this technique, the rapid atrial pacing should be terminated on a trial basis after an appropriate period of time. If the tachyarrhythmia recurs, continuous rapid atrial pacing should be resumed. If the tachyarrhythmia does not recur, usually the atrial fibrillation will convert spontaneously to sinus rhythm within a short period. Occasionally, atrial fibrillation may persist in a patient, and DC cardioversion may be required to obtain sinus rhythm. We have never had to perform continuous rapid atrial pacing to sustain atrial fibrillation for more than 72 hours, the average period of pacing being about 24 hours.

RAPID ATRIAL PACING TO PRODUCE 2:1 ATRIOVENTRICULAR CONDUCTION

In the event of recurrent paroxysmal atrial tachycardia following its interruption with rapid atrial pacing or any other technique,

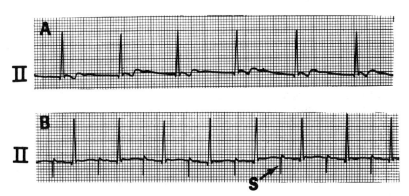

Figure 15.13. EKG lead II recorded from the same patient in both *Panels A and B. Panel A* demonstrates a spontaneous AV junctional rhythm with retrograde AV conduction at a rate of about 65 beat/minute. *Panel B* demonstrates that when atrial pacing at a rate of 90 beat/minute was initiated, 1:1 anterograde AV conduction was obtained. S = stimulus artifact. Reproduced with permission from Waldo and MacLean.[17]

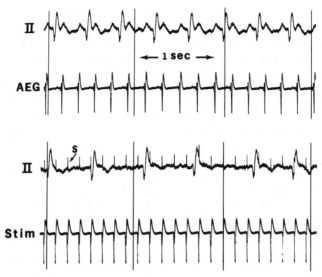

Figure 15.14. The *top panel* shows EKG lead II recorded simultaneously with a bipolar A_{EG} during atrial flutter at a rate of 320 beat/minute with 2:1 AV conduction, producing a ventricular rate of 160 beat/minute. The atrial flutter had been interrupted successfully on several occasions with rapid atrial pacing but it recurred each time. Therefore, as shown in the *bottom panel*, continuous rapid atrial pacing at 450 beat/minute was initiated. Pacing at this rate precipitated and sustained atrial fibrillation and was associated with a slowing of the ventricular response rate to about 120 beat/minute. Digoxin was administered to slow the ventricular response rate further. Quinidine was also administered. Continuous rapid atrial pacing to sustain atrial fibrillation for control of the ventricular rate was required for 26 hours in this patient. Earlier termination of rapid pacing resulted in recurrence of the atrial flutter. When the rapid atrial pacing was finally terminated, atrial fibrillation was transiently present, converting spontaneously to sinus rhythm within several minutes. Time lines are at 1-second intervals. S = stimulus artifact. Reproduced with permission from Waldo et al.[13]

or in the event of ectopic (nonparoxysmal) atrial tachycardia with 1:1 AV conduction in which rapid atrial pacing short of producing atrial fibrillation has not interrupted the rhythm, rapid atrial pacing in the range of 180 to 230 beat/minute can be initiated to slow the ventricular rate by producing a paced atrial tachycardia with a 2:1 AV response[13,17] (Fig. 15.15). Simply by pacing the atria rapidly and taking advantage of functional AV block, the ventricular rate is decreased significantly. We have never had to perform continuous rapid atrial pacing to sustain 2:1 AV conduction for more than 72 hours, the average period of pacing being about 21 hours.

DIAGNOSIS AND TREATMENT OF VENTRICULAR TACHYCARDIAS

Diagnosis

Ventricular tachycardia must always be suspected in the presence of a wide QRS complex tachycardia. The differential diagnosis, of course, includes a supraventricular tachycardia with aberrant ventricular conduction. When the diagnosis is unclear, and if the patient's clinical status permits it, either recording or pacing through the bipolar atrial wire electrodes usually will enable the diagnosis to be established. Recording of a bipolar electrogram may document AV dissociation (Fig. 15.16). In the presence

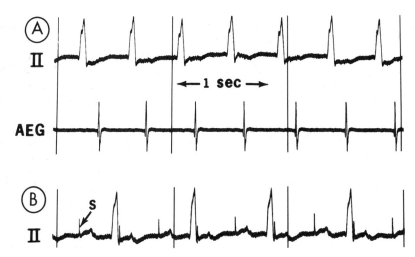

Figure 15.15. *Panel A.* EKG lead II recorded simultaneously with a bipolar AEG demonstrating an ectopic atrial tachycardia at a rate of 140 beat/minute with 1:1 AV conduction. Overdrive atrial pacing suppressed the arrhythmias, but rapid atrial pacing at rates just short of precipitating fibrillation failed to interrupt it. Therefore, as shown in *Panel B*, continuous rapid atrial pacing at a rate of 180 beat/minute was initiated. This produced 2:1 AV conduction with a clinically satisfactory rate of 90 beat/minute. The arrhythmias resolved spontaneously in 24 hours. Time lines are at 1-second intervals. S = stimulus artifact. Reproduced with permission from Cooper et al.[21]

Sequential strips

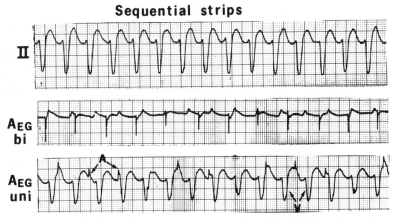

Figure 15.16. The *top tracing* demonstrates a regular, wide QRS complex tachycardia at 130 beat/minute and presents the classic problem of the differential diagnosis of such a tachycardia. A bipolar A$_{EG}$ (*middle tracing*) was then recorded and demonstrated a regular rate of 100 beat/minute, clearly establishing the presence of AV dissociation and making the diagnosis of ventricular tachycardia virtually certain. However, the diagnosis of an AV junctional tachycardia with aberrant ventricular conduction was still possible, though unlikely. The *bottom tracing* demonstrates a unipolar A$_{EG}$ and is presented to illustrate that although the diagnosis of AV dissociation could be made from the unipolar A$_{EG}$, the diagnosis is infinitely easier and more certain from the recording of the bipolar atrial electrogram. A = atrial complex; V = ventricular complex. Reproduced with permission from Waldo et al.[16]

of a wide QRS complex tachycardia with a 1:1 AV relationship, if atrial pacing at a rate just faster than that of the tachycardia results in production of a fusion beat and/or a narrow QRS complex, the diagnosis is established (Fig. 15.17).

Treatment

Either intravenous lidocaine therapy and/or DC cardioversion is generally the treatment of choice for ventricular tachycardia. However, this arrhythmia, when not induced by a spontaneous automatic pacemaker, may be effectively treated by rapid ventricular or even rapid atrial pacing.[17, 18, 27] Atrial pacing will only be successful if 1:1 AV conduction of each atrially-paced beat occurs. Because ventricular tachycardia can also be transiently entrained,[18] the method of pacing is similar to the pacing technique described for Type I atrial flutter (Fig. 15.18). When the situation permits it, pacing at a rate at least 10 beats faster than the spontaneous ventricular rate should be initiated, and after 5 to 30 seconds, pacing should be abruptly terminated. If the ventricular tachycardia has not been interrupted, the pacing should be repeated, increasing the pacing rate by increments of 5 to 10 beat/minute. Generally, pacing at rates between 115 to 125% of the intrinsic rate are required to interrupt the tachycardia, although rates as high or higher than 140% of the intrinsic rate have been reported.[18, 27] Rapid pacing at rates faster than the intrinsic rate of the tachycardia which fail to interrupt the tachycardia have merely transiently entrained it (Fig. 15.18).[18] Thus, as with rapid atrial pacing to interrupt Type I atrial flutter, paroxysmal atrial tachycardia, and ectopic atrial tachycardia, ventricular pacing to interrupt ventricular tachycardia must achieve a critical rate to interrupt the ventricular tachycardia (Fig. 15.18).[17, 18, 27] On occasion, ventricular paired-pacing may be required to interrupt or control this arrhythmia.[17, 18]

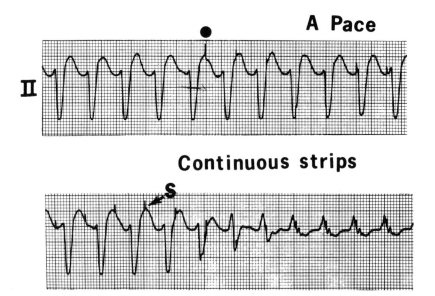

A Pace

Continuous strips

Figure 15.17. EKG lead II recorded from the same patient whose EKG tracing are illustrated in Figure 15.16. The *solid circle* in the *top strip* marks the onset of atrial pacing at a rate just faster than that of the spontaneous tachycardia. The *bottom strip*, which is continuous with the *top strip*, illustrates that the ventricular rate increases to the atrial pacing rate. More important, the appearance of fusion beats (fifth through seventh beats) permits the diagnosis of ventricular tachycardia to be established with certainty. S = stimulus artifact. Reproduced with permission from Waldo et al.[16]

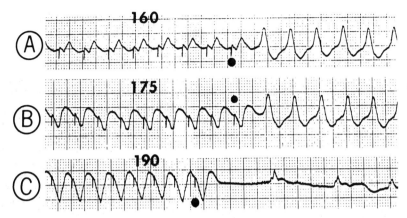

Figure 15.18. *Panels A, B, and C* are recorded from a patient who developed spontaneous ventricular tachycardia at a rate of 150 beat/minute. EKG lead II is recorded throughout. *Panel A* shows the termination of ventricular pacing (*dot*) at a rate of 160 beat/minute, with prompt return of the spontaneous ventricular tachycardia. *Panel B* shows termination of pacing (*dot*) at a rate of 175 beat/minute, with prompt return of the ventricular tachycardia following termination of pacing. In this patient, pacing at 155 beat/minute, 165 beat/minute, and 180 beat/minute also failed to interrupt the tachycardia. *Panel C* shows termination of pacing at a rate of 190 beat/minute with successful interruption of the tachycardia. Note, as illustrated in *Panels A* and *B*, that during periods of transient entrainment of the tachycardia at different pacing rates, there were different degrees of ventricular fusion. Modified from MacLean et al.[18]

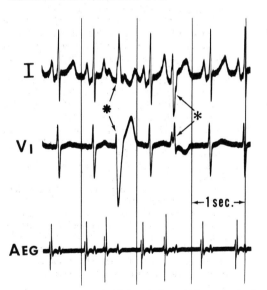

Figure 15.19. EKG leads I and V_1 recorded simultaneously with a bipolar A_{EG} during a sinus rhythm during which premature beats with wide QRS complexes (denoted by a *star* and an *asterisk*), of different morphologies were noted. The simultaneous record-

DIAGNOSIS AND TREATMENT OF EXTRASYSTOLES

Diagnosis

The ability to record a bipolar atrial electrogram is especially helpful in establishing the chamber of origin of a premature beat, particularly when the premature beat is associated with a wide QRS complex and identification of atrial activation in the EKG is uncertain (Fig. 15.19). Also, on occasion, it may be desirable to introduce premature atrial beats by means of the atrial electrodes to establish whether they are associated with aberrant ventricular conduction manifesting a QRS morphology which was previously recorded but which could not be

ing of the A_{EG} readily demonstrated that each wide QRS complex was preceded by a premature atrial beat, thereby demonstrating that the wide QRS complex premature beats resulted from aberrant ventricular conduction of premature atrial beats.

diagnosed as ventricular or supraventricular in origin.

Treatment

Ventricular extrasystoles are often easily suppressed simply by increasing the heart rate either with atrial or ventricular pacing.[16,17] Atrial extrasystoles also may be suppressed simply by increasing the atrial rate with atrial pacing.[17] For some patients in whom it is judged important to suppress the premature atrial beats, it may be necessary to pace the atria at very rapid rates. This usually requires atrial pacing at rates between 180 to 230 beat/minute because these rates are most effective in suppressing the premature atrial beats and also will produce 2:1 AV conduction with a clinically acceptable ventricular rate.[13,16,17]

SUMMARY

The demonstrated safety, efficacy, and ease of utilization of the temporarily-placed epicardial wire electrodes highly recommend their routine use. By having temporary stainless steel wire electrodes available in the postoperative period, the diagnosis of arrhythmias following open heart surgery is greatly facilitated. Furthermore, because of the clinical advantages of cardiac pacing, it becomes the treatment of choice for many, if not most, arrhythmias in the postoperative period.

References

1. Harris PD, Singer DH, Malm JR, et al: Chronically implanted cardiac electrodes for diagnostic, therapeutic, and investigational use in man. *J Thorac Cardiovasc Surg* 54:190, 1967.
2. Harris PD, Malm JR, Bowman FO Jr, et al: Epicardial pacing to control arrhythmias following cardiac surgery. *Circulation* 37(Suppl. 2):178, 1968.
3. Litwak RS, Kuhn LA, Gadboys HL, et al: Support of myocardial performance after open cardiac operations by rate augmentation. *J Thorac Cardiovasc Surg* 56:484, 1968.
4. Woodson RD, Starr A: Atrial pacing after mitral valve surgery, *Arch Surg* 97:894, 1968.
5. Beller BM, Frater RWM, Wulfsohn N: Cardiac pacemaking in the management of postoperative arrhythmias. *Ann Thorac Surg* 6:68, 1968.
6. Hodam RP, Starr A: Temporary postoperative epicardial pacing electrodes. Their value and man-

7. Iwa T, Sugiki K, Todo K, et al: Atrial pacemaker III. *Jpn J Thorac Surg* 24:796, 1971.
8. Waldo AL, Ross SM, Kaiser GA: The epicardial electrogram in the diagnosis of cardiac arrhythmias in the postoperative patient. *Geriatrics* 26:108, 1971.
9. Waldo AL, Vitikainen KJ, Kaiser GA, et al: Atrial standstill secondary to atrial inexcitability (atrial quiescence). *Circulation* 46:690, 1972.
10. Mills NL, Ochsner JL: Experience with atrial pacemaker wires implanted during cardiac operations. *J Thorac Cardiovasc Surg* 66:878, 1973.
11. Pittman DE, Gay TC, Patel II, et al: Termination of atrial flutter and atrial tachycardia with rapid atrial stimulation. *Angiology* 36:784, 1975.
12. Waldo AL, Krongrad E, Kupersmith J, et al: Ventricular paired pacing to control rapid ventricular heart rate following open heart surgery. Observations on ectopic automaticity. Report of a case in a four-month-old patient. *Circulation* 53:176, 1976.
13. Waldo AL, MacLean WAH, Karp RB, et al: Continuous rapid atrial pacing to control recurrent or sustained supraventricular tachycardias following open heart surgery. *Circulation* 54:245, 1976.
14. Waldo AL, MacLean WAH, Karp RB, et al: Entrainment and interruption of atrial flutter with atrial pacing. Studies in man following open heart surgery. *Circulation* 56:737, 1977.
15. Wells JL Jr, Karp RB, Kouchoukos NT, et al: Characterization of atrial fibrillation in man. Studies following open heart surgery. *PACE* 3:965, 1978.
16. Waldo AL, MacLean WAH, Cooper TB, et al: Use of temporarily placed epicardial wire electrodes for the diagnosis and treatment of cardiac arrhythmias following open heart surgery. *J Thorac Cardiovasc Surg* 76:500, 1978.
17. Waldo AL, Maclean WAH: *The Diagnosis and Treatment of Arrhythmias Following Open Heart Surgery. Emphasis on the Use of Epicardial Wire Electrodes.* Futura Publishing Co., Mt. Kisco, NY, 1980.
18. MacLean WAH, Plumb VJ, Waldo AL: Transient entrainment and interruption of ventricular tachycardia. *PACE* 4:358, 1981.
19. Wells JL Jr, MacLean WAH, James TN, et al: Characterization of atrial flutter. Studies in man after open heart surgery using fixed atrial electrodes. *Circulation* 60:665, 1979.
20. MacLean WAH, Cooper TB, Waldo AL: Use of cardiac electrodes in the diagnosis and treatment of tachyarrhythmias. *Cardiovasc Med* 3:965, 1978.
21. Cooper TB, MacLean WAH, Waldo AL: Overdrive pacing for supraventricular tachycardia. A review of theoretical implications and therapeutic techniques. *PACE* 1:196, 1978.
22. Waldo AL, Plumb VJ, Arciniegas JG, et al: Transient entrainment and interruption of the atrioventricular bypass pathway type of paroxysmal atrial tachycardia. A model for understanding and identifying reentrant arrhythmias. *Circulation* 67:73, 1983.
23. Vassalle M: The relationship among cardiac pace-

makers. Overdrive suppression. *Circ Res* 41:269, 1977.

24. Cranefield PF: Paired pulse stimulation and post-extrasystolic potentiation of the heart. *Prog Cardiovasc Dis* 8:446, 1966.

25. Cranfield PF, Hoffman BF: The physiologic basis and clinical implications of paired pulse stimula-tion of the heart. *Dis Chest* 49:561, 1966.

26. Resnikov L: Electrical slowing of the heart and postextrasystolic potentiation. *Med Clin North Am* 54:247, 1970.

27. Fisher JD, Mehra R, Furman J: Termination of ventricular tachycardia with bursts of rapid ventricular pacing. *Am J Cardiol* 41:94, 1978.

CHAPTER 16

DIASTOLIC FUNCTION AND THE HYPERTROPHIED VENTRICLE

MARTIN M. LeWINTER, M.D.

It is now possible to identify the various determinants of the relation between pressure and volume in the diastolic left ventricle. These include intrinsic factors such as passive muscle stiffness, chamber geometry, relaxation rate, ventricular suction, and viscous effects, and extrinsic factors such as the influence of the pericardium, ventricular interaction, "erectile" effects, and heart rate. Changes in diastolic function are important in the pathophysiology of various disorders and may by themselves produce significant pulmonary venous hypertension and apparent shifts in the Frank-Starling relationship. In hypertrophy states significant alterations in diastolic function are known to occur, although the mechanism of these changes is not clear. Further, certain abnormalities in diastolic function in hypertrophic states may be associated with myocardial fibrosis and thus may be a marker of irreversible ultrastructural changes. Thus, in cardiac hypertrophy knowledge of diastolic function may be as important as knowledge of systolic function.

INTRODUCTION

The ability to understand and analyze factors which influence the relationship between pressure and volume in the diastolic left ventricle has increased considerably in the last decade. In this chapter we shall attempt to review what is known about normal diastolic mechanics, the clinical significance of changes in diastolic function, and what is known about diastolic function in hypertrophic states.

Definition

Before proceeding, it is helpful to clearly define several terms which are sometimes used inconsistently.

DIASTOLE

Although diastole is sometimes defined as the time from aortic valve closure to mitral valve closure (or the isovolumic relaxation period plus the ventricular filling period), for the purposes of this discussion diastole will be considered as the time from mitral valve opening to mitral valve closure.

CHAMBER COMPLIANCE

Chamber compliance is the change in diastolic volume occurring in association with a given change in diastolic pressure, or $\Delta V/\Delta P$. Unless specified otherwise, pressure will refer to intracavitary as opposed to transmural pressure. Chamber compliance can be analyzed in what is sometimes termed a *dynamic* fashion, in which $\Delta V/\Delta P$ is measured over some part of or an entire *single diastolic cycle*, or it can be analyzed in what is sometimes termed a *static* fashion, by picking a single point or points during *multiple cardiac cycles* (e.g., at end-diastole or during slow-filling) over a range of pressure and volumes. The static technique is more amenable to animal studies in which pressure and volume may be easily manipulated. The advantage of the latter technique is that a much larger portion of the pressure-volume relation can be described and therefore, if one wishes, more confidently fitted to some mathematical relationship. For most clinical studies, in which only one or perhaps two cardiac cycles is generally available for analysis, the dynamic technique is used. While it is possible to fit portions of a single cycle to a mathematical relationship, this can be done with less confidence using the dynamic technique because only a small portion of the diastolic pressure-volume relation is available for analysis.

CHAMBER STIFFNESS

Chamber stiffness is simply the inverse of chamber compliance, or $\Delta P/\Delta V$.

MUSCLE STIFFNESS

Muscle stiffness is the change in stress occurring in association with a given change in strain in cardiac muscle, or Δ stress/Δ strain. The term *stress* refers to the tension per unit of cross-sectional area of the muscle. The term *strain* refers to the length (l) of a muscle above its length when it is unstressed (lo) or l/lo. Strain may be thought of simply as the percent extension of a muscle above its unstressed length. Stress, strain, and stiffness are easily measured directly in isolated muscle. As will be seen, these variables can be derived in the intact left ventricle from knowledge of pressure, volume, wall thickness, and geometry of the chamber. The significance of *muscle* as opposed to *chamber* stiffness is two-fold. First, muscle stiffness is an intrinsic property of the myocardium whereas chamber stiffness can be influenced by external factors to be discussed later. Second, since both stress and strain are normalized variables, calculation of muscle stiffness allows comparison between different hearts whereas comparing chamber stiffness between different hearts has considerable potential for

error. Analogous to chamber stiffness, in the intact left ventricle muscle stiffness can be derived in a dynamic or static fashion.

MUSCLE COMPLIANCE OR ELASTANCE

These terms are used to indicate the inverse of muscle stiffness, or Δ strain/Δ stress.

PASSIVE CHAMBER OR MUSCLE PROPERTIES

Use of the term "passive" implies that chamber stiffness or compliance or muscle stiffness or elastance is analyzed at a time when filling or lengthening rates are sufficiently slow such that viscous effects which occur at high filling or lengthening rates are inconsequential (these effects will be discussed subsequently). In the intact left ventricle, this generally means that analysis is confined to the so-called slow-filling portion of diastole.

Determinants of the Relationship Between Diastolic Pressure and Volume in the Intact Left Ventricle

The determinants of the relationship between pressure and volume in the diastolic left ventricle can be categorized either as *intrinsic*, those which are a function of the properties of the left ventricular (LV) muscle itself or the geometry of the chamber, or *extrinsic*, meaning all others, for example, the pressure outside the chamber and the duration of diastolic filling time.

INTRINSIC DETERMINANTS

In Figure 16.1 (*top left* and *right*) are shown schematic plots of the relation between LV pressure and volume as a function of time during the isovolumic relaxation period and diastole proper. On the *bottom* is shown the relation between pressure and volume during diastole for two cardiac cycles at differing levels of pressure and volume. During isovolumic relaxation pressure falls precipitously and of course, volume is constant and equal to the end-systolic volume. Beginning at the time of mitral valve opening there is a brief period during which pressure continues to fall but volume begins to increase rapidly. Subsequently, pressure

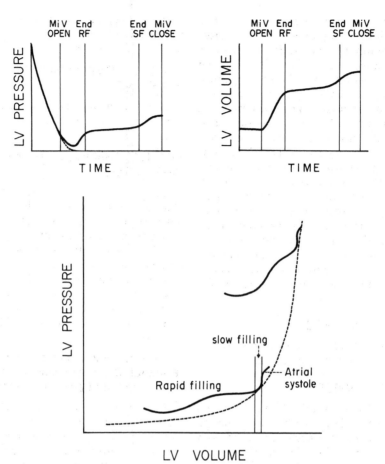

Figure 16.1. Schematic representation shows the relation between LV pressure and time (*top left*), LV volume and time (*top right*) and LV pressure and volume (*bottom*) beginning at time of aortic valve closure and ending at end-diastole. See text for description. LV = left ventricular; MV = mitral valve; RF = rapid filling; SF = slow filling.

also begins to rise rapidly along with volume until both level off fairly abruptly. This period beginning with mitral valve opening during which volume increases rapidly is known as the rapid filling phase. The point at which the rate of pressure and volume increase levels off signals the onset of the slow-filling phase, during which both pressure and volume gradually increase. Finally, with atrial systole there is a second, briefer period during which both pressure and volume rise rapidly until ventricular contraction begins and the mitral valve closes.

Let us first direct our attention to the slow-filling phase of the cardiac cycle. In the bottom of Figure 16.1, the *dashed line* represents the relation between pressure and volume derived from slow-filling phases obtained from a large number of beats encompassing a wide range of pressures and volumes. This, then, is the passive pressure-volume relation of the left ventricle. Note that it is curvilinear, or exponential in form, being relatively flat at low pressures and volumes and almost infinitely steep at high pressures and volumes. The implication of this feature is that passive chamber compliance is not constant but rather a function of the level of pressure and volume, being markedly reduced at high pressures and volumes. The converse is true of chamber stiffness. Also, note that during the slow-filling phase of both of the individual beats shown in the bottom of Figure 16.1, pressure and volume fall on the passive relation but that during rapid filling and atrial systole pressure and volume deviate from the passive relation, a point we shall return to later. Thus, two important determinants of the relation between diastolic pressure and volume are the shape and position of the passive pressure-volume relation and where on this relation the left ventricle is operating. It is important to specify both shape and position because a simple parallel shift in position of the passive pressure-volume relation to either the left or right does not constitute a change in chamber compliance or stiffness; the latter is only altered when the shape of the relation is changed (i.e., it becomes more or less steep). It also follows that since the passive pressure-volume relation is exponential it can be characterized mathematically by its slope and intercept; these would constitute a type of chamber compliance or, conversely, chamber stiffness constants.

As indicated previously, it is also possible to calculate muscle stiffness from data obtained in the intact left ventricle and, if analysis is confined to the slow-filling phase, to derive a passive stiffness relation. The simplest way to calculate the stress component of stiffness in the intact left ventricle is to employ some variation of the La Place relation. For a thin-walled sphere, the La Place relation states that stress in the middle of the wall equals:

$$\frac{\text{Pressure (p)} \times \text{Radius (r)}}{2 \times \text{wall thickness (h)}} \qquad 1$$

Since the shape of the left ventricle is better approximated by an ellipsoid of revolution than a sphere, a geometric term may be added to this relation which reflects the ratio of the semiminor to semimajor (or long) axis of the ventricle. Stress in the midwall at the level of the minor axis in the circumferential direction becomes larger as the shape of the ventricle becomes more ellipsoidal (i.e., as the ratio of the semiminor to semimajor axis decreases) and smaller as the ventricle becomes more spherical (i.e., as the ratio approaches 1). As a practical matter, calcula-

tion of wall stress requires simultaneous measurement of pressure, minor and possibly major axis dimension, and wall thickness. Such data can be obtained from a high quality LV pressure recorded simultaneously with dimensions and wall thickness using techniques such as contrast angiography, echocardiography, or gated computed tomography. There are a number of technical problems inherent in such calculations, however. Diastolic pressure must be of excellent quality (generally obtained with high fidelity, micromanometer tip catheters) because even modest errors in diastolic pressure may result in major errors in wall stress calculations. Further, dimension and wall stress measurements have intrinsic problems with respect to resolution and accuracy using any techniques. Finally, in using the La Place relation, pressure properly refers to distending or transmural pressure rather than intracavitary pressure, so that ideally some measure of the pressure around the heart (e.g., esophogeal pressure) should be obtained and subtracted from the intracavitary pressure. While it should be evident that wall stress calculations have major difficulties, calculation of the strain component of muscle stiffness has an even more fundamental problem. While it is relatively easy to measure circumferential length (i.e., radius) at the level of the semiminor axis, determination of lo, minor axis radius when distending pressure (or stress) is zero, is a formidable task in the intact left ventricle. In animal studies, some approximation of unstressed dimensions can be obtained by employing transient periods of vena caval occlusion to reduce filling to a point such that transmural distending pressure is close to zero. This type of maneuver is of course impossible in clinical studies so that no direct approximation of unstressed dimensions is possible. Passive stress-strain relations, like pressure-volume relations, are exponential in form, and similarly can be characterized by slope and intercept. Therefore, in theory, it should be possible to extrapolate the pressure-volume relation to the zero pressure intercept and calculate an unstressed radius at this volume. Unfortunately, at very low pressure both the passive pressure-volume and stress-strain relations deviate from an exponential relation in an as yet poorly defined fashion,[1] so that such extrapolation is not justified. To overcome this problem, some clinical investigators have taken the approach of extrapolating the pressure-volume relation to some relatively low level of pressure (e.g., 5 mm Hg) at which the relation is known to remain exponential and use a radius calculated at this level of volume instead of a true unstressed radius.[2] Regardless of methodology, it should be obvious that strain calculations, particularly those made from clinical studies, are significantly hampered by this inability to know unstressed dimensions with confidence. Finally, one other limitation of clinical estimates of passive stress-strain and pressure-volume relations should be mentioned. As indicated previously, it is generally possible to have only cardiac cycles obtained over a narrow range of slow-filling pressures and volume in clinical studies; for instance, an angiogram performed at one level of cardiac filling. As can be appreciated from the *bottom* portion of Figure 16.1, only a very small portion of the total pressure-volume (or stress-strain) relation during slow-filling is therefore available for analysis. Consequently, since noise is unavoidably present in this sort of data, prediction of the entire passive pressure-volume or stress-strain relation from a small portion is inherently subject to error.

Based on the previous discussion, it is now possible to describe mathematically how the concept of muscle stiffness is related to chamber stiffness or compliance. We have previously indicated that muscle stiffness = Δ stress/Δ strain. By substituting the equations for stress and strain,

$$\text{muscle stiffness} = \frac{\Delta\left(\dfrac{Pr}{2h}\right)}{\Delta\left(\dfrac{r}{ro}\right)}. \qquad 2$$

By rearrangement,

$$\text{muscle stiffness} \times \Delta\left(\frac{r}{ro}\right) = \Delta\left(\frac{Pr}{2h}\right) \qquad 3$$

If we consider two ventricles which are

identical with respect to volume and internal dimension (radius), wall thickness and unstressed dimension (ro), but differ in muscle stiffness, and increase the internal dimension in both ventricles by the same amount, it should be apparent from the above equations that the change in pressure for an identical change in radius (or volume) will be larger in the ventricle with the greater muscle stiffness. This is because change in radius, as specified previously, is the same in both cases, and change in wall thickness must therefore also be the same by the principle of conservation of mass. Therefore, the only term on the right side of *Equation 2* which can change if muscle stiffness is increased is the change in pressure. If change in pressure is larger for a given change in radius (or volume), this of course means that chamber compliance is reduced and, conversely, chamber stiffness is increased for the ventricle with greater muscle stiffness.

The passive pressure-volume relation can be considered a basic determinant of the relation between diastolic pressure and volume upon which several other intrinsic determinants of this relation are superimposed. Looked at another way, when the ventricle is filling slowly (or passively), its pressure and volume adhere closely to the passive relation (Fig. 16.1). However, as we have seen, during other phases of diastole (rapid filling and atrial systole), pressure and volume deviate from the passive relation in such fashion that pressure is higher than would be predicted from the passive relation. Further, as can be seen in the *bottom* portion of Figure 16.1, during some portions of the rapid filling and atrial systolic phases, ΔP/ΔV may be lower or higher than would be predicted from the passive relation. Several intrinsic determinants of diastolic function may account for these deviations from the passive relation. The first of these is the process of myocardial relaxation. Relaxation in the intact heart is a complex phenomenon and a complete discussion is beyond the scope of this paper. Nonetheless, there has been considerable recent interest in quantifying the relaxation process in the intact heart and one technique which has been employed is calculation of what is termed the time constant of isovolumic pressure fall as an index of relaxation rate.[3,4] As shown in the graph in the *top left* portion of Figure 16.1, LV pressure falls precipitously during the isovolumic relaxation period. In fact, during this period the time course of pressure fall is exponential in nature and therefore can be described by a time constant (T) which is defined as the negative reciprocal of the slope of the natural logarithm of pressure versus time. Relaxation rate would not be a significant determinant of the relation between diastolic pressure and volume if relaxation was essentially complete by the time the mitral valve opens. However, in normal human subjects the magnitude of T is usually in the range of 30 to 40 msec, slow enough that a significant although modest amount of relaxation is still occurring at the time the mitral valve opens. Thus, incomplete relaxation is a factor which tends to increase diastolic pressure at any volume during the very early phase of diastole. This is illustrated by the *dashed line* in Figure 16.1, *top left*, which represents the pressure which would be present in the left ventricle if the mitral valve were not allowed to open, i.e., pressure would be dependent primarily on the relaxation process and would continue to fall exponentially. As can be seen, if relaxation (independent of filling) were the sole determinant of early diastolic pressure, the relaxation process is slow enough that it accounts for a certain amount of the diastolic pressure present. This effect of incomplete relaxation is quite modest in normal subjects but may be a significant determinant of diastolic pressure-volume relations in conditions such as myocardial ischemia where T may be considerably prolonged.

Another intrinsic factor which may influence the diastolic pressure-volume relation in the very early portion of diastole is the phenomenon of ventricular suction.[5,6] Under certain conditions (usually markedly reduced cardiac volume) the pressure recorded in the left ventricle early in diastole may be subatmospheric, a finding which strongly suggests that the left ventricle actively assists its own filling at this time by virtue of suction. Under more physiological conditions, pressure normally declines very

early in diastole while volume increases (Fig. 16.1), exactly the reverse of the behavior which would be expected if the ventricle was filling passively and further evidence of some sort of suction effect. While this area remains somewhat controversial there is now considerable evidence that suction does occur and may be a particularly important mechanism of ventricular filling in situations such as hypovolemia or cardiac tamponade when ventricular volume is markedly reduced. As can be seen in Figure 16.1, to the extent that suction occurs this effect would tend to reduce pressure at any volume.

Another intrinsic factor which influences the relation between pressure and volume during the early portion of diastole is viscous resistance to stretch.[7,8] The LV myocardium displays several types of viscous behavior when it is stretched or lengthened, the most important of which is that the more rapidly it is lengthened the more it resists being lengthened, i.e., it becomes stiffer at rapid lengthening rates. This type of behavior appears to account in part for the deviation from the passive pressure-volume (or stress-strain) relation which occurs during the rapid filling phase, particularly when $\Delta P/\Delta V$ is greater than that which would be predicted from the passive relation. This behavior appears to be dependent not only on lengthening or filling rate but also on the absolute level of pressure or stress, being more important when these are high. Thus, in comparing the two beats shown schematically in the *bottom* of Figure 16.1, the beat at a higher pressure level demonstrates greater deviation from the passive pressure-volume relation. For sake of completeness, two other viscous effects which are easily demonstrated in isolated cardiac muscle should be mentioned. One of these is stress relaxation, or a gradual decline in passive tension which occurs after the muscle is abruptly subjected to an increase in length, and the other is creep, or a gradual increase in length which occurs after the muscle is abruptly subjected to an increase in passive tension. The significance of these viscous phenomena are uncertain in the intact heart, although there is evidence that they occur under certain conditions.[9]

One additional intrinsic factor should be mentioned. This is the end-systolic volume. It should be obvious that end-systolic volume is a critical determinant of diastolic pressure and volume because it is the end-systolic volume which determines the point on the pressure-volume relation at which the subsequent diastole begins. In a sense, end-systolic volume is the link between systole and diastole. The primary determinants of end-systolic volume are ventricular afterload and contractile state. End-systolic volume varies directly with the former and indirectly with the latter. All else being equal, a change in end-systolic volume will result in a similar change in pressure and volume during the subsequent diastole.

EXTRINSIC FACTORS

Certain of the extrinsic factors are those which exert an outside force on the left ventricle. The most obvious of these is the presence of an intact pericardium. It has been repeatedly shown that the normal pericardium can exert a restraining force on filling of the normal heart, including the left ventricle.[10,11] Precisely at what cardiac volume this occurs is unclear, but this effect is certainly important at volumes above the normal physiological range. The influence of an intact pericardium on the passive pressure-volume relation of the left ventricle is illustrated in Figure 16.2. At relatively low volumes the pericardium can accommodate its contents without difficulty; indeed, at these low volumes the pressure-volume relation of the pericardium must fall below that of the heart because the pericardium is obviously larger than the heart while its pressure is generally 0 mm Hg or even negative at these volumes. However, at some point the pericardial pressure-volume relation abruptly increases its slope ($\Delta P/\Delta V$) and pericardial compliance becomes reduced and less than that of the cardiac chambers. This point occurs at a pericardial volume which is less than that which the heart could occupy were it maximally filled in the absence of the pericardium. Thus, as the cardiac volume is increased it reaches a value which corresponds to a pericardial volume at which pericardial compliance markedly decreases. The heart, in a sense,

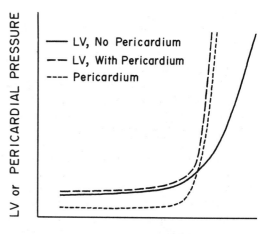

Figure 16.2. Schematic representation shows passive intracavitary pressure-volume relations of the left ventricle with and without an intact pericardium and of the pericardium itself. At the point at which the pressure-volume relation of the heart intersects the pericardial pressure-volume relation, the pericardium becomes the limiting factor for further cardiac filling. See text for further description.

engages the pericardium. At this point, the pericardium exerts a restraining force on the cardiac chambers. A positive intrapericardial pressure is recorded which is reflected as an increase in the intracavitary chamber pressure and in effect the cardiac chambers are competing for space within the pericardial sac. While the transmural filling pressure of the cardiac chambers does not change substantially with the onset of this pericardial effect (because further increases in chamber volume are severely limited), chamber compliance, as defined previously, is reduced because of the large change in intracavitary pressure occurring with small changes in volume. Conversely, in the absence of the pericardium, chamber compliance is increased above the level of volume at which the pericardial restraining effect becomes important. In summary, the presence of an intact pericardium results in a steeper pressure-volume relation of the cardiac chambers (reduced chamber compliance), including the left ventricle.

An intimately-related extrinsic factor which influences the LV pressure-volume relation is diastolic ventricular interaction. For the cardiac ventricles, the term "interaction" refers to the extent that filling of one ventricle influences the pressure-volume relation of the other ventricle.[12, 13] Specifically, as shown in Figure 16.3, as the filling of one ventricle increases, the pressure-volume relation of the contralateral ventricle shifts upward and to the left (i.e., a higher pressure at any volume). There is disagreement as to whether the slope of the pressure-volume relation is steeper (whether chamber compliance is reduced), or if this is merely a parallel shift. Diastolic ventricular interaction is mediated by shifts of the interventricular septum in response to changes in the transseptal pressure gradient and perhaps other mechanical factors. Thus, from the standpoint of the left ventricle, the right ventricular diastolic pressure can be considered as an outside force acting on the

left ventricle through the septum in an analogous fashion as the outside force posed by the pericardium acts on the left ventricular free wall. Diastolic interaction can be readily demonstrated in the absence of the pericardium, but the effect is considerably magnified when the pericardium is intact (see Figure 16.3).[13, 14] The explanation for this relationship between the pericardium and diastolic interaction has to do with the fact that in the absence of the pericardium the LV free wall can expand in response to a leftward septal shift occurring when right ventricular filling increases. However, the intact pericardium may limit LV free-wall expansion under these conditions—the net result is an even larger increase in LV pressure at a given volume due to the combination of septal shifting and increased pericardial restraint to expansion of the free wall.

Diastolic interaction and its close relationship to the pericardium may, at least in part, explain alterations in the LV pressure-volume which occur in clinical situations in which the right heart is dilated, for instance, cor pulmonale and use of positive airway pressure.

Another extrinsic factor which must also be mentioned is the fact that the heart, enclosed in the pericardium, is surrounded by the lungs and the relatively fixed rib cage and chest cavity. Just as the cardiac chambers may compete for space within the pericardial sac, the heart and lungs may similarly compete for space within the thorax. The precise nature of this interplay between the heart and lungs remains uncertain, as does its physiological significance. Again, positive airway pressure may be cited as an example of a maneuver which shifts the LV pressure-volume relation upward and to the left likely because of complex effects on ventricular interaction, the influence of the pericardium, and the interplay between the lungs and the heart.

The amount of blood contained in the heart muscle constitutes an additional extrinsic influence on diastolic pressure and volume. There is reasonably good evidence that an increase in the amount of blood contained in the myocardium results in increases in passive chamber or muscle stiff-

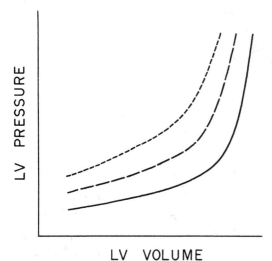

LV VOLUME

Figure 16.3. Schematic representation shows the effects of ventricular interaction. *Solid line* is the LV pressure-volume relation with the right ventricle empty. *Large dashed line* is the pressure-volume relation with the right ventricle filled in the absence of the pericardium. *Small dashed line* is the pressure-volume relation at the same level of right ventricular filling with an intact pericardium. See text for further description.

ness, the so-called erectile property of heart muscle.[15] The physiological importance of this determinant of diastolic pressure and volume is at present uncertain; however, in an area distal to a coronary occlusion a reduction in the erectile effect could potentially be of great significance.

Finally, heart rate may also be considered an extrinsic determinant of pressure and volume during diastole. When heart rate increases, cycle length decreases primarily at the expense of diastole and, in particular, the slow-filling phase. Therefore, by virtue of reduced diastolic filling time, pressure and volume at the end of diastole are reduced as is the average level of diastolic pressure and volume. Changes in heart rate do not specifically alter the relation between pressure and volume, however, only the time available for filling. Increases in heart rate also produce modest increases in inotropic state even when they are not associated with altered antonomic influences (e.g., atrial pacing as opposed to exercise). Therefore, there is also some decrease in end-systolic volume when heart rate increases; the effect of the latter on diastolic pressure and volume have been discussed previously.

CLINICAL SIGNIFICANCE OF ALTERATIONS IN DIASTOLIC FUNCTION

The clinical significance of altered diastolic function falls in a number of areas. While a complete list of these points of significance is beyond the scope of this paper, three of the more important ones are as follows.

First, dyspnea, reflecting pulmonary venous hypertension, is of course one of the most important clinical manifestations of heart disease. It has become apparent that elevation of LV diastolic pressure causing pulmonary venous hypertension sufficient to produce dyspnea can occur due to abnormalities in diastolic function alone or in combination with systolic dysfunction. For example, patients with reduced chamber compliance due to concentric LV hypertrophy in response to aortic valve obstruction or systemic hypertension or patients with

hypertrophic cardiomyopathy may have pulmonary venous hypertension and dyspnea in the absence of detectable systolic dysfunction or even super-normal systolic function.[16,17] Abnormalities of diastolic function in addition to abnormal systolic function may also be responsible for elevated LV diastolic pressure in ischemic heart disease.[18] Second, clinicians routinely depend on assessment of the Frank-Starling relationship in hemodynamic management of patients by relating cardiac output or stroke volume (SV) to the LV filling pressure. As shown in Figure 16.4, depression of systolic function can of course depress the Frank-Starling relation resulting in reduced SV at a given filling pressure. It is less well-appreciated that alterations in diastolic function in the absence of systolic abnormalities can also shift the Frank-Starling relationship. Specifically, if diastolic pressure is higher at a given volume due to alterations in any of the determinants of the LV diastolic pressure-volume relation, this will result in apparent depression of the Frank-Starling reltionship when the cardiac output or SV and filling pressure are used to assess this relationship. The reverse is

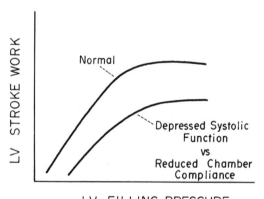

Figure 16.4. Schematic representation shows the Frank-Starling relationship as measured by the relation between filling pressure and stroke work. The Frank-Starling relationship is depressed if systolic function is impaired, but similar apparent depression can occur due to reduced diastolic chamber compliance alone. See text for further description.

true if diastolic pressure is reduced for a given diastolic volume. The reason for these apparent shifts of the Frank-Starling relationship in patients with diastolic dysfunction has to do with the fact that the clinician usually must depend on filling pressure rather than filling volume as an index of preload. Filling volume is a much more accurate index of preload as it relates to muscle or sarcomere length at the fiber level than filling pressure. If the relation between filling volume and filling pressure is altered as a result of diastolic abnormalities but systolic function is normal, the true relation between preload (or diastolic volume) and SV will remain normal in the presence of an abnormal relation between filling pressure and SV. Thus, in patients with abnormal diastolic function it is incorrect to assume that depression of the Frank-Starling relationship (as assessed by filling pressure and SV) necessarily indicates impaired systolic function. Finally, in some ways the most important point of significance in relation to diastolic functional abnormalities is the fact that evidence is now available which indicates that in both pressure and volume overload LV hypertrophy, alterations in passive muscle stiffness may signal the presence of significant fibrosis and identify the patient in whom irreversible changes in myocardial ultrastructure have occurred.[2] While this evidence is at present very preliminary, these findings suggest that determination of muscle stiffness in patients could possibly have a very significant role in decision-making in regard to timing of value replacement, for example.

ALTERATIONS IN DIASTOLIC FUNCTION IN LEFT VENTRICULAR HYPERTROPHY

While it is now possible to identify the various determinants of the diastolic pressure-volume relation and to quantify most of them, analysis of which of these determinants is abnormal in hypertrophic states is very much in a beginning stage. The following will serve to summarize what is known in three forms of LV hypertrophy, concentric hypertrophy due to chronic pressure overload, eccentric hypertrophy due to

chronic volume overload, and hypertrophic cardiomyopathy.

It has long been appreciated that diastolic pressure is increased at a given diastolic volume in concentric hypertrophy due to chronic pressure overload.[2,16] This is, in part, due to the fact that if wall thickness is increased without an increase in internal chamber size or geometry (which is the case in concentric hypertrophy), there is an obligatory decrease in passive chamber compliance even if passive muscle stiffness is unchanged. This situation is depicted schematically in Figure 16.5, in which two ventricles differing in wall thickness begin with the same internal radius and are acutely dilated to the same final radius. It is intuitively obvious that it will require a higher distending pressure to produce the same volume in the thicker walled ventricle and that a larger increase in distending pressure will be required to produce the same increment in volume (i.e., $\Delta P/\Delta V$ will be greater). This can also be demonstrated mathematically, by *Equation 3*. If muscle stiffness and ro are the same in the two ventricles and, by definition $\Delta(r/ro)$ is the same, then $\Delta(Pr/2h)$ must also be equal in the two ventricles. Using the principle of conservation of mass, it can be shown by simple geometric principles, that the change in wall thickness as dilatation occurs in the hypertrophied ventricle is such that the difference in pressure must be larger for the term $\Delta(Pr/2h)$ to remain equal. Thus, if nothing else but wall thickness is different in concentric hypertrophy, passive chamber compliance must be reduced. In addition to this obligatory decrease in chamber compliance, there is also evidence that in some cases of concentric hypertrophy, passive muscle stiffness is also increased.[2,16] This factor would lead to a further decrease in chamber compliance. At present, there is no information available about alterations in other determinants of the diastolic pressure-volume relation, for example, viscous properties, relaxation rate, etc., in pressure overload concentric hypertrophy. There is somewhat more information available in the case of eccentric hypertrophy due to chronic volume overload. By eccentric hypertrophy is meant a situation in which additional sar-

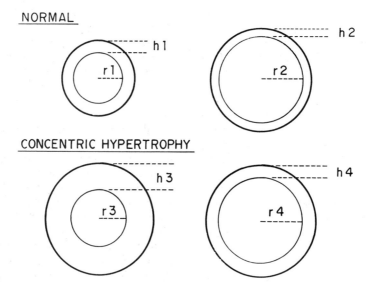

Figure 16.5. Schematic representation shows a normal and concentrically hypertrophied left ventricle. Both ventricles begin at the same internal radius (r1 and r3) and are dilated to the same internal radius (r2 and r4). Because wall thickness is greater in the hypertrophied ventricle, Δ pressure as dilation occurs must be greater in the hypertrophied ventricle (see text). r = internal radius; h = wall thickness.

comeres are added predominantly in series so that chamber volume increases without as large an increase in wall thickness as occurs in concentric hypertrophy. Further, the chronically volume-loaded ventricle generally becomes more spherical in shape (the ratio of major to minor axis decreases). There is also some evidence that passive muscle stiffness is increased in eccentric hypertrophy.[2] However, such calculations are complicated by the fact that the increase in internal radius in relation to wall thickness and the decrease in the major-minor axis ratio would have opposite effects on wall stress, while unstressed ventricular dimensions would be expected to increase by some uncertain amount, thus further confounding strain calculations. As shown in Figure 16.6, it is well documented that the diastolic pressure-volume relation is shifted to the right, in this form of hypertrophy (a lower pressure for a given volume).[19-21] Such observations have been made both from single diastolic cycles or in a static fashion providing a passive pressure-volume relation. Further, there is also evidence that the passive pressure-volume relation is steeper than

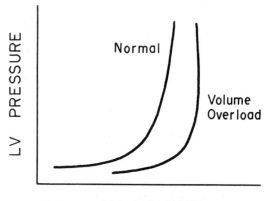

Figure 16.6. Schematic representation shows the passive pressure-volume relation in the normal and chronically volume-overloaded left ventricle. In chronic volume overload, the pressure-volume relation is both shifted to the right and steeper than normal.

normal, i.e., chamber compliance is reduced. Thus, in this form of hypertrophy there would appear to be an unusual combination of changes in the passive pressure-volume relation such that despite the fact that pressure is lower at a given volume (due to the rightward shift), chamber compliance is reduced. The rightward shift in the pressure-volume relation accounts for the observation that diastolic pressure is frequently surprisingly low in chronic regurgitant lesions such as aortic or mitral insufficiency despite markedly increased ventricular volumes. The mechanism of these changes in the passive pressure-volume relation are unclear, but could relate to the aforementioned geometric changes and/or the assumed increase in unstressed dimensions, both of which would tend to reduce the distending pressure needed to achieve a given volume. Similar to the situation with concentric hypertrophy, there is essentially no information in regard to alterations in other intrinsic determinants of the diastolic pressure-volume relation.

The pericardium may also play an important role in diastolic alterations in chronic volume overload hypertrophy. There is good evidence that in acute, severe volume overload lesions (before significant hypertrophy has taken place), the pericardium restrains ventricular filling and is an important cause of increased intracavitary diastolic pressure and reduced chamber compliance.[22, 23] Further, the hemodynamic profile in this condition is frequently very similar to that of constrictive pericarditis.[22] This role of the pericardium is basically identical to that which it performs in the normal heart subjected to acute volume expansion. The resemblance of acute volume overload to constrictive pericardial disease is generally not present in the chronic situation, after eccentric hypertrophy has occurred. Thus, in dogs with chronic volume overload hypertrophy due to a systemic arteriovenous fistula we have demonstrated that the influence of the pericardium on the diastolic pressure-volume relation is markedly reduced compared to acute volume overload.[23] One obvious and generally assumed explanation for the fact that the pericardium can accommodate the large, chronically volume-loaded heart more easily than the smaller, acutely volume-loaded heart is that the pericardium increases in size. While the pericardium is capable of a modest amount of simple stretch, however, this is probably not enough to account for the sizeable increases in pericardial volume which would be required to accommodate a volume-loaded heart which may be 50 to 100% larger than normal. We have recently obtained evidence that the pericardial pressure-volume relation is markedly shifted to the right in experimental chronic volume overload in association with increases of pericardial surface area of up to 50% and increases in pericardial mass.[24] The latter observations suggest that the pericardium undergoes either hypertrophy and/or hyperplasia in response to chronic volume overload and that this may be an important mechanism whereby the influence of the pericardium on the LV pressure-volume relation is reduced. Because of the relation of the pericardium to ventricular interaction, these findings also imply that interaction may be a less important determinant of the LV pressure-volume relation in the chronically volume-loaded heart. While extrapolation of these results obtained in experimental animal preparations to the clinical situation must be made with caution, they do demonstrate that the pericardium is capable of considerable adaptation to chronic stretch and that its influence on left ventricular diastolic pressure-volume relations may be sizeably altered.

In the case of hypertrophic cardiomyopathy, it is now clear that abnormalities in diastolic function are extremely important.[17] Chamber compliance appears to be markedly reduced in this disorder. This is, in part, due to the markedly increased wall thickness in relation to internal radius, i.e., the same considerations apply here as in concentric hypertrophy. Whether muscle stiffness is altered in this condition is unknown, and stress-strain analysis would be particularly difficult because of the frequently asymmetric nature of the hypertrophy. As with other hypertrophic states, there is virtually no information about other intrinsic determinants of diastolic pressure and volume, except that there is evidence that relaxation is impaired and could be a significantly more important determinant of diastolic pressure and volume than in the normal left ventricle. Interestingly, calcium channel blockers appear to reverse this abnormality of relaxation and, at the same time, lower diastolic pressure.

In summary, while there is considerable descriptive information about alterations in the LV diastolic pressure-volume relation in hypertrophic states, the precise mechanisms involved and which of the determinants of this relation are altered are largely unknown and constitute a fertile area for future investigation.

References

1. Glantz SA: Computing indices of diastolic stiffness has been counter productive. *Fed Proc* 39:162, 1980.
2. Hess OM, Schneider, J, Koch R, et al: Diastolic function and myocardial structure in patients with myocardial hypertrophy. *Circulation* 63:360, 1981.
3. Weiss JL, Frederiksen JW, Weisfeldt ML: Hemodynamic determinants of the time-course of fall in canine left ventricular pressure. *J Clin Invest* 58:751, 1976.
4. Karliner JS, LeWinter MM, Engler RL, et al: Pharmacologic and hemodynamic influences on the rate of isovolumic left ventricular relaxation in the normal conscious dog. *J Clin Invest* 60:511, 1977.
5. Tyberg JV, Keon WJ, Sonnenblik EH, et al: Mechanics of ventricular diastole. *Cardiovasc Res* 4:423, 1970.
6. Sabbah HN, Stein PD: Pressure-diameter relations during early diastole in dogs; Incompatability with the concept of passive left ventricular filling. *Circ Res* 48:357, 1981.
7. Rankin JS, Arentzen CE, McHale PA, et al: Viscoelastic properties of the diastolic left ventricle in the conscious dog. *Circ Res* 41:37, 1977.
8. Pouleur H, Karliner JS, LeWinter MM, et al: Diastolic viscous properties of the intact left ventricle. *Circ Res* 45:410, 1979.
9. LeWinter M, Engler R, Pavelec R: Time-dependent shifts of the left ventricular pressure-dimension relationship. *Circ Res* 45:641, 1979.
10. Glantz SA, Misbach GA, Moores WY, et al: The pericardium substantially affects the left ventricular pressure-volume relationship in the dog. *Circ Res* 42:422, 1978.
11. Shirato K, Shabetai R, Bhargava V, et al: Alteration of the left ventricular diastolic pressure-segment length relation produced by the pericardium. *Circulation* 57:1191, 1978.
12. Taylor RR, Covell JW, Sonnenblick EH, et al: Dependence of ventricular distensibility on filling of the opposite ventricle. *Am J Physiol* 213:711, 1967.
13. Janicki JS, Weber KT: The pericardium and ventricular interaction, distensibility, and function. *Am J Physiol* 38:H494, 1980.
14. Pabson J, Permutt S: The role of the pericardium in diastolic interdependence of the right and left ventricles. *Fed Proc* 37:778, 1978.
15. Vogel WM, Apstein CS, Briggs LL, et al: Acute alterations in left ventricular diastolic chamber stiffness: Role of the "erectile" effect of coronary arterial pressure and flow in normal and damaged hearts. *Circ Res* 51:465, 1982.
16. Peterson KL, Tsuji J, Johnson AD, et al: Diastolic left ventricular pressure-volume and stress-strain relations in patients with valvular aortic stenosis and left ventricular hypertrophy. *Circulation* 58:77, 1978.
17. Sanderson JE, Gibson DG, Brown DJ, et al: Left ventricular filling in hypertrophic cardiomyopathy: An angiographic study. *Br Heart J* 39:661, 1977.
18. Paulus WJ, Serizawa T, Grossman W: Altered left ventricular diastolic properties during pacing-induced ischemia in dogs with coronary stenoses. *Circ Res* 50:218, 1982.
19. Gault JH, Covell JW, Braunwall E, et al: Left ventricular performance following correction of free aortic regurgitation. *Circulation* 42:773, 1970.
20. McCullough WH, Covell JW, Ross J Jr: Left ventricular dilatation and diastolic compliance changes during chronic volume overloading. *Circulation* 54:943, 1972.
21. LeWinter MM, Engler R, Karliner JS: Enhanced left ventricular shortening in conscious dogs with chronic volume overload. *Am J Physiol* 238:H126, 1980.
22. Bartle SH, Hermann HJ: Acute mitral regurgitation in man. Hemodynamic evidence and observations indicating an early role for the pericardium. *Circulation* 36:839, 1967.
23. LeWinter MM, Pavelec R: Influence of the pericardium on left ventricular end-diastolic pressure-segment relations during early and later stages of experimental chronic volume overload in dogs. *Circ Res* 50:501, 1982.
24. Freeman G, LeWinter MM: Pericardial adaptations during chronic cardiac dilatation in dogs. *Circ Res* 54:294, 1984.
25. Bonow RO, Rosing DR, Bacharach SL, et al: Effects of verapamil on left ventricular systolic function and diastolic filling in patients with hypertrophic cardiomyopathy. *Circulation* 64:787, 1981.

CHAPTER 17

CORONARY ARTERY DISEASE AND NONCARDIAC SURGERY

JULIE A. SWAIN, M.D.

With the advent of vascular reconstructive surgery and the increasing use of coronary artery bypass, the patient with atherosclerotic vascular disease can often expect to have an increased life expectancy and a more normal lifestyle. The patient with coronary artery disease who needs a noncardiac operation, especially vascular surgery, presents a dilemma. Peripheral vascular reconstructive surgery used to be neglected because the life expectancy of a patient with coronary disease was poor. The increased awareness of the significance of coronary artery disease, as well as better diagnostic methods, have improved the treatment of these patients.

The coexistence of coronary disease and other conditions may affect the outcome of noncardiac operations. While this is most evident for vascular surgery, this includes any type of major surgery, such as pulmonary resections and major abdominal procedures. Patients with atherosclerotic vascular disease have a high incidence of associated coronary artery disease.[1] Likewise, the major mortality in vascular surgery is due to coronary artery disease. Another important consequence of the coexistence of these diseases are that the results of coronary artery bypass can be compromised by severe peripheral vascular disease, especially carotid lesions.

It has long been recognized that patients with coronary artery disease have a greater mortality from procedures requiring general anesthesia.[2] The operative risk depends on the severity of the coronary disease, the type of operative procedure, the severity of a patient's previous myocardial infarction (MI), and the interval between the infarction and the operation.[3]

The following will outline the risk data for patients with coronary artery disease and present the data related to staged and concurrent coronary artery bypass operations and the noncardiac procedure.

Several large-scale studies in the 1950s and 1960s showed that the risk of general anesthetic in the overall population was greater for those patients with coronary artery disease.[4–8] These mortality statistics can now be questioned in light of recent advances in anesthetic and pharmacological treatment in the patient with coronary disease. Because the older data on general anesthetics in coronary patients are suspect because of advances in anesthesia, a recent study by Tarhan[3] showed in two separate study groups in 1972 and 1978 that there was no difference in reinfarction rate or mortality. This indicates that new anesthetic techniques have had a relatively small impact on this morbidity and mortality.

What is known is that patients who suffer an MI with general anesthesia have a higher mortality. A series of studies by the Mayo Clinic[9] followed patients undergoing noncardiac surgery who had had a previous MI. When the noncardiac procedure was performed less than 3 months after MI, there was a 27% reinfarction rate with 69% of these patients dying from their reinfarction. When the surgical procedure was withheld until 3 or 6 months after infarction, there was an 11% reinfarction rate. When the procedure was separated from the MI by a time period longer than 6 months, a 5% reinfarction rate remained. This is several times higher than that of the general population undergoing general anesthesia.

Patients undergoing vascular reconstructive procedures have a higher incidence of cardiac-related morbidity and mortality. This is due to several factors. Patients with diffuse peripheral vascular atherosclerotic occlusive disease also have a greater chance of having coronary atherosclerosis. Also, major vascular surgery leads to increased blood loss and more afterload changes than general surgical procedures. Several studies have shown that a major cause of operative mortality for abdominal aortic aneurysm resection and carotid endartectomy is MI.[10-13] Similarly, late followup on patients undergoing these two procedures have shown that the major mortality is related to cardiac causes. Thompson et al.[10] demonstrated that 52% of the late deaths in a large series of carotid endarterectomies were due to cardiac causes.

Therefore, by being able to identify the patient with coronary artery disease, one might be able to diminish the cardiac morbidity and mortality by treatment of the coronary artery disease.

Preliminary screening of all preoperative vascular patients should include a history for cardiac disease. In 1981, the Cooperative Coronary Artery Surgery Study (CASS) outlined the angiographic findings of coronary disease relating to the symptoms of definite angina, probable angina, and nonspecific chest pain.[14] All patients with unstable angina or previous MIs were excluded. In men with definite angina there was a 93% incidence of significant coronary artery disease. In women with definite angina the incidence was 72%. Significant coronary disease was defined as greater than 70% stenosis in one vessel or greater than 50% stenosis in the left main coronary artery.

The CASS study revealed that noninvasive diagnosis for left main or triple-vessel disease was suggested by several noninvasive tests. This included ST segment depression during exercise, ischemia in the recovery period from exercise, decreased blood pressure with exercise, a positive stress isotope study, and decreased ejection fraction on venticulography. However, the number of false-negatives in this study varied from 0 to 17% for each of these tests. Therefore, the conclusion of the CASS study was that "in older patients with a high prevalence of left main or three-vessel coronary disease, the large number of undetected patients may warrant angiography regardless of the (noninvasive) test results."

The Cleveland Clinic is conducting a study to address the problem of the vascular surgery patient with coronary artery disease.[15] All patients admitted to undergo an abdominal aortic aneurysm resection, aortofemoral reconstruction, femoropopliteal bypass, or carotid endarterectomy, undergo preoperative coronary angiography. In the first 100 patients with abdominal aortic aneurysms, 31 have undergone coronary artery bypass with no mortality. In a similar study, Tomatis et al.[1] in 1972 performed coronary angiography on 100 selected patients prior to vascular surgery. Fifty percent of these patients were found to have significant coronary artery disease. In light of these statistics, a careful diagnostic workup, including noninvasive tests and possibly including coronary angiography, is indicated in patients who are to undergo vascular surgery. By identifying patients with coronary artery disease preoperatively, the opportunity exists to decrease the morbidity and mortality associated with general anesthesia and noncardiac surgery in these patients.

In patients with known coronary artery disease, the dilemma of treating both coronary artery disease and other noncardiac disease is presented. In patients with mild to moderate coronary artery disease, pharmacological management including beta-blockers and calcium channel antagonists may be adequate. With the increasing interest in angioplasty, some patients may be candidates for percutaneous transluminal coronary angioplasty prior to their vascular surgical procedure. In the patient with severe coronary artery disease, several options are present. The data previously presented indicate that when these patients are untreated they have an unacceptably high morbidity and mortality from cardiac disease during their noncardiac operative procedure. Therefore, definitive treatment must be undertaken. Definitive treatment currently is regarded as coronary artery bypass surgery. This can either be staged, such that the coronary bypass is performed before the vascular procedure, or the vascular procedure (such as carotid endarterectomy) may take precedence, in which case it is followed by the coronary bypass surgery; or both procedures can be performed concurrently.

If coronary artery bypass surgery is performed in the presence of vascular disease, there are several possible complications. When an abdominal aortic aneurysm is present, this may rupture secondary to transient hypertension in the perioperative period. Likewise, there is a hypercoagulable state after bypass and this in combination with transient hypotension may precipitate thrombosis of the aneurysm. Also, the altered perfusion from the aortic cannulation may create distal embolization. In the patient with carotid stenosis, a cerebrovascular accident may be precipitated by changes in perfusion pressure (either hyper- or hypotension) or by distal embolization.

There have been several studies of patients who have prior coronary bypass and then undergo an operative procedure.[16–20] These data suggest that patients with prior coronary bypass have a lower risk of mortality from MI than the unselected population. In addition to decreasing the cardiac morbidity and mortality during the operative procedure, the patients with prior coronary bypass have a better long-term outlook. The study by Crawford et al.[19] showed that late deaths occurred in only 13% of the patients. The study by McCollum et al.[20] included only those patients followed longer than 5 years. There was a 3% long-term mortality in these patients which can be compared to an expected 25% long-term mortality.

The final class of patients to consider are those patients with either severe or unstable coronary artery disease accompanied by severe peripheral vascular disease. In these patients, doing the vascular procedure first would place them in jeopardy for MI,[10–13] but performing the vascular procedure first may put them at risk for morbidity secondary to vascular complications.[21] By doing a combined coronary bypass and noncardiac procedure, presumably one could decrease the myocardial and vascular complications, obviate the need for a second anesthetic, and decrease the number of nosocomial infections and other postoperative complications, such as pulmonary embolism. Advocates of combined procedures point out that there would be a lower total cost, less discomfort, and presumably, a faster recovery.[22]

Several series have demonstrated that combined coronary bypass and noncardiac procedures can be done safely.[22–29] Most of the procedures were vascular, however, several lung resections and gastrointestinal operations have been combined with coronary bypass. However, combined procedures may lead to complications. Because coronary bypass patients must be heparinized, bleeding through implanted grafts or suture lines may be increased. The increased length of the procedures may lead to pulmonary and infection complications. Combining a bowel procedure with an implanted foreign body, such as a cardiac valve or Dacron graft, might be complicated by seeding infection.

In the patient with stable coronary artery disease who is to undergo major, noncardiac surgery, pharmacological treatment with beta-blocking agents and calcium antagonists preoperatively, combined with careful anesthetic technique, may be all that is required. However, some patients may be candidates for percutaneous transluminal coronary angioplasty to diminish the risk of postoperative cardiac complications. In the patient with severe coronary artery disease who needs elective vascular surgery, a staged procedure may be contemplated where a coronary artery bypass is performed followed by the vascular procedure at a later date. Current data seem to indicate that waiting 6 weeks to 3 months when possible between operations is optimum. The most life-threatening conditions occur when a patient has severe unstable coronary artery disease combined with unstable vascular disease such as severe carotid stenosis or expanding abdominal aortic aneurysm. In these cases, it seems warranted to consider a combined approach during one operative procedure to correct both the coronary and vascular lesions.

References

1. Tomatis LA, Fierens EE, Verbrugge GP: Evaluation of surgical risk in peripheral vascular disease by coronary arteriography: A series of 100 cases. *Surgery* 71:429, 1972.
2. Tarhan S, Moffitt EA, Taylor WF, et al: Myocardial infarction after general anesthesia. *JAMA* 22:1451, 1972.
3. Tarhan S: Risk of anesthesia in patients with heart disease. *Cleve Clin Q* 48:50, 1981.
4. Dana JB, Ohler RL: Influence of heart disease on surgical risk. *JAMA* 162:878, 1956.
5. Arkins R, Smessaert AA, Hicks RG: Mortality and morbidity in surgical patients with coronary artery disease. *JAMA* 190:485, 1964.
6. Nachlas MM, Abrams SJ, Golberg MM: The influence of arteriosclerotic heart disease on surgical risk. *Am J Surg* 101:447, 1961.
7. Etsten B, Proger S: Operative risk in patients with coronary heart disease. *JAMA* 159:845, 1955.
8. Alexander S: Surgical risk in the patient with arteriosclerotic heart disease. *Surg Clin North Am* 48:513, 1968.
9. Steen PA, Tinker JH, Tarhan S: Myocardial reinarction after anesthesia and surgery. *JAMA* 239:2566, 1978.
10. Thompson JE, Austin DJ, Patman RD: Carotid endarterectomy for cerebrovascular insufficiency: Long-term results in 592 patients followed up to thirteen years. *Ann Surg* 172:663, 1970.
11. Hertzer NR, Lees CD: Fatal myocardial infarction following carotid endarterectomy. *Ann Surg* 194:212, 1981.
12. Young AE, Sandberg GW, Couch NP: The reduction of mortality of abdominal aortic aneurysm resection. *Am J Surg* 134:585, 1977.
13. Sundt TM, Sandok BA, Whisnant JP: Carotid endarterectomy. Complications and preoperative assessment of risk. *Mayo Clinic Proc* 50:301, 1975.
14. Chaitman BR, Bourassa MG, Davis K, et al: Angiographic prevalence of high-risk coronary artery disease in patient subsets (CASS). *Circulation* 64:360, 1981.
15. Coronary angiography. In: *Surgery Practice News*, p 1, January, 1982.
16. Mahar LJ, Steen PA, Tinker JH, et al: Perioperative myocardial infarction in patients with coronary artery disease with and without aorta-coronary artery bypass grafts. *J Thorac Cardiovasc Surg* 76:533, 1978.
17. Edwards WH, Mulherin JL, Walker WE: Vascular reconstructive surgery following myocardial revascularization. *Ann Surg* 187:653, 1978.
18. Scher KS, Tice DA: Operative risk in patients with previous coronary artery bypass. *Arch Surg* 111:807, 1976.
19. Crawford ES, Morris GC Jr, Howell JF, et al: Operative risk in patients with previous coronary artery bypass. *Ann Thorac Surg* 26:215, 1978.
20. McCollum CH, Garcia-Rinaldi R, Graham JM, et al: Myocardial revascularization prior to subsequent major surgery in patients with coronary artery disease. *Surgery* 31:302, 1977.
21. Javid H, Tufo HM, Najafi H, et al: Neurological abnormalities following open-heart surgery. *J Thorac Cardiovasc Surg* 58:502, 1969.
22. Korompai FL, Hayward RH, Knight WL: Noncardiac operations combined with coronary artery bypass. *Surg Clin North Am* 62:215, 1982.
23. Mehigan JT, Buch WS, Pipkin RD: A planned approach to coexistent cerebrovascular disease in coronary artery bypass candidates. *Arch Surg* 112:1403, 1977.
24. Urschel HC, Razzuk MA, Gardner MA: Management of concomitant occlusive disease of the carotid and coronary arteries. *J Thorac Cardiovasc Surg* 72:829, 1976.
25. Bernhard VM, Johnson WD, Peterson JJ: Carotid artery stenosis. Association with surgery for coronary artery disease. *Arch Surg* 105:837, 1972.
26. Okies JE, MacManus Q, Starr A: Myocardial revascularization and carotid endarterectomy: A combined approach. *Ann Thorac Surg* 23:560, 1977.
27. Morris GC Jr, Ennix CL Jr, Lawrie GM, et al: Management of coexistent carotid and coronary artery occlusive atherosclerosis. *Cleve Clin Q* 45:125, 1978.
28. Dalton ML, Parker TM, Mistrot JJ, et al: Concomitant coronary artery bypass and major noncardiac surgery. *J Thorac Cardiovasc Surg* 75:621, 1978.
29. Reis RL, Hannah H III: Management of patients with severe, coexistent coronary artery and peripheral vascular disease. *J Thorac Cardiovasc Surg* 73:909, 1977.

CHAPTER 18

PERIOPERATIVE VASODILATOR THERAPY

JAMES D. WISHEART, B.Sc., M.Ch., F.R.C.S.

In 1964, Ross and Braunwald[1] demonstrated the adverse effect of acute elevation of arterial pressure on left ventricular (LV) performance in patients with a diseased myocardium. Subsequently, vasodilator therapy has become established in the treatment of patients with LV failure, in whom it achieves improved systemic hemodynamics, better ventricular function, and in certain circumstances, a more favorable balance of oxygen demand and supply to the myocardium. The high incidence of hypertension associated with coronary artery grafting led to the application of vasodilator therapy to surgery. This is a critical review of the present knowledge of the effects of vasodilator therapy in surgical patients. Vasodilator drugs dilate systemic arterioles, pulmonary arterioles, and veins.

The range of vasodilator drugs include hydralazine, which is nearly a pure arteriolar dilator, and at the other extreme, nitroglycerine, which in low doses is a nearly pure venous dilator. Most vasodilator agents including sodium nitroprusside and higher-dose nitroglycerine are both arteriolar and venous dilators.

The primary effect of the action of these drugs is to reduce systemic vascular resistance and thus reduce arterial pressure. These drugs reduce venous tone, increase venous capacitance, and thus decrease the cardiac filling pressures. They also reduce pulmonary vascular resistance and thus reduce pulmonary artery pressure. The secondary or indirect effects in certain circumstances are to increase the stroke volume (SV) because of the reduction in afterload. By the reduction in cardiac filling pressure, the vasodilators reduce the diastolic pressure and dimension of the ventricles and also therefore, the systolic dimensions of the ventricles. In certain circumstances, vasodilators improve the balance of oxygen supply and demand to the myocardium, particularly in the subendocardium. Vasodilators prevent or control crises of elevation of pulmonary vascular resistance in children.

PHYSIOLOGICAL CHANGES OCCURRING AT AND AFTER CARDIOPULMONARY BYPASS

In order to place the effects of vasodilator drugs in their perioperative setting, we need to recognize the physiological changes which occur as a result of cardiopulmonary bypass and which influence systemic arteriolar tone, venous tone, myocardial oxygen demand and supply, and pulmonary arteriolar tone.

Systemic Arteriolar Tone and Stroke Volume

During and after cardiopulmonary bypass an increase in systemic vascular resistance due to arteriolar vasoconstriction has been widely observed and has both humoral and neural causes.[2–13] During cardiopulmonary

217

bypass arteriolar vasoconstriction may lead to impaired or nonhomogeneous tissue perfusion. In the postoperative period following the correction of valvular and congenital abnormalities, arteriolar constriction will increase arterial pressure and afterload, and will lead to a decrease in SV.[14-17] There will be an increase in LV systolic wall tension and in LV end-diastolic pressure and volume. This deterioration in both the systolic and diastolic function of the left ventricle may contribute to an imbalance of oxygen supply and demand to the myocardium.

Whereas systemic hypertension may follow other forms of heart surgery in less than 10% of cases, after coronary artery surgery it is likely to occur in 50% or more cases. Hypertension following coronary artery surgery is associated with an increase in systemic vascular resistance, but in contrast to valve and congenital patients the SV may be increased due to more effective ventricular performance. The level of hypertension may threaten to produce surgical bleeding, however more significant is its potential for increasing myocardial oxygen demand in patients who are already subject to myocardial ischemia.[18-21]

The Venous Tone

When considering the cardiovascular system attention is usually focused on the heart and the arterial circulation. As a result the dynamic role of the venous system in the regulation of the circulation is less well appreciated. The venous system normally contains 70 to 80% of the total blood volume and by its ability to make rapid adjustments in its capacity, it ensures that the central blood volume is maintained at a level appropriate for proper filling of the ventricles. Control of venous capacity is not by local metabolic changes as in arterioles, but chiefly by sympathetic action on the smooth muscle of the veins.[22]

Following open heart surgery it was demonstrated by Reid and his colleagues[23] in 1967, that there was increased venomotor tone leading to reduced venous capacitance. This was associated with a reduced total blood volume while the central blood volume was maintained and the cardiac filling pressure increased.[24] Making similar observations in 1982[25], Doty et al. observed that venous capacitance was reduced by the general effects of the operation and not chiefly by cardiopulmonary bypass itself. This observation is consistent with the fact that the mechanisms for controlling arteriolar and venous smooth muscle are different, and that increases in arteriolar tone and in venous tone do not necessarily occur in parallel as two facets of generalized changes in vaso motor activity.

It may be of major importance that there is a reduction in venous capacitance and total blood volume following cardiopulmonary bypass. First, an incompletely filled venous system may mean that its dynamic role in regulating the circulation cannot be maintained, in the face of such common postoperative events as hemorrhage, spontaneous arteriolar and venous dilation and dysrhythmias. Second, elevation of venous tone may elevate ventricular filling pressures beyond the top of the LV function curve in certain patients.

Myocardial Oxygen Demand and Supply

The physiological determinants of oxygen demand for the myocardium are heart rate, LV systolic wall tension, determined by LV systolic pressure and LV size, and myocardial contractility. Myocardial oxygen supply is determined chiefly by diastolic time per minute which in turn is inversely related to the heart rate, diastolic arterial pressure, less the diastolic ventricular pressure, and oxygen content of the blood and the position of the oxygen dissociation curve.[26-30]

Commonly-used and easily-derived indices of oxygen demand are the tension-time-index and the rate-pressure product. An index of oxygen supply is the diastolic-pressure-time-index.

A common error is to consider oxygen demand or oxygen supply in isolation. It is not sufficient to say that some physiological or pharmacological manipulation reduces oxygen demand or that alternately, it increases oxygen supply; it is necessary to consider the balance of demand and supply. For instance, many interventions which reduce oxygen demand, also reduce oxygen supply—therefore it is the final balance which determines the benefit to the patient.

How do these changes in vascular tone following cardiopulmonary bypass influence oxygen demand and supply? Increases in arteriolar tone and in ventricular dimension may lead to increased oxygen demand due to an increase in LV systolic wall tension. Increases in ventricular filling pressure associated with increased venous tone and increases in heart rate, will both reduce oxygen delivery while any increase in heart rate will increase oxygen demand. On the other hand, the increased diastolic arterial pressure associated with arteriolar vasoconstriction may increase oxygen supply. Thus, the effect of open heart surgery on the blood vessels tends to alter the balance, leading to an excess of demand over supply.

Pulmonary Arteriolar Tone

The state of the pulmonary arterioles is chiefly of relevance following the correction in infants and young children of those congenital abnormalities associated with increased pulmonary vascular resistance and a labile pulmonary vascular bed. All the neural and humoral factors influencing systemic arterioles are present and a number of additional factors are recognized although our knowledge in this area is somewhat inadequate. An acute increase in pulmonary vascular resistance due to pulmonary arteriolar constriction may occur with a decrease in arterial oxygen tension, a decrease in pH, with anxiety or pain, with respiratory inadequacy, fighting the ventilator, etc. This increase in the afterload of the right ventricle can lead to acute right ventricular failure and critical deterioration in the condition of the child.

PERIOPERATIVE VASODILATOR THERAPY

The potential scope of this chapter includes the preoperative control of arterial pressure in dissections of the aorta; the preoperative management of LV failure, with or without the balloon pump, the use of vasodilators on bypass to ensure uniform cooling and rewarming, to control perfusion pressure and to maintain homogeneous tissue perfusion and many other topics, including the need for adequate monitoring if vasodilator drugs are to be used properly. However, the use of vasodilator therapy will be considered only in relation to its effect on systemic and pulmonary hemodynamics, and on myocardial function throughout the operative period. The use of vasodilators will be discussed with the following emphases: the heart as a pump and the ability of vasodilators to improve and stabilize the cardiac output by their action on arterioles and veins; the balance of oxygen demand and supply to the LV myocardium—can vasodilators help maintain a proper balance? and the prevention and treatment of episodic rises in pulmonary vascular resistance in children.

The Heart as a Pump

ARTERIOLAR TONE IN ADULTS

In 1980 Marco studied a group of patients following valve replacement and used hydralazine as a pure arteriolar dilator.[31] Systemic vascular resistance together with arterial pressure fell but left atrial pressure remained stable. With this constant LV filling pressure, and reduced afterload, stroke index increased from 26.9 to 34.0 ml/M^{-2}. In 1972 Kouchoukos et al.[32] studied the effects of reducing arterial pressure within hours of surgery for valve replacement. Trimethaphan was used, which is both an arteriolar and venous dilator; it reduced both arterial and left atrial pressures. In patients whose LV function was impaired (mean left atrial pressure = 25 mm Hg) the stroke index increased from 17 to 20 ml/M^{-2} and the left atrial pressure fell from 25 to 16 mm Hg. In those with good LV function (mean left atrial pressure = 10 mm Hg), the stroke index actually fell from 30 to 25 ml/M^{-2} and the left atrial pressure fell from 10 to 6 mm Hg. (Fig. 18.1).

The distinction in the response to vasodilator therapy which Kouchoukos et al.[32] made between those with and without LV failure is a most important observation which has been confirmed by a number of other studies in a variety of circumstances.

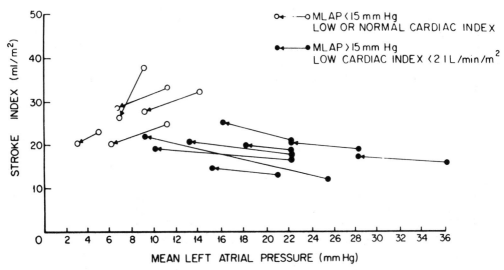

Figure 18.1. Effect of trimethaphan infusion is shown after open heart surgery on stroke index and left atrial pressure in two groups of patients: those with a mean left atrial pressure under 15 mm Hg and over 15 mm Hg. Reproduced with permission from Kouchoukos et al.[32]

In 1977 Roberts et al.[29] showed that sodium nitroprusside is effective in controlling hypertension following coronary surgery and that it will increase SV only in those with impaired LV function. LV filling pressure fell, and the heart rate rose in all patients: however the heart rate was higher in those with a low LV filling pressure. More recently Campbell and his colleagues[33] from Glasgow studying a group of patients after coronary artery surgery in whom we believe that the left atrial pressure was low found a significant increase in heart rate after the administration of sodium nitroprusside. These studies indicate that agents which are both arteriolar and venous dilators will reduce both the arterial pressure and also the LV filling pressure. In patients with good LV function this would seem to cause them to move to the left and downward along a LV function curve resulting in a reduced stroke index with a lower LV filling pressure[34, 35] (Fig. 18.2A); in addition there may be an increase in heart rate. On the other hand patients with impaired LV function benefit from this maneuver in as much as they either move to the left, that is, to a better position, on a function curve of a failing left ventricle, or else they move to a

more favorable LV function curve. In either case they achieve a higher SV with a lower LV filling pressure (Fig. 18.2B). These relationships are well illustrated in a slightly different way in Figure 18.3[36] which shows how pure venodilators simply move the position to the left along a LV function curve; a pure arteriolar dilator shifts the position to a more favorable curve, and an agent like sodium nitroprusside or prazocin achieves a combination of these two effects.

ARTERIOLAR TONE IN CHILDREN

Appelbaum and colleagues[37] studied children under 18 months of age within 3 hours of surgery for the correction of congenital abnormalities. They found that an infusion of sodium nitroprusside caused arterial and left atrial pressure and systemic vascular resistance to fall, while cardiac index rose from 1.92 to 2.25 L/minute^{-1}M^{-2}. When the LV filling pressure was restored there was a further increment in cardiac index to 2.71 L/minute^{-1}M^{-2} without a significant rise in arterial pressure or systemic vascular resistance. Thus the vasodilator created a "preload reserve" which when used achieved the further increase in cardiac index (Fig. 18.4).[38] This illustrates the principle that

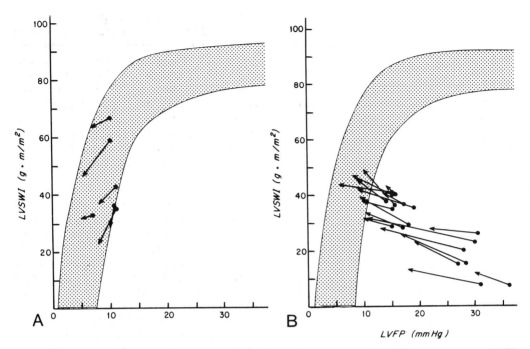

Figure 18.2. LV stroke work index (*LVSWI*) is plotted against LV filling pressure (*LVFP*) before and during intraoperative nitroprusside administration: (*A*) to seven patients with coronary artery disease and normal LV function; (*B*) to 18 patients with coronary artery disease and chronic LV dysfunction. All patients demonstrated improvement of LV function. Each *dot* presents control values, while the *arrowhead* represents values obtained during nitroprusside administration. Reproduced with permission from Lappas et al.[34]

afterload should be minimized and preload maximized, or optimized.

In 1979 Benzing et al.[39] showed that by adding an inotropic agent to the sodium nitroprusside a further significant incremental increase in cardiac output could be achieved.

An interesting report came from Williams et al.[40] from the Mayo Clinic who investigated nine patients after the Fontan procedure (that is, right atrial to pulmonary artery bypass) when cardiac output is critically dependent on the level of pulmonary vascular resistance. They used dopamine (7.5 $\mu g/kg^{-1}minute^{-1}$), sodium nitroprusside (up to 5 $\mu g/kg^{-1}minute^{-1}$) both alone and in combination. They demonstrated the ability of sodium nitroprusside to reduce pulmonary vascular resistance from 375 to 169 dynes/second/cm^{-5}/M^{-2} and, to increase the cardiac output in these unusual circum-stances from 1.98 to 2.57 liters/min-$ute^{-1}M^{-2}$.

Thus we may conclude that in patients with poor LV function vasodilators lead directly to an improvement in cardiac performance; if the principle of minimum afterload and maximum or optimum preload is maintained, and the preload reserve fully utilized, then a further improvement in cardiac performance will be achieved. In patients with good LV function it will be necessary to manipulate both preload and afterload (or even add an ionotrope) to improve performance; maintenance of the filling pressures may also be necessary to prevent a tachycardia in this group.

VENOUS TONE

Nitroglycerine in low doses acts by relaxing the smooth muscle of the venous wall leading to pooling of blood in the venous

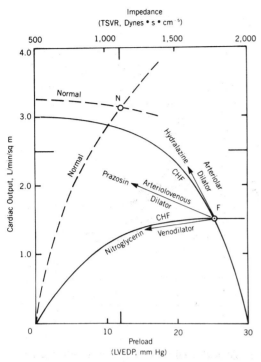

Figure 18.3. The relationship of LV preload (*LVEDP*) and aortic impedance (*TSVR*) to cardiac output is shown in normal and failing left ventricle. In normal heart (*Point N*), cardiac output is principally regulated by changes in preload (left-to-right ascending *broken line* relating LVEDP to cardiac output; alterations in impedance are of minor importance (left-to-right horizontal *broken line* relating TSVR to cardiac output. In contrast, in failing heart (*Point F*) with congestive heart failure (*CHF*), cardiac output is principally regulated by changes in impedance (right-to-left ascending *unbroken line* relating TSVR to cardiac output; alterations in preload are of minor importance (depressed left-to-right *horizontal line* relating LVEDP to cardiac output). In failing heart, pure arteriolodilator, hydralazine hydrochloride, raises lowered cardiac output markedly with mild decline of elevated LVEDP (*vertical arrow from Point F*); balanced arteriolovenous dilator, prazosin hydrochloride, raises lowered cardiac output and decreases elevated LVEDP considerably (*diagonal arrow from Point F*); and pure venodilator, sublingual

system and a reduction in preload. Miller et al.[41] in 1975 found in nonsurgical patients with failing left ventricles that administration of sodium nitroprusside reduced forearm venous tone and that forearm venous volume increased. The fall in venous tone correlated well with a reduction in end-diastolic volume. Reduction in the diastolic size of the ventricle leads to reduction in the systolic size of the ventricle, and thus both systolic wall tension and oxygen requirement fall.

Gall et al.[42] have shown in patients following mitral valve replacement that administration of nitroglycerine in moderate doses beginning less than 1 hour after surgery achieves a dramatic increase in venous capacitance from 0.5 to 2.0 units. It also reduces peripheral resistance and left atrial pressure, with a modest rise in cardiac output.

There were similar findings[42] in patients given nitroglycerine following coronary artery surgery, when venous capacitance dramatically increased. Another group had actual postoperative hypertension, treated by sodium nitroprusside which brought the total peripheral resistance, cardiac index, and left atrial pressure close to the levels produced by nitroglycerine, but it failed to increase venous capacitance from control levels. This demonstrates the more powerful venodilator effect of glyceryl trinitrate. Kaplan[50] and others have shown that venodilatation will reduce LV pressure and volumes and therefore both reduce myocardial oxygen need and improve supply.

While the controversy regarding the relative merits of pure arterial dilation, mixed arterial and venous dilation, or strong venodilation has not yet been resolved, it is important to bear in mind that both arteriolar constriction and venous constriction are involved in the overall vasoconstrictive responses which influence blood flow follow-

nitroglycerin, decreases elevated LVEDP markedly with little or no improvement of lowered cardiac output (*horizontal arrow from Point F*). Reproduced with permission from Mason et al.[36]

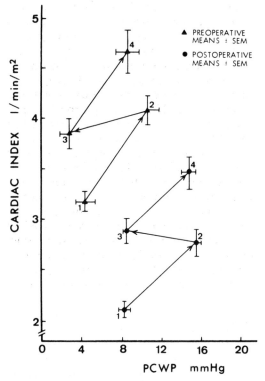

CARDIAC INDEX l/min/m²

PCWP mmHg

▲ PREOPERATIVE
   MEANS ± SEM
● POSTOPERATIVE
   MEANS ± SEM

Figure 18.4. The maximum effects of preload elevation, afterload reduction and preload restoration on cardiac index pre- and postoperatively are shown. Stages 1 show the relationship between CI and pulmonary capillary wedge pressure (*PCWP*) initially, stages 2 after maximum volume loading, stages 3 after maximum vasodilation with nitroprusside and stages 4 after preload restoration during constant nitroprusside infusion. Nitroprusside produced highly significant upward movements of the LV function curves both pre- and postoperatively. Reproduced with permission from Meretoja and Laaksonen.[38]

ing cardiac operations. Vasodilators designed to return the circulation to normal should achieve the desired effect on the whole cardiovascular system.

Myocardial Function

The effect of vasodilators on the myocardial oxygen demand and supply ratio in any individual patient is the most fundamentally important part of this whole discussion. Theoretically we recognize that vasodilators acting on arterioles and veins will reduce myocardial oxygen demand by reducing LV systolic wall tension: on the other hand demand may be increased by increases in heart rate, and supply decreased by a reduced arterial diastolic pressure: supply will be improved by the decrease in LV diastolic pressure. What actually happens? We must recognize that detailed knowledge of myocardial oxygen demand and supply in the individual patient is very limited. There are a number of imperfect ways by which myocardial oxygen demand and supply may be observed in different circumstances.

Global myocardial blood flow and oxygen use may be measured; unfortunately, global measurements fail to reflect the purely local changes which occur in any type of regional ischemia. Regional myocardial blood flow or oxygen utilization may be measured or estimated indirectly. Indices may be derived from systemic hemodynamic data, such as the rate pressure product or the diastolic pressure time index.

In 1974 Rowe and Henderson[43] studied the effects of sodium nitroprusside in dogs. They observed that global coronary blood flow increased and coronary vascular resistance decreased; reduced oxygen extraction resulted in a higher coronary sinus oxygen content and tension. Hess et al.[44] in 1983 made a similar series of observations in dogs, and in addition observed that sodium nitroprusside caused an increase in the ratio of epicardial to endocardial blood flow (Fig. 18.5) i.e., diverted blood to the outer one-third where it almost certainly was not needed; glyceryl trinitrate did not have this effect. This could mean that the increase in blood flow with sodium nitroprusside was largely epicardial, or that the global measurement, which fails to reflect regional areas of lower flow, was disproportionately influenced by the high epicardial flows. In either instance the global parameters must be received critically.

Attempts were made to observe the effects of sodium nitroprusside and glyceryl trinitrate in an acutely ischaemic area in dogs by DaLuz and his colleagues[45] in 1975 and Chiariello et al.[46] in 1976. DaLuz et al.[45]

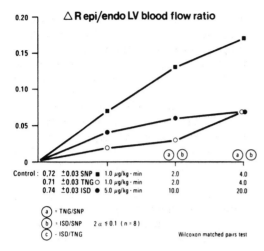

Figure 18.5. Changes are shown in the epicardial/endocardial LV blood flow ratio (Δ R epi/endo) in dogs after 10-minute infusion of sodium nitroprusside and glyceryl trinitrate at doses of 1, 2, and 4 mμcg/kg^{-1}/minute^{-1} and isosorbide dinitrate at 5, 10, and 20 mμcg/kg/minute. Comparison with initial values (control, x ± s$_x$); Δ values = x̄. Reproduced with permission from Hess et al.[44]

reported that in dogs with acute ischemia, sodium nitroprusside increased the regional venous outflow from the ischemic area. However, Chiariello et al.[46] also studying dogs, found that sodium nitroprusside decreased blood flow to the region of ischemia whereas glyceryl trinitrate increased blood flow to this area. In addition, glyceryl trinitrate increased the endo- to epicardial blood flow ratio. Alongside these dynamic observations he noted that the ST segment on the EKG tended to be elevated with sodium nitroprusside and not with glyceryl trinitrate. Mann et al.[47] in 1977 studied patients with coronary artery disease and also demonstrated that sodium nitroprusside reduced myocardial blood flow to the ischemic region whereas glyceryl trinitrate increased it. Other investigators, notably Flaherty et al.[48] and Kaplan and Jones[49] have consistently observed that abnormalities of the ST segments are improved by nitroglycerine whereas this is not always the case with sodium nitroprusside (Fig. 18.6).

The final way of observing the effects of vasodilator drugs upon the myocardium is to look at the various indices of myocardial oxygen demand and supply. Miller et al.[41] in 1975 using sodium nitroprusside in patients with coronary artery disease noted that the LV tension-time index decreased from 3300 to 2600 and that the LV end-diastolic volume index decreased from 113 to 92 (Fig. 18.7). He also noted that the heart rate tended to be higher in patients with a low LV end-diastolic pressure. This observation was noted in the study from Glasgow by Campbell et al.[33], where administration of sodium nitroprusside to patients following coronary artery surgery resulted in an increase in the rate pressure product due to elevation of the heart rate, and therefore an increase in myocardial oxygen demand. It is important to remember that the

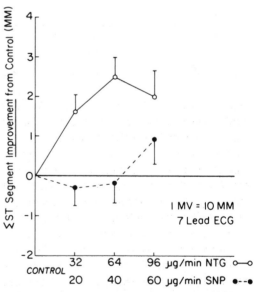

Figure 18.6. Summation of ST-segment improvement from control values is shown for both nitroglycerin and sodium nitroprusside in patients having coronary artery surgery. Nitroglycerin significantly improved the ST segment at all doses. With the two smaller doses of sodium nitroprusside the ST-segment depression was unchanged. Reproduced with permission from Kaplan and Jones.[49]

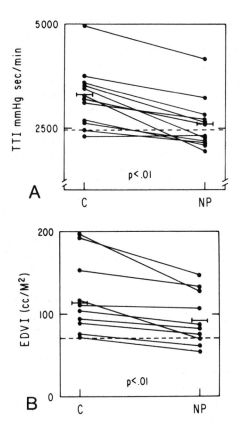

Figure 18.7. The effect of nitroprusside in chronic ischemic heart disease on two indices of myocardial oxygen consumption is shown. *Panel A*, tension time index (*TTI*) and *Panel B*, end-diastolic volume index (*EDVI*). *Dashed horizontal lines* represent upper limits of normal. Reproduced with permission from Miller et al.[41]

unthinking use of sodium nitroprusside in patients without a failing heart and with a low LV filling pressure, can lead to an increased heart rate with an increase in myocardial oxygen demand and possibly not even an increase in SV. This can be prevented by maintaining the LV filling pressure at an adequate level which will both increase the SV and reduce oxygen demand by preventing the tachycardia. Kaplan and Jones,[49] in a number of studies on patients with coronary artery disease undergoing surgery and prior to bypass, found that both sodium nitroprusside and nitroglycerine reduced the rate pressure product and the

tension-time index (Fig. 18.8). The diastolic arterial pressure (coronary artery perfusion pressure) is an index of oxygen supply to the myocardium, and Kaplan and Jones found this was reduced more with sodium nitroprusside than with nitroglycerine.

The evidence, therefore, indicates that in patients with coronary artery disease, glyceryl trinitrate is the superior drug. This is demonstrated by the bulk, although not all, of the evidence from studies of dogs with acute ischemia, by studies of the ST segments in patients as well as laboratory animals, and by the study of the various indices of myocardial oxygen demand and supply. The reasons for the superiority would seem to be related to the following observations. Glyceryl trinitrate is a less powerful arteriolar dilator and maintains arterial diastolic pressure, and therefore, coronary perfusion pressure better than sodium nitroprusside.

The mode of action of the two drugs on the coronary arteries would appear to be different. It is widely believed that sodium nitroprusside may dilate resistance vessels as it does in the systemic circulation, and this would have the consequence of producing a "steal" syndrome and the diversion of blood away from the ischemic areas

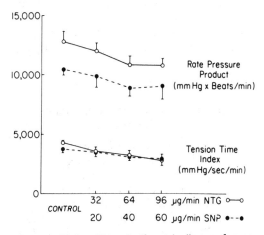

Figure 18.8. Two indirect indices of myocardial oxygen demand are decreased by nitroglycerin and sodium nitroprusside in patients having coronary artery surgery. Reproduced with permission from Kaplan and Jones.[49]

where there is a high fixed resistance to blood flow. Alternately, with minimal effect on resistance arterioles in the coronary system, glyceryl trinitrate is believed to dilate the conductance vessels and in particular the intercoronary artery collaterals. This would result in an improved perfusion pressure and therefore, delivery of blood to the whole myocardium including the ischemic area. As a result of improving, or preventing ischemia in the LV myocardium, it is believed that LV diastolic compliance improves.[50,51] Thus, adequate volume filling of the left ventricle can be achieved at a lower LV filling pressure. This, in turn, will lead to further improvement in perfusion and oxygenation of the inner one-third. Both systolic and diastolic ventricular function will benefit.

Thus it would appear that sodium nitroprusside and nitroglycerine have broadly similar effects on systemic hemodynamics and on reducing myocardial oxygen demand. In coronary patients, the effect of glyceryl trinitrate upon myocardial blood flow and oxygen supply to potentially ischemic areas would seem to be significantly better than sodium nitroprusside; thus, it should be used in coronary artery surgery, particularly prior to bypass. If complete revascularization is achieved, postoperative hypertension may be more easily controlled with nitroprusside. In the absence of complete revascularization glyceryl trinitrate should be used throughout and after the operation.

Pulmonary Vascular Resistance in Children

Although the mythology about pulmonary vascular resistance following corrective open heart surgery in children is substantial, the documentation is meager. The first reports of postoperative pulmonary hypertensive crises leading to hypoxemia and right heart failure, appeared as recently as 1979 when Weller et al.[52] reported three cases of documented pulmonary hypertensive crises treated with tolazoline, the histamine agonist and alpha-adrenergic antagonist. Tolazoline used as a pulmonary (and of course systemic) arteriolar dilator has a number of quite severe side-effects, notably stimulation of gastric secretions, by its histamine agonist properties. Sodium nitroprusside is valuable as an alternative pulmonary vasodilator.

Applebaum et al.[37] studied 16 infants under 18 months of age in the intensive care unit after surgery. They all had low cardiac output, with high systemic vascular resistance and arterial pressures. Sodium nitroprusside infusion had the predicted effects on arterial blood pressure, cardiac output, left atrial pressure, and systemic vascular resistance. In addition, it caused a reduction of right atrial pressure from 12.5 to 9.8 mm Hg, pulmonary artery pressure from a mean of 29 to 20 mm Hg, and pulmonary vascular resistance from 8.6 to 4.3 units M^{-2}.

The study by Stephenson and associates[53] included a subgroup with elevated pulmonary artery pressure who were treated with sodium nitroprusside and dopamine both alone and in combination. The systemic hemodynamics changed as previously described, and the elevated pulmonary vascular resistance was reduced by sodium nitroprusside from 547 to 298 dynes/second/cm^{-5}.

THE USE OF VASODILATORS ON BYPASS

We might ask whether the use of vasodilators in the latter part of cardiopulmonary bypass with the perfused, beating and nonworking heart, and while coming off bypass, has any influence on the rate or completeness of the recovery of the myocardium from the preceding ischemic period, or on eventual ventricular performance. Will the balance of oxygen supply and demand to the myocardium be improved during the recovery period? It could be argued that the use of vasodilators would improve the oxygen supply/demand ratio, and therefore would improve the recovery of the myocardium, particularly the inner one-third from ischemia, even when it had been protected with cardioplegia. If this could be achieved, then one would anticipate improved myocardial function and reduced myocardial damage following surgery. There is a reported reduction in the incidence of postoperative dysrhythmias following the use of vasodilators at this stage,[54] but there is virtually no other direct information bearing on this question.

As a crude clinical observation, it seems to be easier to institute vasodilator therapy while still on bypass than afterward. Presumably this is because there is an assured blood flow during the initiation of therapy. It seems that having started vasodilator therapy on bypass, it is easier to establish a stable state early afterward. This could be because vasodilation produces stability because it reduces vasomotor lability from the time of withdrawal of cardiopulmonary bypass and after the withdrawal. It is also possible that with the adjunctive use of inotropes and/or maintenance of adequate filling pressure as required, one would expect an improvement in cardiac output immediately after bypass. It is possible that venodilation means that there is more likely to be an adequate circulating volume occupying the venous capacitance vessels, and therefore, their ability to make dynamic adjustments to the circulatory system would be restored immediately after bypass. Finally, it could be possible because the pulmonary vascular bed is also stabilized.

Again, there is little information which might be used to confirm or refute these suggestions.

CONCLUSIONS

The physiological consequences of cardiopulmonary bypass tend to lead to a reduction in SV and a possibly adverse balance of oxygen demand and supply. Postoperative hypertension may be controlled by vasodilator drugs. In patients with poor LV function, vasodilator drugs will enhance SV and improve the balance of oxygen demand and supply to the myocardium. In patients with good LV function, SV may only be increased if the filling pressure is maintained; this may also prevent a tachycardia.

In patients with coronary artery disease, glyceryl trinitrates are superior to sodium nitroprusside in preventing regional myocardial ischemia and should be used in the early stages of coronary artery surgery in anticipation of complete revascularization, and throughout if revascularization is incomplete. Maintenance of venous capacitance with vasodilator drugs enables the dynamic regulation of the circulation to be restored. The level of pulmonary vascular resistance may be controlled and stabilized. Used judiciously, vasodilators may reduce SV and increase oxygen demand if the increase in heart rate is not controlled.

References

1. Ross J, Braunwald E: The study of left ventricular function in man by increasing resistance to ventricular ejection with angiotensin. *Circulation* 29:739, 1964.
2. Replogle R, Levy M, DeWall RA, et al: Catecholamine and serotonin response to cardiopulmonary bypass. *J Thorac Cardiovasc Surg* 44:638, 1962.
3. Bailey DR, Miller ED, Kaplan JA, et al: The Renin-Angiotensin-Aldosterone system during cardiac surgery with morphine—nitrous oxide anesthesia. *Anesthesiology* 42:539, 1975.
4. Taylor KM, Jones JV, Walker MS, et al: The cortisol response during heart-lung bypass. *Circulation* 54:20, 1976.
5. Taylor KM, Wright GS, Reid JM, et al: Comparative studies of pulsatile and non-pulsatile flow during cardiopulmonary bypass. II The effects on the adrenal secretion of cortisol. *J. Thorac Cardiovasc Surg* 75:574, 1978.
6. Taylor KM, Morton IJ, Brown JJ, et al: Hypertension and the renin-angiotensin system following open heart surgery. *J Thorac Cardiovasc Surg* 74:840, 1977.
7. Taylor KM, Bain WH, Russel M, et al: Peripheral vascular resistance and angiotensin II levels during pulsatile and non-pulsatile cardiopulmonary bypass. *Thorax* 34:594, 1979.
8. Taylor KM, Brannan JJ, Bain WH, et al: Role of angiotensin II in the development of peripheral vasoconstriction during cardiopulmonary bypass. *Cardiovasc Res* 13:269, 1979.
9. Taylor KM, Casals J, Morton JJ, et al: Haemodynamic effects of angiotensin blockade after cardiopulmonary bypass. *Br Heart J* 41:380, 1979.
10. Philbin DM, Coggins CH, Wilson N, et al: Antidiuretic hormone levels during cardiopulmonary bypass. *J Thorac Cardiovasc Surg* 73:145, 1977.
11. Philbin DM, Levine FH, Emerson CW, et al: Plasma vasopressin levels and urinary flow during cardiopulmonary bypass in patients with valvular heart disease. Effect of pulsatile flow. *J Thorac Cardiovasc Surg* 78:779, 1979.
12. Hine IP, Wood WG, Mainwaring-Burton RW, et al: The adrenergic response to surgery involving cardiopulmonary bypass, as measured by plasma and urinary catecholamine concentrations. *Br J Anaes* 48:355, 1976.
13. Hoar PF, Hickey RF, Ullyot DJ: Systemic hypertension following myocardial revascularization. A

method of treatment using epidural anaesthesia. *J Thorac Cardiovasc Surg* 71:859, 1976.

14. Rastelli GC, Kirklin JW: Hemodynamic state early after replacement of aortic valve with ball-valve prosthesis. *Surgery* 61:873, 1967.

15. Austen WG, Corning HB, Moran JM, et al: Cardiac hemodynamics immediately following aortic valve surgery. *J Thorac Cardiovasc Surg* 51:461, 1966.

16. Rastelli GC, Kirklin JW: Hemodynamic state early after prosthetic replacement of mitral valve. *Circulation* 34:448, 1966.

17. Austen WG, Corning HB, Moran JM, et al: Cardiac hemodynamics immediately following mitral valve surgery. *J Thorac Cardiovasc Surg* 51:468, 1966.

18. Estafanous FG, Tazari RC, Buckley S, et al: Arterial hypertension in immediate post-operative period after valve replacement. *Br Heart J* 40:718, 1978.

19. Estafanous FG, Tazari RC: Systemic arterial hypertension associated with cardiac surgery. *Am J Cardiol* 46:685, 1980.

20. Roberts AJ, Niarches AP, Subramanian VA, et al: Systemic hypertension associated with coronary artery bypass surgery. Predisposing factors, haemodynamic characteristics, humoral profile and treatment. *J Thorac Cardiovasc Surg* 74:846, 1977.

21. Hanson EL, Kane PB, Askanazi J, et al: Comparison of patients with coronary artery or valve disease: Intraoperative differences in blood volume and observations of vasomotor response. *Ann Thorac Surg* 22:343, 1976.

22. Shepherd JT, Vanhoutte PM: Role of the venous system in circulatory control. *Mayo Clin Proc* 53:247, 1978.

23. Reid DJ, Digerness S, Kirklin JW: Changes in whole body venous tone in surgical patients. *Surg Gynecol Obstet* 125:1212, 1967.

24. Cleland J, Pluth JR, Tauxe WN, et al: Blood volume and body fluid compartment changes soon after closed and open intracardiac surgery. *J Thorac Cardiovasc Surg* 52:698, 1966.

25. Doty DB, Montanaro GD, Carter JG, et al: Vasomotor dynamics associated with cardiac operations. II. Effect of cardiopulmonary bypass on venous tone. *J Thorac Cardiovasc Surg* 83:732, 1982.

26. Buckberg GD: Subendocardial ischaemia after cardiopulmonary bypass. *J Thorac Cardiovasc Surg* 64:669, 1972.

27. Hoffman JIE, Buckberg GD: Pathophysiology of subendocardial ischaemia. *Br Med J* 1:76, 1975.

28. Buckberg GD: Left ventricular subendocardial necrosis. *Ann Thorac Surg* 24:379, 1977.

29. Waller JL, Kaplan JA, Jones EL: Anesthesia for coronary revascularization. In Kaplan JA (ed): *Cardiac Anesthesia*, Vol. I. New York, Grune & Stratton, 1979.

30. Braunwald E: Control of myocardial oxygen consumption: Physiologic and clinical considerations. *Am J Cardiol* 27:416, 1971.

31. Marco JD, Standeven JW: Afterload reduction with hydralazine following valve replacement. *J Thorac Cardiovasc Surg* 80:50, 1980.

32. Kouchoukos NT, Sheppard LC, Kirklin JW: Effect of alterations in arterial pressure on cardiac per-

formance early after open intracardiac operations. *J Thorac Cardiovasc Surg* 64:563, 1972.

33. Campbell CS, Wallwork J, Taylor KM, et al: The haemodynamic effects of sodium nitroprusside following cardiopulmonary bypass: A clinical study. *J Cardiovasc Surg* 23:41, 1982.

34. Lappas D, Lowenstein E, Waller J, et al: Haemodynamic effects of nitroprusside infusion during coronary artery operation in man. *Circulation* 54(Suppl 3):4, 1976.

35. Flaherty J, Magee PA, Gardiner TL, et al: Comparison of intravenous nitroglycerine and sodium nitroprusside for treatment of acute hypertension developing after coronary artery bypass surgery. *Circulation* 65:1072, 1982.

36. Mason DT, Awan NA, Joye JA, et al: Treatment of acute and chronic congestive heart failure by vasodilator—afterload reduction. *Arch Intern Med* 140:1577, 1980.

37. Appelbaum A, Blackston EH, Kouchoukos NT, et al: Afterload reduction and cardiac output in infants early after intra-cardiac surgery. *Am J Cardiol* 39:445, 1977.

38. Meretoja OA, Laaksonen VO: Hemodynamic effects of preload and sodium nitroprusside in patients subjected to coronary bypass surgery. *Circulation* 58:815, 1978.

39. Benzing GI, Helmsworth JA, Schreiber JT, et al: Nitroprusside and epinephrine for treatment of low output in children after open-heart surgery. *Ann Thorac Surg* 27:523, 1979.

40. Williams DB, Kiernan PD, Schaff HV, et al: The hemodynamic response to dopamine and nitroprusside following right atrium-pulmonary artery bypass (Fontan procedure). *Ann Thorac Surg* 34:51, 1982.

41. Miller RR, Vismara LA, Zelis R, et al: Clinical use of sodium nitroprusside in chronic ischaemic heart disease. *Circulation* 51:328, 1975.

42. Gall WE, Clarke WR, Doty DB: Vasomotor dynamics associated with cardiac operations I. Venous tone and the effects of vasodilators. *J Thorac Cardiovasc Surg* 83:724, 1982.

43. Rowe GG, Henderson RH: Systemic and coronary haemodynamic effects of sodium nitroprusside. *Am Heart J* 87:83, 1974.

44. Hess W, Bruckner JB, Patschke D, et al: The effects of glyceryl trinitrate, isorbide dinitrate and sodium nitroprusside on haemodynamics, coronary blood flow and myocardial oxygen consumption—An experimental study. *Intensive Care Med* 9:53, 1983.

45. Da Luz PL, Forrester JS, Wyatt HL, et al: Haemodynamic and metabolic effects of sodium nitroprusside on the performance and metabolism of regional ischaemic myocardium. *Circulation* 52:400, 1975.

46. Chiariello M, Gold HK, Leinbach RC, et al: Comparison between the effects of nitroprusside and nitroglycerine on ischaemic injury during acute myocardial infarction. *Circulation* 54:766, 1976.

47. Mann T, Cohn PF, Holman L, et al: Effect of nitroprusside on regional myocardial blood flow in coronary artery disease. Results in 25 patients and

comparison with nitroglycerine. *Circulation* 57:732, 1978.

48. Flaherty JT, Reid PR, Kelly DT, et al: Intravenous nitroglycerine in acute myocardial infarction. *Circulation* 51:132, 1975.

49. Kaplan JA, Jones EL: Vasodilator therapy during coronary artery surgery: Comparison of nitroglycerin and nitroprusside. *J Thorac Cardiovasc Surg* 77:301, 1977.

50. Kaplan JA: "Nitrates." In Kaplan JA (ed): *Cardiac Anesthesia*, Vol 2. *Cardiovascular Pharmacology*. New York, Grune & Stratton, 1983.

51. Curling PE, Kaplan JA: Indications and uses of intravenous nitroglycerine during cardiac surgery. *Angiology* 33:302, 1982.

52. Weller J, George BL, Muilder DG, et al: Diagnosis and management of postoperative pulmonary hypertensive crisis. *Circulation* 60:1640, 1979.

53. Stephenson LW, Edmunds HL Jr, Raphaely R, et al: Effects of nitroprusside and dopamine on pulmonary arterial vasculature in children after cardiac surgery. *Circulation* 60(Suppl):104, 1979.

54. Arom KV, Angaran DM, Lindsay WG, et al: Effect of sodium nitroprusside during the rayback period of cardiopulmonary bypass on the incidence of postoperative arrhythmias. *Ann Thorac Surg* 34:307, 1982.

CHAPTER 19

PERIOPERATIVE USES OF INOTROPIC DRUGS

JACK D. COPELAND, M.D.

Nearly all of the nonphysiological conditions created by heart operations requiring cardiopulmonary bypass have been implicated in the genesis of postoperative low cardiac output.[1,2] Continuous nonpulsatile perfusion, microembolization and poor perfusion of capillary beds may cause multiple organ failure after 2 to 3 hours of cardiopulmonary bypass. Crossclamping the aorta causes irreversible myocardial ultrastructural damage if extended for over 30 minutes at normothermic temperatures. Lowering the myocardial temperature by topical or central cooling forestalls irreversible damage for several hours. Regardless of the technique of preservation or the crossclamp period, it is likely that all techniques cause some damage to the myocardium resulting in postoperative depression of cardiac function. Kirklin et al.[3] has suggested that myocardial necrosis (focally scattered or subendocardial) causes postoperative low output syndromes and is responsible for postoperative elevation of the creatine phosphokinase MB band. Our observations of scattered foci of subendocardial necrosis on early (less than 7 post-transplant days) cardiac biopsies following heart transplantation in the absence of cardiac rejection support this theory.

One mechanism for scattered necrosis in open heart procedures may be air embolism, especially to the right coronary orifice and distribution of the right coronary artery. Even if considerable time is spent with maneuvers to remove air, complete and consistent freedom from air embolism may be a physical impossibility. Capillary "air locks" may result in scattered foci of necrosis most likely in the subendocardium, the most distal part of the myocardial capillary bed. Transmural or subendocardial myocardial infarction, known to occur in 4 to 7% of coronary artery bypass operations, may also be a mechanism for myocardial injury and thus exacerbate pre-existing dysfunction and any global injury which occurs.

The effects of intraoperative damage are as varied as the etiologies, but they all fall into the category of myocardial dysfunction. Such dysfunction, if associated with necrosis of 40% or more of left ventricular (LV) myocardium[4,5] may cause death.

Short of death, the physiological abnormalities related to myocardial dysfunction range from minimal vasoconstriction with oliguria to "cardiogenic shock" characterized by severe vasoconstriction, hypotension (systolic <80 mm Hg), severe oliguria, and lactic acidosis. Early recognition of cardiac dysfunction and institution of appropriate inotropic therapy may salvage a considerable number of patients.

THE DIAGNOSIS OF LOW OUTPUT SYNDROME

Commonly-used monitoring techniques such as arterial, central venous, and pulmonary arterial or left atrial pressure measurements in combination with serial thermodilution cardiac outputs provide a considerable amount of information for identification of the patient requiring inotropic support. More basic information such as cardiac rate and rhythm, body temperature, peripheral perfusion, urine output, arterial pH and blood gases, and careful examination of the patient by a perceptive physician who continues to return frequently to the bedside may add a great deal more to the information necessary for making critical decisions.

Serial patient evaluation should include a careful physical examination of the pupils, heart, lungs, skin, venous pulsations, abdomen, and extremities. Only a limited neurological exam need be done in the anesthetized patient immediately following surgery. But a very careful examination of the hands and feet may be more important than any objective data. Residents are instructed always to check the feet looking for five signs for estimating cardiac output: (a) quality of pulses, (b) skin temperature, (c) skin color, (d) capillary refill, and (e) venous filling.

Aside from evaluating cardiac surgical patients at the bedside, the current state of the art dictates that the physician anticipate which patient may be a higher risk and therefore need inotropic therapy. In order to anticipate, the physician must have a clear and detailed appreciation of the patient's preoperative condition, risk category, anesthetic management, and operation. For instance, patients with severe chronic mitral stenosis and atrial fibrillation preoperatively almost uniformly need inotropic support after mitral valve replacement (Table 19.1). Similarly, patients with dilated ventricles and or low ejection fractions (<.4) from mitral regurgitation, aortic stenosis or regurgitation, or previous myocardial infarction rarely do well without inotropic support. Congenital repairs which leave the patient with a large right ventricular outflow patch and some pulmonic insufficiency nearly always cause enough right ventricular dysfunction to decrease cardiac output and thus require inotropic support.

Quantitative measurements, clinical signs, and anticipation are necessary for early diagnosis of low output syndrome. Several important facts are also helpful. Renal and cerebral blood flows autoregulate down to a mean arterial pressure of 60 mm Hg below which they fall linearly with pressure. Thus, minimally acceptable mean arterial pressure in adults is 60 mm Hg. In children, this value may be slightly lower. A cardiac index of less than 2 liter/minute/M^2 places the patient at markedly increased risk as does a systemic vascular resistance greater than 2100 dynes/second/cm^{-5}.[6]

Table 19.1.
Conditions Commonly Requiring Postoperative Inotropic Support

Valvular: Chronic mitral stenosis; dilated left ventricle from mitral regurgitation, aortic stenosis or regurgitation; severe ventricular hypertrophy from aortic stenosis, chronic hypertension, coarctation or idiopathic hypertrophic subaortic stenosis

Coronary: Ejection fraction <.4 due to previous myocardial infarction; LV aneurysm repair; mitral regurgitation or ventricular septal defect from previous myocardial infarction

Congenital: Tetralogy of Fallot with large right ventricular outflow patch, atrioventricular canal with residual mitral or tricuspid regurgitation, large ventricular septal defect in association with small left ventricle

Length of Cardiopulmonary Bypass: >2 hours

Length of Aortic Crossclamp time: >1.5 hours

Anesthetic and Operative Management: Low blood pressure during induction and prebypass periods

THE TYPICAL LOW-OUTPUT PATIENT

The typical patient requiring inotropic therapy separates from cardiopulmonary bypass without difficulty. Arterial pressure is high for several hours and vasoconstricted, cool, pulseless, pale lower extremities with poor capillary refill and poor venous filling are seen (Table 19.2). The patient's temperature is low initially and climbs slowly from the 35°C range to 39°C while the extremities remain cool and constricted. Cardiac index is below 2 liter/minute/M^2 and systemic vascular resistance is greater than 1500 dynes/second/cm^{-5}. In patients not requiring inotropic support, levels of endogenous catecholamines fall to normal within 20 minutes after discontinuation of cardiopulmonary bypass[8, 9] and by 4 to 8 hours, postoperative sympathetic tone decreases and the extremities begin to vasodilate progressively with a drop in core temperature and increasing peripheral warmth and arterial pulsations. Other signs of improved perfusion also become apparent (urine output, color, capillary refill, etc.). In the case of low-output syndrome, progressive distal vasodilation is not observed, consequently the cool vasoconstricted areas cannot provide a means for dissipation of

body heat and the core temperature remains elevated and often rises to the 40°C range. In these patients, cardiac index remains uniformly low and systemic vascular resistance elevated. If the patient has not yet been started on inotropic therapy and/or vasodilators this picture is an unequivocal indication. One would hope, however, to have observed the trend toward continued constriction, falling blood pressure, decrease in pulse pressure (usually a pulse pressure less than 25 mm Hg is an indication of low output, less than 20 mm Hg is borderline for survival), and failure of systemic pressure to rise in the face of optimum filling pressures. A central venous pressure of 15 mm Hg is usually optimum as is a pulmonary artery wedge pressure of 14 to 18 mm Hg. Exceeding these loading pressures often results in pulmonary and dependent edema and hepatomegaly.

EFFECTS OF INOTROPES ON THE CONTRACTILE MECHANISM

The five commonly used inotropic medications include the catecholamines, norepinephrine and epinephrine, and three sympathomimetic agents, isoproterenol, dopamine, and dobutamine. They differ in avidity of binding to the beta-myocardial receptors and in arrythmogenic, chronotropic, and peripheral effects. Structurally, they are quite similar and their mechanism of stimulating increased cardiac contractility (inotropic effect) is identical (Table 19.3).

The myocardium contracts by virtue of myofilaments which "slide" past each other thereby reducing the length the sarcomere. Simultaneous reduction of sarcomere length in millions of sarcomeres results in cardiac contraction (Fig. 19.1). Calcium facilitates this mechanism by binding to troponin on the actin (thin) filaments which then allows the actin and myosin (thick) filaments to interact.

These five inotropes bind to beta-receptors on a myocardial cell membrane which in turn stimulate adenyl cyclase to increase levels of cyclic adenosine monophosphate (AMP) which facilitates influx of calcium through calcium channels. The increase in intracellular calcium makes more calcium

Table 19.2.
Typical Findings in Patients Requiring Inotropic Therapy Postcardiopulmonary Bypass

1. Anticipation (see Table 19.1)
2. Hypotension: mean arterial pressure <70 mm Hg in adults, <60 mm Hg in children; systolic arterial pressure <90 mm Hg in adults, <70 mm Hg in children
3. Narrow pulse pressure (<30 mm Hg)
4. Urine output 30 cc/hour in adults, <1 cc/kg/hour in children
5. Five signs in feet: pale, cool, pulseless, poor capillary refill, absent venous filling
6. Persistent hyperthermia
7. Low cardiac index (<2.4 liter/min/M^2)
8. High systemic vascular resistance (>1500 dynes·sec·cm^{-5})
9. Metabolic acidosis
10. Agitation

available for binding to troponin and in this way improves sarcomere shortening.[10, 11] Calcium given by bolus or infusion may cause similar improvement, but this effect is usually limited to several minutes and becomes less apparent when the serum calcium rises above the normal range.

Each of these inotropes produces a unique clinical response. Therefore, they are not interchangeable. The more powerful the agent (norepinephrine, epinephrine) the more skill, perseverance, and experience are needed to administer the agent and the more likely a combination with vasodilator therapy may be necessary.

Choosing among the available inotropes for postcardiac surgical therapy should be based upon the needs of the patient. Blind

Table 19.3.
Structure, Action, and Relative Potency of the Commonly Used Inotropes

	STRUCTURE	ACTION	MECHANISM	RELATIVE CARDIAC* POTENCY	HEART RATE* INCREASE (BEATS/MINUTE)	BLOOD PRESSURE* INCREASE (mm Hg)
Norepinephrine	HO–⟨⟩–CH CH$_2$ NH$_2$ / OH	Direct	Beta Receptor Stim.	50	16	22
Epinephrine	HO–⟨⟩–CH CH$_2$NH / OH CH$_3$	Direct	''	100 +	16 +	15 +
Isoproterenol	HO–⟨⟩–CH CH$_2$ NHCH /CH$_3$ \CH$_3$	Direct	''	100	33	– 19
Dopamine	HO–⟨⟩–CH$_2$ CH$_2$ NH$_2$	Stimulates Norepinephrine Release	''	1	6	27
Dobutamine	HO–⟨⟩–CH$_2$ CH$_2$ NH CH CH$_2$ CH$_2$–⟨⟩–OH / CH$_3$	Direct	''	4	8	16

from Tuttle, RR, Mills. J based upon dose to raise contractile tension by 50%
*author's estimate

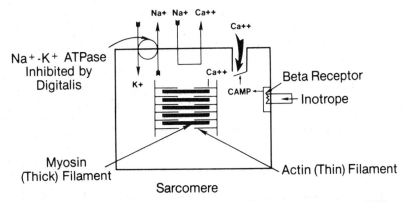

Figure 19.1. Digitalis preparations ("digitalis") block sodium-potassium ATPase causing increased intracellular sodium and decreasing calcium loss by Na$^+$-Ca^{++} countertransport thus increasing Ca^{++} available for calcium binding to troponin (on actin filament) permitting interaction between actin and myosin. Catecholamines and sympathomimetic agents binding at the beta-receptor increase levels of cyclic AMP which promotes calcium influx through calcium channels making Ca^{++} more available for binding to troponin. Figure based on Scholz[10] and Weber.[11]

dependence on one agent or another for all situations may deprive the patient of his optimal chance for survival. Thus, the patient with a low or normal heart rate, vasoconstriction, and low cardiac output is ideally suited for treatment with isuprel, whereas the tachycardiac, dilated patient with oliguria should be treated with dopamine.

PHYSIOLOGY OF INOTROPIC THERAPY

Frank-Starling curves describe a relationship between cardiac function and filling pressure. As the filling pressure increases, cardiac output increases to a plateau. If the heart is overfilled cardiac output decreases (Fig. 19.2). Inotropic stimulation of the normal heart results in supernormal cardiac outputs at all levels of preload. Myocardial depression results in subnormal cardiac outputs over the range of preloads. Inotropic stimulation of the depressed heart returns its function curve toward normal usually causing simultaneous increase in cardiac output and decrease in preload.

Similar function curves can be generated by using increasing concentrations of inotropes. In a comparison of dobutamine and dopamine, we obtained curves for each of these agents at infusion rates of 2.5, 5.0, and 7.5 μg/kg/minute (Fig. 19.3)[12] in patients after coronary artery bypass grafting.

These curves show a rise in stroke volume (SV) at nearly constant preload (wedge pressure) with infusion of dobutamine. In contrast, SV rose little after the initial dose of

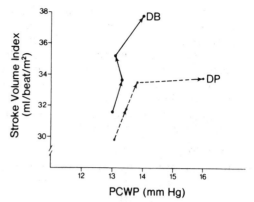

Figure 19.3. Modified LV function curves for each drug plotting pulmonary capillary wedge pressure (*PCWP*) and stroke volume index are shown. (*DB* = dobutamine; *DP* = dopamine.)

dopamine 2.5 μg/kg/minute while the wedge pressure rose considerably and the rise of wedge pressure was associated with a rise in afterload (mean arterial pressure). No attempt was made to maintain preload by addition of volume. Therefore with dopamine, the minimal rise in SV was obtained by increasing LV resting wall tension (preload) and systemic vascular resistance (afterload). In contrast, the rise in SV with dobutamine was associated with constant preload and a slight fall in afterload.

Ross[13] and co-workers have used the force-velocity relationship to further describe the normal, depressed and inotrope-stimulated heart (Fig. 19.4). Each of the curves shown is at a constant preload, with the magnitude of preload increasing as indicated by the *arrow*. Thus, at a given afterload (*x*), the depressed heart has the lowest preload and velocity of contraction (SV-*a*). At that same afterload, increasing the preload results in an increased SV (*b*). The preload may be increased thus increasing SV until the Frank-Starling limit is reached. This may still be less than the SV (*a*) of a normal heart at the same afterload x (*c*) and considerably less than the SV of an inotrope-stimulated heart (*d*). Note that the inotrope-stimulated heart functions at a higher preload than the depressed or normal heart which is another way of saying that

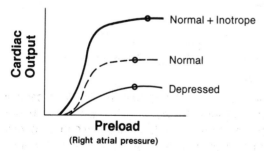

Figure 19.2. Family of Starling curves for depressed, normal, and inotrope stimulated hearts is shown.

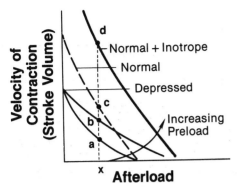

Figure 19.4. Force-velocity relationships in depressed, normal, and inotrope stimulated hearts are shown. Note that each curve represents a constant preload and that preload increases as indicated by the *arrow*. Reproduced with permission from Ross.[13]

at greater preloads it generates greater cardiac outputs.

It is also of interest that increasing afterload along any of the constant preload lines results in a drop in SV, or an "afterload mismatch." Thus, treatment of patients with pressors in the absence of volume loading (preload increase) decreases SV and cardiac output.

A schematic representation of the circulation (Fig. 19.5, after Guyton[14]) may help explain some of the changes seen with administration of inotropes. The amount of blood returning to the heart (venous return, *a.*) must equal the amount of blood leaving the heart (cardiac output, *b.*). The relation between the forces shows:

$$Cardiac\ Output = Venous\ Return$$
$$= \frac{Afterload - Preload}{Resistance}$$

Drugs which increase the cardiac output with no change in afterload drop the resistance and may drop the preload. These are positive inotropes. Pressors which cause an increase in resistance (afterload) drop the cardiac output. Vasodilators which drop the resistance may increase the cardiac output if the afterload is not also simultaneously decreased.

Under conditions of constant resistance, increases in afterload with respect to pre-

load increase cardiac output. Increase of preload unaccompanied by increased afterload decreases cardiac output.

COMPARISON: DOPAMINE, DOBUTAMINE, AND OTHER INOTROPES

We have recently completed a study of dopamine and dobutamine in patients after coronary artery bypass (Table 19.4).[12] Dobutamine in increasing doses caused an increase in cardiac index and SV without significantly changing heart rate, blood pressure, wedge pressure, or systemic vascular resistance. Dopamine raised cardiac index, but at the expense of an increased blood pressure, wedge pressure, and systemic vascular resistance. Our conclusion was that dopamine acts as a vasopressor even at doses less than 10 mg/kg/minute. Since it increased afterload, heart rate, and myocardial contractility while dobutamine increased only contractility it must increase myocardial oxygen consumption more than dobutamine. Dobutamine, on the other hand, raises cardiac index by acting as an inotrope increasing SV without increasing afterload and LV end-diastolic pressure.

The most common postoperative scenario is the normotensive vasoconstricted patient with high normal heart rate. Dobutamine may be more helpful in this situation.

Others have also found dobutamine to be effective after cardiopulmonary bypass[15, 16] in augmenting cardiac output without significantly elevating heart rate. For patients with ventricles which were neither volume- nor pressure-loaded preoperatively, as in our study, cardiac output increases in the

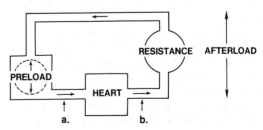

Figure 19.5. A schematic representation of the circulatory system is shown. Reproduced with permission from Guyton.[14]

Table 19.4.
Summary of Hemodynamic Data for All Patients*

Variables†	Control	Dose (μg/kg/min)		
		2.5	5.0	7.5
Dobutamine (N = 10)				
HR (beat/min)	87.6 ± 12.4	88.2 ± 13.4	92.1 ± 13.6	93.4 ± 17.5
MAP (mm Hg)	79.4 ± 5.3	81.8 ± 4.7	82.4 ± 6.0	92.4 ± 15.3
PCWP (mm Hg)	13.0 ± 2.2	13.3 ± 2.9	13.1 ± 4.2	14.0 ± 3.7
CI (liter/min/M²)	2.7 ± 0.6	2.9 ± 0.6	3.2 ± 0.6‡	3.4 ± 0.8‡·§
SVI (ml/min/M²)	31.6 ± 8.7	33.7 ± 10.0	35.1 ± 8.6	37.8 ± 11.4‡
PVR (resistance units)	30.7 ± 7.5	29.5 ± 7.6	26.8 ± 6.1	28.1 ± 7.2
Dopamine (N = 10)				
HR (beat/min)	96.3 ± 13.4	96.3 ± 12.7	98.2 ± 12.2	99.8 ± 15.1
MAP (mm Hg)	80.4 ± 5.4	81.6 ± 9.1	85.1 ± 9.7	94.1 ± 12.1‡
PCWP (mm Hg)	13.0 ± 3.4	13.4 ± 4.1	13.9 ± 4.6	16.0 ± 5.4‡
CI (liter/min/M²)	2.8 ± 0.4	2.9 ± 0.6	3.2 ± 0.6‡	3.3 ± 1.8‡
SVI (ml/min/M²)	29.7 ± 6.6	31.7 ± 8.2	33.5 ± 8.7	33.8 ± 10.1
PVR (resistance units)	29.4 ± 4.9	28.7 ± 6.2	27.4 ± 5.9	30.0 ± 6.8§

* Data shown as group mean ± 1 standard deviation.
† HR = heart rate; MAP = mean arterial pressure; PCWP = pulmonary capillary wedge pressure; CI = cardiac index; SVI = stroke volume index; PVR = peripheral vascular resistance (resistance units = MAP/CI).
‡ $p < 0.05$ versus control.
§ $p < 0.05$ versus previous dose.

face of falling systemic and pulmonary vascular resistances with dobutamine.[17] Dobutamine was also found to be more helpful than dopamine in ventricles which were volume-loaded preoperatively (mitral or aortic regurgitation), but not significantly better in hearts which were pressure-loaded (aortic stenosis).

Favorable results after cardiopulmonary bypass have been reported with dopamine when compared to isuprel.[18] An increase in cardiac output and a decrease in systemic vascular resistance were noted with both drugs, but heart rate was more markedly elevated with isuprel.

Additional studies of other inotropes have failed to establish that the catecholamines or isuprel are superior to dobutamine. Dopamine has been demonstrated to cause stimulation of vascular receptors in renal, mesenteric, coronary, and cerebral circulation resulting in increased blood flow to these areas.[19] In man, the major benefit derives from the renal effects, and on our service, dopamine is most often reserved for

this purpose. Dobutamine has been used most often as our first-line drug because it is associated with positive inotropic action but not with significant increase in heart rate or afterload. Myocardial oxygen consumption may be less with dobutamine than with other inotropes and patients with infarcts or ischemia may therefore benefit. When prevention of extention of an infarct is a major consideration,[20, 21] intra-aortic balloon counterpulsation and dobutamine may be of value.

FIRST- AND SECOND-LINE AGENTS FOR LOW OUTPUT SYNDROME

The following description of the five agents considered in this chapter divides them into first- and second-line agents in order to: (a) facilitate choosing among these agents and (b) separate them into agents which are easier to use (first-line) from drugs which require more attentive supervision (second-line) (also see Table 19.5).

Table 19.5.
Clinical Indications for Inotropes in Adults*

	Cardiac Index	Heart Rate	Vascular Tone	Urine Output	Central Venous Pressure	Combination Agent(s)
Isuprel	<2.4 liter/minute/M^2	<110	Constricted	<30 cc/hour	≥15 mm Hg	Dopamine, epinephrine
Dopamine	Any	Any	Any	<30 cc/hour	12 to 15 mm Hg	Dobutamine, nitroprusside, isuprel
Dobutamine	<2.4 liter/minute/M^2	Not >130	Constricted	Any	≥15 mm Hg	Dopamine, epinephrine
Norepinephrine	<2.4 liter/minute/M^2	Any	Dilated	>30 cc/hour	≥15 mm Hg	Regitine
Epinephrine	<2.4 liter/minute/M^2	Not >130	Constricted	Any	≥15 mm Hg	Nitroprusside, dobutamine

* Clinical variables which are favorable for use of specific inotropes, i.e. isuprel is best used in patients with cardiac <2.4, heart rate <110 constricted vascular tone, low urine output (<30 cc/hour), and venous pressure of 15.

First-Line Agents

ISOPROTERENOL

Isoproterenol, a powerful inotrope and chronotrope and peripheral vasodilator, is best used in low output vasoconstricted patients with heart rates under 110/minute and adequate preload. The dose range is 1 to 4 μg/minute (.25 to 4 μg/min in children) with a dilution of 4 mg/1000 cc 5% dextrose in water (D5W) (4 μg/cc) and a usual starting rate of 15 cc/hour or 1 μg/minute (4 cc/hour in children). Start isoproterenol slowly (.25 to .5 mg/min) to prevent tachycardia and sudden vasodilatation. Raise the dose until the desired inotropic effect is obtained or the heart rate exceeds 120/minute (adults) or 160/minute (children). Simultaneous volume replacement is required to prevent hypotension. Dopamine (5 to 7.5 μg/kg/min) may be added to isoproterenol therapy to cause a mild pressor effect and maintain adequate urine output. Epinephrine may be added (1 to 4 μg/min) when an inadequate inotropic effect is obtained with isuprel alone. One must, however, be aware of the potential additive chronotropic effects of these two agents.

DOPAMINE

Dopamine, after cardiac surgery is only a moderately good inotrope and becomes a pressor at doses of ≥ 10 μg/kg/minute (adults) and about ≥ 5 μg/kg/minute (children). It is useful because it does not increase heart rate until the dose exceeds 5 μg/kg/minute and it is associated with increased blood flow in the kidneys (dopaminergic receptors) and urine output. The starting dose range is 2.5 to 5 μg/kg/minute obtained with a dilution of 800 mg/liter D5W (800 μg/cc). One should generally not exceed 10 μg/kg/minute unless used in combination with vasodilator.

We nearly always use dopamine primarily to increase renal blood flow in addition to another agent for inotropic support. Since neither dopamine nor dobutamine have prominent chronotropic effects this is a favorable combination, particularly when inadequate inotropic response obtained with 10 μg/kg/minute of dopamine addition of dobutamine (5 to 30 μg/kg/min) may be helpful. Nitroprusside (.1 to 1 μg/kg/min) may counteract the pressor effects of dopamine. A careful titration of each drug must be done for this to be effective. An optimal preload maintenance is vital with central venous pressure of 15 mm Hg or pulmonary artery wedge pressure of 14 to 18 mm Hg in adults, or central venous pressure of 10 mm Hg in children. Combination with isoproterenol (1 to 4 μg/min) may be helpful in situations where increase in cardiac output or heart rate is desirable and not satisfactorily abtained with dopamine alone.

DOBUTAMINE

Dobutamine is a powerful inotrope with activity similar to isoproterenol but without the chronotropic effect. It has little effect on heart rate until the dose approaches 10 μg/kg/minute and causes increasing peripheral vasodilatation as the dose is increased. We use a dose of 2.5 to 30 μg/kg/minute and a dilution of 1000 mg/liter D5W (1000 μg/cc).

In the patient with persistent constricted low output, already receiving dobutrex, low-dose dopamine (2.5 to 5 μg/kg/minute) may raise the blood pressure slightly and maintain a reasonable urine output (30 cc/hour in adults or 1 cc/kg/hour in children). Epinephrine at 1 to 4 μg/minute should be used in addition to high-dose dobutamine when further increase in cardiac output is necessary to prevent lactic acidosis. Table 19.5 lists clinical situations in which inotropes are indicated.

Second-Line Agents

NOREPINEPHRINE

Norepinephrine is a pressor causing intense vasoconstriction. It is best used in vasodilated patients (systemic vascular resistance < 1000 dynes/sec/cm^{-5}) with normal cardiac and urine outputs. A dose of .5–4 μg/minute in a standard dilution 4 mg/1000 cc D5W (4 μg/cc) run at 15 cc/hour in combination with phentolamine (equal concentration) increases cardiac output and renal blood flow[22] in a shock preparation.

EPINEPHRINE

Epinephrine at low doses (1 to 2 μg/min) dilates peripherally and at higher doses (4 μg/min) vasoconstricts. Because it is a potent inotrope and chronotrope and causes decrease in renal blood flow, it is seldom used as first-line drug. We reserve epinephrine for patients who cannot be stabilized with isuprel, dopamine, or dobutamine. Our usual dose is 1 to 8 μg/minute (.25 to 2 μg/hour in children) obtained by diluting 4 mg/1000 cc D5W (4 μg/cc) and administering at a starting rate 15 cc/hour (1 μg/min) (4 cc/hour is .25 μg/min in children). We nearly always use epinephrine in combination with nitroprusside to counter the peripheral constricting effect. Our method is to start epinephrine then add nitroprusside and enough volume to maintain preload. Our goal is to maintain blood pressure and preload and increase cardiac output with a resulting reduction in resistance. Epinephrine is occasionally added to ongoing dobutamine therapy when we find inadequate cardiac output and continuing low output syndrome in face of considerable dobutamine dosage (30 μg/kg/min). In this situation we consider using Lasix 20 to 40 mg, or Lasix plus mannitol (.5 gm/kg), and/or dopamine (2.5 to 5 mg/kg/min) to maintain urine output.

GENERAL POLICIES IN THE USE OF INOTROPES

If the mean arterial pressure rises above 100 mm Hg in adults or 80 mm Hg in children, we add nitroprusside, .1 to 1 μg/kg/minute starting dose, and titrate the dose higher to maintain what seems to be an ideal mean arterial pressure of 80 to 90 mm Hg in adults[23] and 60 to 75 mm Hg in children.

When combination therapy with these first-line agents fails, we turn to epinephrine to bring blood pressure into physiological range (mean arterial pressure = 60 mm Hg) then add nitroprusside and volume therapy concomitantly to maintain optimal preload with maintenance of arterial pressure.

Failure of this combination in the absence of a surgically remedial problem such as cardiac tamponade is usually associated with a grave prognosis. In most cases, if intra-aortic balloon therapy has not already been instituted it is started and LV assist must be considered.

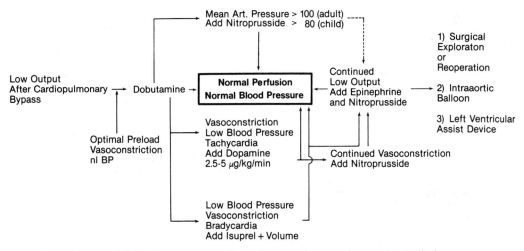

Figure 19.6. Treatment options for postbypass low output all shown.

Digitalis

Digitalis preparations are often used in postoperative patients, but seldom thought to have inotropic effects equal to any of the previously discussed inotropes. Potential toxicity and absence of second to second control obtainable with intravenous infusions make digitalis of limited use. Transition from the inotropes discussed in this chapter to digitalis therapy as intravenously-infused inotropic medications are tapered is an important aspect of postoperative care after the heart has begun to return to normal function.

Amrinone

Amrinone, a new agent under clinical investigation, apparently acts by a mechanism different from the sympathomimetic inotropes and therefore may be of additional benefit to low output post-cardiopulmonary bypass patients. Preliminary evidence suggests that this agent inhibits the degradation of cyclic AMP by inhibiting the enzyme phosphodiesterase.[24] The resulting elevation in cyclic AMP increases availability of calcium for binding to actin thus allowing the actin and myosin filaments to interact.

The usual intravenous dose of 1.5 to 3.5 μg/kg/minute has been effective in increasing cardiac output in patients with end-stage cardiac disease. In potential cardiac recipients, we have seen improvement when other intravenous inotropes including sympathomimetics and digitalis glycosides have failed.

Further clinical trials will be necessary before this agent is proven valuable in postoperative patients.

TREATMENT OPTIONS FOR POSTBYPASS-LOW OUTPUT SYNDROME

Our approach to the usual patient in low output after cardiopulmonary bypass is tailored to the usual findings: normal heart rate, vasoconstriction, low to low-normal cardiac output, oliguria, and normal to low-normal blood pressure in whom optimal preloading has failed to improve the situation. We start with dobutamine and follow the general schema outlined in Figure 19.6 treating hypertension with nitroprusside and continuing low output with the addition of other inotropes. We generally turn to other first line agents before resorting to epinephrine and nitroprusside a combination which we believe is more powerful, but more fraught with potential problems.

References

1. Copeland JG, Griepp RB, Stinson EB, et al: Long term follow up after isolated aortic valve replacement. *J Thorac Cardiovasc Surg* 74:875, 1977.
2. Salomon NW, Stinson EB, Griepp RB, et al: Patient related risk factors as predictors of results following mitral valve replacement. *Ann Thorac Surg* 24:519, 1977.
3. Kirklin JW, Conti VR, Blackstone EH: Prevention

of myocardial damage during cardiac operations. *N Engl J Med* 301:135, 1979.

4. Scheidt S, Aschei MR, Killip T: Shock after acute myocardial infarction. *Am J Cardiol* 26:556, 1970.

5. Page DL, Caulfield JB, Kastor JA, et al: Myocardial changes associated with cardiogenic shock. *N Engl J Med* 285:133, 1971.

6. Norman JC, Cooley DA, Igo SR, et al: Prognostic indices for survival during post cardiotomy intra-aortic balloon pumping. *J Thorac Cardiovasc Surg* 74:709, 1977.

7. Tuttle RR, Mills J: Dobutamine: development of a new catecholamine to selectively increase cardiac contractility. *Circ Res* 36:185, 1975.

8. Reves JG, Karp RB, Buttner EE, et al: Neuronal and adrenomedullary catecholamine release in response to cardiopulmonary bypass in man. *Circulation* 66:49, 1982.

9. Tan CK, Glisson SN, El-Etr AA, et al: Levels of circulating norepinephrine and epinephrine before, during, and after cardiopulmonary bypass in man. *J Thorac Cardiovasc Surg* 71:928, 1976.

10. Scholz H: Pharmacological actions of inotropic agents. *Eur Heart J* 4(Suppl A):161, 1983.

11. Weber KT: New hope for the failing heart. *Am J Med* 72:665, 1982.

12. Salomon NW, Plachetka JR, Copeland JG: Comparison of dopamine and dobutamine following coronary artery bypass grafting. *Ann Thorac Surg* 33:48, 1982.

13. Ross J: Afterload mismatch and preload reserve: a conceptual framework for the analysis of ventricular function. *Prog Cardiovasc Dis* 18:255–264, 1976.

14. Guyton AC: *Textbook of Medical Physiology.* Philadelphia, W.B. Saunders Co., 1976, p. 297–310.

15. Sakamoto T, Yamada T: Hemodynamic effects of dobutamine in patients following open heart surgery. *Circulation* 55:525, 1977.

16. Lewis GRJ, Poole Wilson PA, Angerpointer TA, et al: Measurement of the circulatory effects of dobutamine, a new inotropic agent, in patients following cardiac surgery. *Am Heart J* 95:301, 1978.

17. DiSesa VJ, Brown E, Mudge GH, et al: Hemodynamic comparison of dopamine and dobutamine in postoperative volume loaded pressure loaded and normal ventricles. *J Thorac Cardiovasc Surg* 83:256, 1982.

18. Hollaway EL, Stinson EB, Derby GC, et al: Action of drugs in patients early after cardiac surgery. *Am J Cardiol* 35:656, 1975.

19. Goldberg LI: Dopamine—clinical uses of an endogenous catecholamine. *N Engl J Med* 291:701, 1974.

20. Maroko PR, Jenkshus JR, Sobel BE, et al: Factors influencing infarct size following coronary artery occlusion. *Circulation* 43:67, 1971.

21. Wantanake T, Covell JW, Maroko PR, et al: Effects of increased arterial pressure and positive inotropic agents on the severity of myocardial ischemia in the acutely depressed heart. *Am J Cardiol* 30:371, 1972.

22. Argenta LC, Kirsch MM, Bove EL, et al: A comparison of the hemodynamic effects of inotropic agents. *Ann Thorac Surg* 22:50, 1976.

23. Stinson EB, Holloway E, Derby G, et al: Control of myocardial performance early after open heart operations by vasodilator treatment. *J Thorac Cardiovasc Surg* 73:523, 1977.

24. Algeo S, Nolan PE, Fenster PE: Amrinone: A new therapy for heart failure. *Drug Therapy* (in press).

CHAPTER 20

DIGITALIS AND DIGITALIS TOXICITY

D. C. CHUNG, M.D.

Digitalis refers to a group of drugs of natural origin which has both a positive inotropic action on the contractile myocardium and a negative dromotropic action on the conducting tissue of the heart. Although the discovery of digitalis has been attributed to Sir William Withering, who published the treatise entitled, "An account of the foxglove and some of its medical uses: with practical remarks on dropsy and other diseases" in 1785, the therapeutic values and toxic properties of these agents were well known to the Romans and Chinese in biblical times.

Since the time of Withering, pure cardiac glycosides have replaced crude preparations and digoxin has become the fourth most frequently prescribed drug, and digitoxin the 16th most frequently described drug in the United States.[1] Despite their popularity, the role of digitalis in therapeutics has given rise to much controversy. The controversies regarding digitalis therapy are related to its narrow therapeutic ratio. Its use in the treatment of congestive heart failure has been challenged repeatedly during this century, first by the diuretics and lately by the vasodilators.

The digitalis preparations are used for prophylaxis against postoperative supraventricular tachyarrhythmias. This has generated heated arguments in the field of thoracic and cardiac surgery. There is no clear concensus as to whether these drugs should be withdrawn from surgical patients before surgery.

In the following sections the controversies related to digitalis are examined and the topic of cardiotoxicity reviewed.

THE ROLE OF DIGITALIS IN HEART FAILURE

Heart failure may be defined as the pathological state in which the heart fails to circulate blood at a rate required to meet the metabolic demands of the body. When systemic and pulmonary congestions are present, the syndrome is called congestive heart failure. However, undue emphasis should not be placed on the adjective "congestive." Heart failure should be regarded as a continuum ranging from simple ventricular dysfunction on the one end to frank congestion together with low cardiac output on the other.[2]

Irrespective of etiology, the treatment of heart failure should be directed toward (a) the removal of the precipitating cause; (b) the correction of the underlying organic cause; and (c) the improvement of circulatory dynamics by decreasing cardiac work, enhancing cardiac output, and reducing congestion. In practical terms, improvement in circulatory dynamics can be achieved through bed rest, a moderate degree of salt abstention, and the use of diuretics, vasodilators, and digitalis.

Although digitalis glycosides have a positive inotropic action that is unique among these three groups of agents, some authors have suggested the use of diuretics or vasodilators in heart failure without regard to the adequacy of digitalization.[3, 4] A review of the effects of these three groups of agents on cardiac performance might clear this confusion.

Diuretics and Cardiac Performance

In cardiac failure, the heart functions on a lower ventricular function curve (Fig. 20.1). Salt and water retention are compensatory mechanisms. As salt and water are retained, ventricular filling pressure (i.e., preload) rises and ventricular function is improved along this lower curve according to the Frank-Starling mechanism. When salt and water retention is excessive, however, congestive symptoms will appear and ventricular performance can be represented by *Point A*.

Diuretics have no effect on the position of the ventricular function curve of the failing heart. By promoting renal excretion of salt and water, diuretics decrease preload. As a result, ventricular performance retreats from *A* to *B* (Fig. 20.1). Since the upper end of the ventricular function curve is almost flat, congestion is relieved but stroke volume (SV) is relatively unchanged. Although diuretics ameliorate edema and congestion, they do not improve myocardial efficiency

or cardiac output. Consequently, the low cardiac output state of congestive heart failure persists and congestion will recur with time.[5]

There is one other disadvantage in using diuretics alone for the treatment of heart failure. Modern diuretics are powerful agents; if an over-vigorous diuresis is allowed to occur, preload will decline to even lower values and ventricular function diminish further to *Point C* with a large fall in SV (Fig. 20.1). Tachycardia with or without orthostatic hypotension following the administration of a diuretic should be regarded as the sign of an adverse circulatory response.

Vasodilators and Cardiac Performance

The effects of vasodilators on the performance of the failing heart are illustrated in Figure 20.2. Unlike diuretics, vasodilators do have a profound influence on the position of the ventricular function curve of the failing heart. This is achieved through lowering of systemic vascular resistance (i.e., afterload). By decreasing afterload, a *pure arterial* vasodilator lowers the impedance that resists ventricular ejection and improves the performance of the failing heart from *Point A* to *B*. As a result of the rise in ventricular output, renal perfusion improves

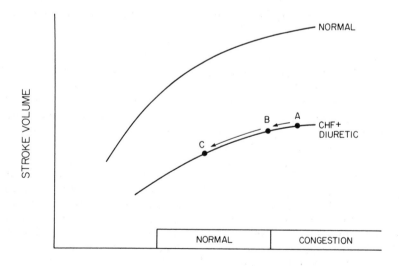

Figure 20.1. The effects of diuretics on cardiac performance are shown.

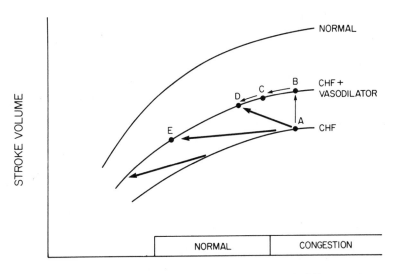

STROKE VOLUME

NORMAL

CONGESTION

LEFT VENTRICULAR FILLING PRESSURE

Figure 20.2.   The effects of vasodilators on cardiac performance are shown.

and renal excretion of salt and water increases. Therefore there is a simultaneous fall in preload together with the alleviation of congestive symptoms, while SV settles at *Point C*. But all commonly used vasodilators have mixed actions on both arterial resistance and venous capacitance vessels. These *mixed-action* vasodilators will cause an additional fall in ventricular filling pressure as a result of venous pooling; and ventricular performance will retreat from *Point C* to *D*. The actual improvement in ventricular function following the administration of a mixed-action agent is, therefore, represented by the *arrow AD*. Since SV and cardiac output improve while systemic vascular resistance falls, blood pressure will remain unchanged.

Like diuretics, vasodilators can cause adverse circulatory changes. If an excessive fall in preload is allowed to occur, ventricular performance will retreat further along the ventricular function curve to *Point E* with a fall in stroke output (Fig. 20.2). This fall in SV will be even more alarming at the lower end of the ventricular function curve. Therefore hemodynamics variables should be monitored closely following the administration of vasodilators. An increase in heart rate and the onset of orthostatic hy-

potension should be regarded as signs of an adverse response.

Digitalis and Cardiac Performance

The most well-known circulatory effect of digitalis glycosides is their positive inotropic action. Traditionally it was thought that a threshold serum or myocardial concentration was necessary for their therapeutic effect—hence the recommendation of a "digitalizing" or loading dose when initiating treatment. But this has been shown to be incorrect. A positive inotropic effect is seen even with small doses of digitalis, and myocardial contractility increases linearly as a function of dose.[6,7]

The effects of digitalis on ventricular function is represented in Figure 20.3. By virtue of their positive inotropic action, digitalis glycosides improve the performance of the failing heart from *Point A* to *B* and eliminate the dependence on compensatory mechanisms to maintain cardiac output and blood pressure normal. With cardiac output improved, renal perfusion is increased and renal excretion of salt and water is more efficient. As a result of diuresis, ventricular filling pressure falls, congestive symptoms abate, and the improvement in ventricular function is represented by the *arrow AC*.

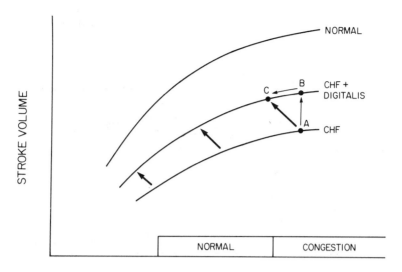

Figure 20.3. The effects of digitalis on cardiac performance are shown.

Unlike diuretics and vasodilators, digitalis glycosides do not have a direct effect on preload. Improvement in ventricular performance is seen along the entire length of the ventricular function curve following the administration of digitalis, although improvement at the lower end of this curve is necessarily smaller (Fig. 20.3).

The salutary effects of diuretics in the treatment of heart failure are mediated through the reduction of preload and those of vasodilators through the reduction of both afterload and preload. That is, diuretics and vasodilators are unloading agents. Both groups of agents can cause adverse circulatory changes through an excessive fall in preload and should be used with caution. The salutary effects of digitalis, on the other hand, are achieved through a unique positive inotropic action. Other than the newly introduced amrinones,[8,9] digitalis glycosides are the only orally active inotropic agents available. Both the ease of administration and the once-daily dose schedule has served to encourage compliance of the patient. It is these pharmacodynamic and pharmacokinetic properties that have made digitalis the mainstay in the pharmacological treatment of chronic heart failure. Although diuretics and vasodilators have found their niche as well, the usefulness of digitalis will remain

for the foreseeable future.[10,11] The glycosides are most beneficial to patients in whom ventricular function is impaired by chronic myocardial ischemia or by an excessive load due to arterial hypertension, aortic stenosis or regurgitation, mitral regurgitation, or congenital heart disease[12]; they are less satisfactory in cardiomiopathies, myocarditis, beriberi heart disease, and cor pulmonale; and they are of little value in mitral stenosis with sinus rhythm, constrictive pericarditis, or cardiac tamponade, and in the so-called high-output failures associated with thyrotoxicosis and sinus rhythm, severe anemia, arterial venous fistula, and Padget's disease of bone.

Although the role of digitalis in chronic heart failure is unchallenged, the usefulness of digitalis in patients who are experiencing acute and transient cardiac dysfunction in the perioperative period is questionable. Acute cardiac dysfunction during the operation and in the postoperative period is frequently due to myocardial depression, myocardial damage, or acute changes in afterload and/or preload. In these situations the institution of hemodynamic monitoring is indicated; the infusion of dopamine or dobutamine with or without nitroprusside or nitroglycerine intravenously by titration is a more controllable method of supporting cardiac function; and counterpulsation should be used in patients who are in cardiogenic shock following acute myocardial infarction or cardiac operations. It must be stressed that underlying and precipitating causes of cardiac dysfunction can coexist in the perioperative period. Some of the more important precipitating factors are infection, infarction, fever, arrhythmias, arterial hypertension, anemia, and fluid overload. A precipitating cause either can be prevented or corrected more readily than the underlying organic cause. It should be identified and eliminated.

PROPHYLACTIC DIGITALIZATION IN SURGICAL PATIENTS

The prophylactic use of drugs, be it antibiotics or digitalis, has always been controversial. The expressed goal of prophylactic digitalization is to reduce the incidence of cardiac complications, mostly supraventricular tachyarrhythmias, in the postoperative period. In the last 40 years a large volume of evidence, both in favor of and against prophylactic digitalization, has accumulated. In this section a summary of both sides of the argument is presented first, before judgment is passed.

Prevention of Cardiac Complication after Thoracic Surgery

Some of the earliest and strongest arguments in favor of prophylactic digitalization came from the area of thoracic surgery. A high incidence of supraventricular tachyarrhythmias (predominantly atrial fibrillation and atrial flutter) soon after pneumonectomy and other noncardiac thoracic operations was first reported in several articles that appeared in the 1940s and 1950s. These articles[13–18] were largely case reports or limited studies, hinting at the beneficial effects of prophylactic digitalization. It was not until 1961 that the more comprehensive retrospective study of Wheat and Burford[19] appeared. In this review of 439 patients who were 55 years of age or older, these authors found that the incidence of postoperative cardiac arrhythmias was 23% in patients who were not digitalized and only 12% in

those who received prophylactic digitalis. This difference was statistically significant ($p < .01$). Atrial fibrillation was by far the most common complication, and the majority of these arrhythmias occurred within 72 hours after surgery.

They found that the incidence of arrhythmias increased with age. Arrhythmias occurred in 12% of patients 55 to 59 years of age; in 20% of patients 60 to 64 years of age; in 24% of patients 65 to 69 years of age; and in 28% of patients 70 years or older.

Burford and Wheat[19] found that prophylactic digitalization reduced the incidence of cardiac arrhythmias in all age groups. The reduction was from 14 to 6% in patients 55 to 59 years of age; from 23 to 13% in patients 60 to 64 years of age; from 26 to 18% in patients 65 to 69 years of age; and from 46 to 10% in patients over 70 years of age.

The incidence of arrhythmias was also influenced by the type of operation. The incidence was 26% following pneumonectomy, 25% following esophagectomy, and only 21% following lobectomy.

Prophylactic digitalization also reduced the incidence of supraventricular arrhythmias in two surgical groups: from 29 to 15% in those who had pneumonectomy, and from 28 to 9% in those who had esophagectomy; but it was without effect on those who had lobectomy.

On this basis these authors recommended that all patients over 60 years of age, in whom a major intrathoracic resection is contemplated, should be digitalized routinely preoperatively. These findings of Wheat and Burford[19] were confirmed later by the retrospective study of Shields and Ujiki[20] and that of Burman.[21] While Shields and Ujiki[20] found that the incidence of atrial fibrillation and flutter in patients who were digitalized before surgery was only one-fifth of that in patients who were not (2.7% in predigitalized patients versus 14% in nondigitalized patients), Burman[21] reported that the incidence of supraventricular tachyarrhythmias and congestive heart failure in predigitalized patients (4.2%) was only one-third of that in nondigitalized patients

(14%). Authors of both studies also reported lower general mortality as well as specific mortality related to cardiac complications in patients who were digitalized prophylactically. As a result of these reports, prophylactic digitalization of patients in the geriatric age group has become standard practice of many thoracic surgeons.

Prophylactic digitalization of thoracic surgical patients would not be a controversy if there had not been evidence to the contrary reported by Juler et al.[22] In their retrospective study, these authors reviewed a total of 563 patients following noncardiac thoracic surgery—395 without preoperative digitalization and 168 with routine prophylactic digitalization. The average age of these patients was 36 years old; the average age of the predigitalized group was 10 years older than that of the nondigitalized group.

They found the incidence of cardiac arrhythmias and congestive heart failure in patients who were digitalized preoperatively was nearly 3.5 times than in patients who were not digitalized (14.8% in predigitalized patients versus 4.3% in nondigitalized patients). This difference was not subjected to statistical analysis.

More specifically, the incidence of supraventricular tachyarrhythmias, cardiac arrest, premature ventricular contractions, and congestive heart failure was 10.7%, 1.8%, 1.8%, and 0.6%, respectively, in the predigitalized group, and 1.8%, 0.8%, 0%, and 1.8%, respectively, in the nondigitalized group.

While mortality due to heart failure was higher in the nondigitalized group (1.5% in nondigitalized patients versus 0.6% in predigitalized patients), mortality due to cardiac arrhythmias was higher in the predigitalized group (4.1% in predigitalized patients versus 1.5% in nondigitalized patients). In summary, mortality due to cardiac complications in the predigitalized group was more than 2.5 times that in the nondigitalized group.

These authors concluded that prophylactic digitalization offered no protection against cardiac arrhythmias in thoracic surgical patients. In fact, they suggested that digitalis cardiotoxicity could have been the cause of some arrhythmias in their patients who were given digitalis prophylactically. However, this study and that of Wheat and Burford are not exactly comparable. Patients in this study are younger and are without history of heart disease. Furthermore, the average age of patients who were digitalized prophylactically was 10 years older than those who were not. Since the incidence of postoperative cardiac arrhythmias following thoracic surgery increases with age, this factor may be partly responsible for the increase in incidence of cardiac arrhythmias found in the predigitalized group.

PREVENTION OF SUPRAVENTRICULAR TACHYARRHYTHMIAS AFTER CARDIAC SURGERY

The practice of prophylactic digitalization in cardiac surgical patients did not come into vogue until the 1960s. But unlike noncardiac thoracic surgery, there was little published evidence to show that prophylactic digitalization was beneficial in cardiac surgical patients. The case in favor of prophylactic digitalization to prevent cardiac arrhythmias or congestive heart failure after cardiac surgery was argued largely on theoretical grounds.[23-28] In the days when the majority of operations performed was correction of valvular or congenital abnormalities, prophylactic digitalization was indeed a logical argument. However, most of the cardiac operations performed today are revascularization of coronary arteries. Therefore this issue should be re-examined. Indeed there are several recent reports on this topic—some in favor of, and the others against, prophylactic digitalization.

The first report in favor of digitalization was that of Johnson et al.,[29] who studied prospectively 120 patients assigned randomly into a nondigitalized control group of 66 patients and a prophylactically digitalized experimental group of 54 patients. Physicians who were in charge of these patients in this study were not blinded to these assignments, and propranolol was discontinued routinely in all patients before their operation. In order to avoid potential digitalis cardiotoxicity, the authors did not fully digitalize the experimental group and the average serum digoxin level of these patients was only 0.75 ng/ml.

They found the incidence of supraventricular tachyarrhythmias was more than 4.5 times higher in the control than in the experimental group (26% in nondigitalized patients versus 5.6% in predigitalized patients). This difference was statistically significant ($p < .01$).

The incidence of premature ventricular contractions was also higher in the control group (26% in nondigitalized patients versus 18.5% in predigitalized patients), but the difference was not statistically significant. At no time was there any evidence of toxic arrhythmias in the experimental group.

There was no difference between the mortality rate of these two groups of patients.

These authors concluded that prophylactic digitalization was effective in the prevention of postoperative supraventricular tachyarrhythmias after coronary artery revascularization; this beneficial effect was seen even when the patients were not fully digitalized. In fact, these authors warned against regimens aimed at full digitalization because of the everpresent potential of toxicity. This beneficial effect of prophylactic digitalization was confirmed by the study of Csicsko et al.[30] who digitalized their patients in the immediate postoperative period, and by that of Johnson's colleagues[31] who repeated the study in patients in whom propranolol was no longer discontinued.

The first report against digitalization was also a prospective study, involving 140 patients assigned randomly to a control group of 79 patients and a digitalized experimental group of 61 patients.[32] As in the study of Johnson et al.,[29] these authors did not use a full digitalizing dose of digoxin and the serum level varied between 0.47 and 1.16 ng/ml in the digitalized experimental group.

The incidence of supraventricular arrhythmias in the experimental group was almost 2.5 times higher than that in the control group (27.8% in the predigitalized versus 11.4% in the nondigitalized group).

This difference was statistically significant ($p < .05$).

The incidence of premature ventricular contractions was also higher in the experimental group (20% in the predigitalized versus 11% in the nondigitalized group), but this difference was not statistically significant.

In addition to these findings, the authors reported that digoxin had to be withdrawn in four of the 61 patients in the experimental group because of toxic arrhythmias. Naturally they recommended against prophylactic digitalization in patients having coronary artery revascularization surgery. This negative correlation between the prophylactic use of digitalis and the incidence of postoperative supraventricular tachyarrhythmias was also observed in the earlier study of Pintor and Magri[33] on patients who had mitral valvuloplasty; the ineffectiveness of digitalis in the prevention of supraventricular tachyarrhythmias after coronary artery bypass surgery was also reported by Roffman and Fieldman,[34] who found that the incidence of this complication was equal in nondigitalized (28.2%) and predigitalized patients (28.9%).

In addition to the evidence presented, there have been other arguments put forth in support of prophylactic digitalization.

Many intravenous and inhalation anesthetic agents are myocardial depressants, and digitalis is the ideal drug to counteract the circulatory depressant effects associated with anesthesia.

The metabolic response to surgery always imposes an additional load on the heart. This extra load is increased even further in the presence of complications (e.g., fever, anemia, and sepsis). Under these circumstances, digitalis is the ideal drug for increasing cardiac reserve.

It is true that digitalis can reverse the myocardial depressant effects of thiopental[35] and halothane[36]; it is also true that digitalis can increase cardiac reserve in selected surgical patients[37-40]; but the necessity for prophylactic digitalization is largely unsubstantiated. For each of the arguments cited above, there is a counterargument. Anesthetics with minimal myocardial depressant effects are available. In any case, a mild to moderate degree of myocardial depression by anesthetics in patients with normal ventricular function decreases myocardial work and myocardial oxygen consumption; this is of benefit particularly to patients with ischemic heart disease.[41, 42] As for increasing myocardial reserve in patients not in heart failure, a metabolic cost has to be paid by the heart for this practice. Digitalization, by increasing the myocardial contractility of patients with normal cardiac function, increases myocardial oxygen consumption of the heart[43, 44] without any improvement in circulatory dynamics. This is a potent argument against prophylactic digitalization in a population 5% of which has overt or cover chronic myocardial ischemia.

Conflicting evidence and arguments concerning the effectiveness of digitalis in the prevention of postoperative supraventricular tachyarrhythmias have been presented. As yet no definitive conclusion can be drawn. Short of a large-scale prospective double-blind study, this controversy is not likely to be settled. However, in addition to the question of effectiveness, two other questions must be answered: (a) the adequacy of the regimens used in prophylactic digitalization and (b) the seriousness of postoperative supraventricular tachyarrhythmias.

In the prophylactic use of medications not only the proper agent should be chosen, but also an effective dose should be used. Therefore, it is important to determine the adequacy of the dose used in preoperative digitalization. This was indeed the approach of Selzer and Walter,[45] who examined 53 patients who were originally in sinus rhythm but developed atrial fibrillation after mitral valve surgery. Since digitalization decreases the rate of ventricular response in supraventricular tachyarrhythmias, they used this rate as an index of the adequacy of the dose.

They found at the onset of atrial fibrillation, the ventricular response was 120 to 200 beat/minute (mean = 163 beat/min) in patients who were not digitalized in the preoperative period; it was 115 to 174 beat/minute (mean = 138 beat/min) in those who were only partially digitalized; and it was 80 to 170 beat/minute (mean = 121 beat/min) in those who were "fully digitalized" by the "average-dose" technique.

Although the ventricular rate was slower in patients digitalized prophylactically, a large dose of digitalis was required to control the ventricular rate at the onset of atrial fibrillation in 50% of the so-called "fully digitalized" patients.

These authors concluded that judging the adequacy of digitalization in patients who have sinus rhythm and are not in heart failure is imprecise. In their hands the average-dose technique had only a 50% chance of attaining adequate digitalization—an exercise with a success rate not dissimilar to the flip of a coin.

An inadequate dose is likely the cause behind many of the failures in using digitalis to prevent postoperative supraventricular tachyarrhythmias, and yet the average-dose technique is the only option in prophylactic digitalization. This practical difficulty in attaining full digitalization of the patient in the preoperative period without pushing him into toxicity is in fact the strongest argument against prophylactic digitalization.

The third question concerns the seriousness of supraventricular tachyarrhythmias in the postoperative period. So far there is no evidence that these arrhythmias can cause harm, provided that the ventricular rate is controlled. This is the age of intensive care units, telemetered monitors, and potent intravenous inotropes and antiarrhythmic agents; supraventricular tachyarrhythmias can be brought under control rapidly with verapamil[46–48] before ill effects on circulatory dynamics are sustained. Careful observation of the patient during the operation and in the postoperative period, as well as decisive actions at the first sign of crisis, is a real alternative to the indiscriminant use of digitalis.

WITHDRAWAL OF DIGITALIS PRESURGICALLY

Whether digitalis should be withdrawn before surgery is another controversy. But unlike prophylactic digitalization, there is no published evidence on this subject, be it in favor of or against this practice. A sampling of current anesthetic monographs has yielded conflicting opinions. Kaplan and Dunbar[49] are against withdrawal; Garman and Fogdall[50] are in favor of withdrawal; Tinker[51] is in favor of withdrawal only before major abdominal, vascular, cardiac, or thoracic operations. None of these authors quoted supporting evidence. In the practice of cardiology, it has been the custom to leave a patient on digitalis for life once he is started on the medication. Although it has been shown that digitalis may be withdrawn in some patients after they have recovered from the acute stage of heart failure, it is impossible to identify these individuals short of a trial withdrawal. The perioperative period is certainly not the appropriate time to institute such a trial. The current philosophy with all medications is against withdrawal before surgery, so long as the dose and effects are optimal—and digitalis should not be an exception. But digitalis preparations do have a narrow therapeutic index; many factors can enhance the sensitivity of the heart to digitalis in the perioperative period. Surgical patients on digitalis should be monitored closely for signs of cardiotoxicity.

Digitalis Cardiotoxicity

Toxicity is a common side-effect of digitalis therapy affecting one-fifth to one-quarter of all treated patients.[52, 53] There are some indications that myocardial sensitivity to the toxic effects of cardiac glycosides is increased in the 24 hours immediately following cardiopulmonary bypass.[54] It may be related to potassium loss as a result of diuresis accompanying hemodilution techniques used in perfusion,[55] a disequilibrium between serum and myocardial digitalis levels following the onset of extracorporeal circulation,[54] and a higher than usual myocardial digitalis concentration in patients were digitalized recently (e.g., in prophylactic digitalization) as opposed to those who are on maintenance therapy.[56]

Digitalis intoxication affects many systems and cardiotoxicity can be fatal. The manifestations of systemic toxicity are listed in Table 20.1. These manifestations are nonspecific in nature; noncardiac symptoms are more common with digitalis leaf than with pure preparations, but *they do not always precede cardiotoxicity*. In fact von Capeller et al.[57] reported that cardiac arrhythmias were the first evidence of digitalis toxicity in nearly 30% of the patients.

Cardiac arrhythmias associated with intoxication can be quite diverse in nature—premature ventricular contractions, heart blocks, supraventricular tachyarrhythmias, sinus bradycardia, sinoatrial arrest and block, and atrial or ventricular fibrillation. In a survey of 10 published reports, Irons and Orgain[58] observed that no single arrhythmia is pathognomonic of digitalis intoxication, but ventricular ectopy (particularly bigemini) and various degrees of heart blocks are more common than others (Table 20.2). More than one type of arrhythmia

Table 20.1.
Systemic Manifestations of Digitalis Toxicity

Gastrointestinal—anorexia, nausea, vomiting, diarrhea, abdominal discomfort
Neuropsychiatric—malaise, headache, paresthesia, neuralgia, confusion, convulsion, anxiety, depression, psychosis
Ophthalmic—yellow/green vision, photophobia, halos, light flashes, scotomata, blurring
Dermatological—rashes, gynecomastia
Cardiac—arrhythmias, increase in severity of heart failure

Table 20.2.
Common Arrhythmias Associated with Digitalis Toxicity[58]

Heart blocks	34%
Ventricular bigemini	24%
Multifocal ventricular premature beats	16%
Nodal tachycardia	13%
Atrial tachycardia	10%
Atrial fibrillation	10%
Ventricular tachycardia	10%

can coexist in the same patient. It should be emphasized that the gradual downward slopping of the ST segment and inversion of the T-wave seen in digitalized patients (described vividly by Dubin as Salvador Dali's mustache) are due to nonspecific changes in repolarization (the so-called digitalis effect) and are not indications of digitalis toxicity.

FACTORS ENHANCING CARDIOTOXICITY

Many factors increase the sensitivity of the heart to the arrhythmogenic effect of digitalis.[59] They include hypokalemia,[60, 61] hypomagnesemia,[60, 62] hypercalcemia,[63] hypoxemia,[64] chronic respiratory disease,[65] old age,[66] myocardial ischemia,[67] hypothyroidism,[68, 69] beta-adrenergic stimulation,[70] and DC countershock.[71] If the patient is on digoxin, renal failure[72–74] and concurrent therapy with quinidine,[75, 76] verapamil,[77–79] or diazepam[80] also have the potential of enhancing toxicity; if the patient is on digitoxin, hepatic failure and withdrawal of enzyme-inducing agents[81] are other factors to be considered. It can be seen that many changes and iatrogenic measures associated with surgery also can increase the risk of toxicity in the perioperative period. They include fluid and electrolyte loss or translocation, myocardial damage, renal dysfunction, hepatic dysfunction, ventilation/perfusion inequalities, induced diuresis, catecholamine infusion, and defibrillation or cardioversion.

THE USE OF SERUM CONCENTRATION ASSAY

Due to the nonspecificity of the systemic and cardiac manifestations of digitalis toxicity, attempts have been made to improve the diagnosis of toxicity by the assay of serum concentration. Radioimmunoassay of digoxin[82] or digitoxin[83] serum concentration is now a well-established technique. The therapeutic concentration of digoxin is between .5 and 2.5 ng/ml; in the range of 2 to 3 ng/ml the therapeutic and toxic concentrations overlap. The therapeutic serum concentration of digitoxin is between 10 and 35 ng/ml and therapeutic and toxic concentrations overlap in the range of 30 to 45 ng/ml. Owing to this large degree of overlap between therapeutic and toxic levels, serum concentration should not be used as the sole criteria in the diagnosis of digitalis toxicity. Clinical acumen should be exercised in the evaluation of potentially toxic patients, and disappearance of toxic manifestations following withdrawal is the only confirmatory test.

THE MANAGEMENT OF CARDIOTOXICITY

The principle of treatment of cardiotoxicity is relatively straightforward and should include the withdrawal of digitalis and diuretics, the correction of hypokalemia, and the identification and elimination of other correctable factors which can enhance digitalis toxicity. If the patient is hemodynamically stable and there is no evidence of ventricular irritability, this approach is usually sufficient. In general toxicity will subside in 2 to 3 days and the dose of digitalis, diuretics, and potassium supplement can be adjusted at the end of this period.

In the presence of hemodynamic instability and/or ventricular irritability, however, more aggressive treatment is necessary. Naturally, digitalis and diuretics should be withdrawn and factors enhancing toxicity eliminated. *Potassium* can protect the heart against digitalis cardiotoxicity[84] and serum level should be increased to the upper limits of normal when toxic tachyarrhythmias or premature ventricular contractions are present. A number of antiarrhythmic agents are also effective. *Lidocaine* is the drug of choice in the treatment of digitalis-induced ventricular irritability.[85, 86] In therapeutic concentrations it reduces the enhanced automaticity of subsidiary pacemakers without affecting myocardial contractility and AV conduction. *Diphenylhydantoin* is another agent which reduces ventricular irritability without affecting contractility.[87, 88] It also suppresses supraventricular arrhythmias induced by digitalis and has the added advantage of enhancing AV conduction which is slowed by digitalis. It is the drug of choice in the treatment of toxic supraventricular tachyarrhythmias with or without AV block.

Propranolol is also effective in the treatment of both ventricular and supraventricular arrhythmias induced by digitalis,[89] but it can depress myocardial contractility and prolong AV conduction. Therefore, it is contraindicated in the presence of congestive heart failure or heart block, unless other supportive measures are instituted. Being less effective than lidocaine or diphenylhydantoin in the treatment of digitalis-induced ventricular tachycardias, it should not be regarded as a first-line drug. *Procainamide* is also a popular agent in the treatment of ventricular arrhythmias and some supraventricular arrhythmias, but its usefulness in the treatment of digitalis-induced tachyarrhythmias has largely been superseded by other agents. However, some authors still find it useful in the treatment of some toxic arrhythmias, particularly paroxysmal atrial tachycardia with block in the absence of hypokalemia.[90] *Cardioversion* for toxic tachyarrhythmias is highly controversial and is usually contraindicated because even more severe and bizarre ventricular arrhythmias have occurred after countershock.[91] But DC countershock is sometimes necessary in tachyarrhythmias refractory to drug therapy. It is a desperate measure and should be undertaken only after all correctable factors have been eliminated. When it is essential to proceed, low energy levels and small-graded increments should be employed.[92] Lidocaine or diphenylhydantoin should be given immediately before cardioversion to suppress ventricular irritability often seen after cardioversion in digitalized patients.[93, 94] If propranolol is used instead of lidocaine or diphenylhydantoin, the prophylactic placement of a transvenous pacemaker is indicated.

When bradyarrhythmias or AV block is present, potassium should *not* be administered unless hypokalemia can be demonstrated. This is because potassium itself can delay AV conduction. *Atropine*, by antagonizing the vagomimetic effects of digitalis on the SA and AV nodes often can restore normal sinus rhythm with one to one AV conduction. When atropine is unsuccessful, the placement of a transvenous pacemaker should be considered.[95]

References

1. Gosselin RA: *National Prescription Audit.* 9th Ed. Gosselin, Ambler, Pennsylvania, 1972.
2. Spann JF, Hurst JW: The recognition and management of heart failure. In Hurst JW (ed): *The Heart.* McGraw-Hill, New York, 1982, p. 407.
3. Dimitroff SP, Lewis RC, Thorner MC, et al: Oral mercurial diuretics: Mercumatilin in the treatment of congestive heart failure. *Am Heart J* 49:407, 1955.
4. Lemberg L: Digitalis in congestive heart failure. *Arch Intern Med* 138:451, 1978.
5. Batterman RC: The status of mercurial diuretics for the treatment of congestive heart failure. *Am Heart J* 42:311, 1951.
6. Klein M, Nejad NS, Lown B, et al: Correlation of the electrical and mechanical changes in the dog heart during progressive digitalization. *Circ Res* 29:635, 1971.
7. Kim YI, Noble RJ, Zipes DP: Dissociation of the inotropic effect of digitalis from its effect on atrioventricular conduction. *Am J Cardiol* 36:459, 1975.
8. LeJemtel TH, Keung E, Sonnenblick EH, et al: Amrinone: A new non-glycosidic, non-adrenergic cardiotonic agent effective in the treatment of intractable myocardial failure in man. *Circulation* 59:1098, 1979.
9. Baim DS, McDowell AV, Cherniles J, et al: Evaluation of a new bipyridine inotropic agent—milrinone—in patients with severe congestive heart failure. *N Engl J Med* 309:748, 1983.
10. Tobin JR: The treatment of congestive heart failure. *Arch Intern Med* 138:453, 1978.
11. Sodums MT, Walsh RA, O'Rourke RA: Digitalis in heart failure. *JAMA* 246:158, 1981.
12. Cohn JN: Indications for digitalis therapy. *JAMA* 229:1911, 1974.
13. Bailey CC, Betts RH: Cardiac Arrhythmias following pneumonectomy. *N Engl J Med* 229:356, 1943.
14. Currens JH, White PD, Churchill ED: Cardiac arrhythmias following thoracic surgery. *N Engl J Med* 229:360, 1943.
15. Massie E, Valle AR: Cardiac arrhythmias complicating total pneumonectomy. *Ann Intern Med* 26:231, 1947.
16. Krosnick A, Wasserman F: Cardiac arrhythmias in the older age group following thoracic surgery. *Am J Med Sci* 230:541, 1955.
17. Cerney CI: The prophylaxis of cardiac arrhythmias complicating pulmonary surgery. *J Thorac Surg* 34:105, 1957.
18. Cohen MG, Pastor BH: Delayed cardiac arrhythmias following non-cardiac thoracic surgery. *Dis Chest* 32:435, 1957.
19. Wheat MW Jr, Burford TH: Digitalis in surgery: extension of classical indications. *J Thorac Cardiovasc Surg* 41:162, 1961.
20. Shields TW, Ujiki GT: Digitalization for prevention of arrhythmias following pulmonary surgery. *Surg Gynecol Obstet* 126:743, 1968.
21. Burman SO: The prophylactic use of digitalis before thoracotomy. *Ann Thorac Surg* 14:359, 1972.
22. Juler GL, Stemmer EA, Connolly JE: Complications

of prophylactic digitalization in thoracic surgical patients. *J Thorac Cardiovasc Surg* 58:352, 1969.

23. Willman VL, Cooper T, Hanlon CR: Prophylactic and therapeutic use of digitalis in open-heart operations. *Ann Surg* 80:860, 1960.

24. Dreifus LS, Rabbino MD, Watanabe Y, et al: Arrhythmias in the postoperative period. *Am J Cardiol* 12:431, 1963.

25. Burman SO: Digitalis and thoracic surgery. *J Thorac Cardiovasc Surg* 50:873, 1965.

26. Braunwald E, Mason DT, Ross J Jr: Studies on the cardiocirculatory actions of digitalis. *Medicine* 44:233, 1965.

27. Bristow JD, Griswold HE: The use of digitalis in cardiovascular surgery. *Prog Cardiovasc Dis* 7:387, 1965.

28. Wynands JE, Sheridan CA, Batra MS, et al: Coronary artery disease. *Anesthesiology* 33:260, 1970.

29. Johnson LW, Dickstein RA, Fruehan CT, et al: Prophylactic digitalization for coronary artery bypass surgery. *Circulation* 53:819, 1976.

30. Csicsko JF, Schatzlein MH, King RD: Immediate postoperative digitalization in the prophylaxis of supraventricular arrhythmias following coronary artery bypass. *J Thorac Cardiovasc Surg* 81:419, 1981.

31. Parker FB Jr, Greiner-Hayes C, Bove EL, et al: Supraventricular arrhythmias following coronary artery bypass. *J Thorac Cardiovasc Surg* 86:594, 1983.

32. Tyras DH, Stothert JC Jr, Kaiser GC, et al: Supraventricular tachyarrhythmias after myocardial revascularization: A randomized trial of prophylactic digitalization. *J Thorac Cardiovasc Surg* 77:310, 1979.

33. Pintor PP, Magri G: Digitalis and mitral surgery. *Cardiology* 55:34, 1970.

34. Roffman JA, Fieldman A: Digoxin and propranolol in the prophylaxis of supraventricular tachydysrhythmias after coronary artery bypass surgery. *Ann Thorac Surg* 31:496, 1981.

35. Goldberg AH, Maling HM, Gaffney TE: The effect of digoxin pretreatment on heart contractile force during thiopental infusion in dogs. *Anesthesiology* 22:975, 1961.

36. Shimosato S, Etsten B: Performance of digitalized heart during halothane anesthesia. *Anesthesiology* 24:41, 1963.

37. Talmage EA: The role of ouabain in myocardial insufficiency during anesthesia and surgery. *Am J Cardiol* 6:747, 1960.

38. Bille-Brahe NE, Engell HC, Sorensen MB: Acute postoperative digitalization of patients with arteriosclerotic heart disease after major surgery. *Acta Anaesthesiol Scand* 24:501, 1980.

39. Bille-Brahe NE, Engell HC, Sorensen MB: Prophylactic digitalization preoperatively of patients with arteriosclerotic heart disease. *Surg Gynecol Obstet* 152:183, 1981.

40. Pinaud MLJ, Blanloeil YAG, Souron RJ: Preoperative prophylactic digitalization of patients with coronary artery disease—a randomized echocardiographic and hemodynamic study. *Anesth Analg* 62:865, 1983.

41. Bland JHL, Lowenstein E: Halothane-induced decrease in experimental myocardial ischemia in the non-failing canine heart. *Anesthesiology* 45:287, 1976.

42. Verrier ED, Edelist G, Consigny PM, et al: Greater coronary vascular reserve in dogs anesthetized with halothane. *Anesthesiology* 53:445, 1980.

43. Covell JW, Braunwald E, Ross J Jr, et al: Studies on digitalis. XVI. Effects on myocardial oxygen consumption. *J Clin Invest* 45:1535, 1966.

44. DeMots H, Rahimtoola SH, Kremkau EL, et al: Effects of ouabain on myocardial oxygen supply and demand in patients with chronic coronary artery disease. *J Clin Invest* 58:312, 1976.

45. Selzer A, Walter RM: Adequacy of preoperative digitalis therapy in controlling ventricular rate in postoperative atrial fibrillation. *Circulation* 34:119, 1966.

46. Singh BN, Ellrodt G, Peter CT: Verapamil: A review of its pharmacological properties and therapeutic uses. *Drug* 15:169, 1978.

47. Antman EM, Stone PH, Muller JE, et al: Calcium channel blocking agents in the treatment of cardiovascular disorders. *Ann Intern Med* 93:875, 1980.

48. Lazzara R, Scherlag B: Treatment of arrhythmias by blocking slow current. *Ann Intern Med* 93:919, 1980.

49. Kaplan JA, Dunbar RW: Anesthesia for noncardiac surgery in patients with cardiac disease. In Kaplan JA (ed): *Cardiac Anesthesia.* Grune & Stratton, New York, 1979, p. 383.

50. Garman JK, Fogdall RP: The prebypass period. In Ream AK, Fogdall RP (eds): *Acute Cardiovascular Management—Anesthesia and Intensive Care.* Lippincott, Philadelphia, 1982, p. 402.

51. Tinker JH: Anesthesia for patients with ischemic heart disease. In Brown BR (ed): *Anesthesia and the Patient With Heart Disease.* F. A. Davis, Philadelphia, 1980, p. 74.

52. Beller GA, Smith TW, Abelmann WH, et al: Digitalis intoxication: A prospective clinical study with serum level correlations. *N Engl J Med* 284:989, 1971.

53. Evered DC, Champman C: Plasma digoxin concentrations and digoxin toxicity in hospital patients. *Br Heart J* 33:540, 1971.

54. Morrison J, Killip T: Serum digitalis and arrhythmia in patients undergoing cardiopulmonary bypass. *Circulation* 47:341, 1973.

55. Chamberlain DA: The influence of cardiopulmonary bypass on plasma digoxin concentrations. In Storsteon O (ed): *Symposium on Digitalis.* Glydendal Norsk Forlag, Oslo, 1973.

56. Krasula RW, Hastreiter AR, Levitsky S, et al: Serum, atrial, and urinary digoxin levels during cardiopulmonary bypass in children. *Circulation* 49:1047, 1974.

57. von Capeller D, Copeland GD, Stern TN: Digitalis intoxication: A clinical report of 148 cases. *Ann Intern Med* 50:869, 1959.

58. Irons GV Jr, Orgain ES: Digitalis-induced arrhythmias and their management. *Prog Cardiovasc Dis* 8:539, 1966.

59. Chung EK, Chung LS: Factors modifying the effi-

cacy of digitalis. In Chung EK (ed): *Controversy in Cardiology—The Practical Clinical Approach.* Springer-Verlag, New York, 1976, p. 85.

60. Kleiger RD, Seta K, Vitale JJ, et al: Effects of chronic depletion of potassium and magnesium upon the action of acetylstrophanthidin on the heart. *Am J Cardiol* 17:520, 1966.

61. Steiness E, Olesen KH: Cardiac arrhythmias induced by hypokalaemia and potassium loss during maintenance digoxin therapy. *Br Heart J* 38:167, 1976.

62. Seller RH: The role of magnesium in digitalis toxicity. *Am Heart J* 82:551, 1971.

63. Nola GT, Pope S, Harrison DC: Assessment of the syngergistic relationship between serum calcium and digitalis. *Am Heart J* 79:499, 1970.

64. Beller GA, Smith TW: Toxic effects of ouabain during normoxia and hypoxia in intact conscious dogs. *Circulation* 45:129, 1972.

65. Green LH, Smith TW: The use of digitalis in patients with pulmonary disease. *Ann Intern Med* 87:459, 1977.

66. Hermann GR: Digitoxicity in the aged: recognition, frequency, and management. *Geriatrics* 21:109, 1966.

67. Rahimtoola SH, Gunnar RM: Digitalis in acute myocardial infarction: help or hazard? *Ann Intern Med* 82:234, 1975.

68. Frye RL, Braunwald E: Studies on digitalis. III. The influence of triiodothyronine on digitalis requirements. *Circulation* 23:376, 1961.

69. Doherty JE, Perkins WH: Digoxin metabolism in hypo- and hyperthyroidism: Studies with tritiated digoxin in thyroid disease. *Ann Intern Med* 64:489, 1966.

70. Becker DJ, Nonkin PM, Bennett LD, et al: Effect of isoproterenol in digitalis cardiotoxicity. *Am J Cardiol* 10:242, 1962.

71. Castellanos A Jr, Lemberg L, Cenurion MJ, et al: Concealed digitalis-induced arrhythmias unmasked by electrical stimulation of the heart. *Am Heart J* 73:484, 1967.

72. Steiness E: Renal tubular secretion of digoxin. *Circulation* 50:103, 1974.

73. Doherty JE, Bissett JK, Kane JJ, et al: Tritiated digoxin: Studies in renal disease in human subjects. *Int J Clin Pharmacol Ther Toxicol* 12:89, 1975.

74. Gault MH, Jeffrey JR, Chirito E, et al: Studies of digoxin dosage, kinetics and serum concentrations in renal failure and review of the literature. *Nephron* 17:161, 1976.

75. Hager WD, Fenster P, Mayersohn M, et al: Digoxin-quinidine interactions: pharmacokinetic evaluation. *N Engl J Med* 300:1238, 1979.

76. Bigger JT Jr, Leahey EB Jr: Quinidine and digoxin—An important interaction. *Drugs* 24:229, 1982.

77. Pedersen KE, Dorph-Pedersen A, Hvidt S, et al: Digoxin-verapamil interaction. *Clin Pharmacol Ther* 30:311, 1981.

78. Schwarts JB, Keefe D, Kates RE, et al: Acute and chronic pharmacodynamic interaction of verapamil and digoxin in atrial fibrillation. *Circulation* 65:1163, 1982.

79. Klein HO, Kaplinsky E: Verapamil and digoxin: Their respective effects on atrial fibrillation and their interaction. *Am J Cardiol* 50:894, 1982.

80. Castillo-Ferrando JR, Garcia M, Carmona J: Digoxin level and diazepam. *Lancet* 2:368, 1980.

81. Solomon HM, Reich S, Spirt N, et al: Interactions between digitoxin and other drugs in vitro and in vivo. *Ann NY Acad Sci* 179:362, 1971.

82. Smith TW, Butler VP Jr, Haber E: Determination of therapeutic and toxic serum digoxin concentrations by radioimmunoassay. *N Engl J Med* 281:1212, 1969.

83. Smith TW: Radioimmunoassay for serum digitoxin concentration: methodology and clinical experience. *J Pharmacol Exp Ther* 175:352, 1970.

84. Chung DC: Anaesthetic problems associated with the treatment of cardiovascular disease: I. Digitalis toxicity. *Can Anesth Soc J* 28:6, 1981.

85. Hilmi KI, Regan TJ: Relative effectiveness of antiarrhythmic drugs in treatment of digitalis-induced ventricular tachycardia. *Am Heart J* 76:365, 1968.

86. Mason DT, Spann JF Jr, Zelis R, et al: The clinical pharmacology and therapeutic applications of the antiarrhythmic drugs. *Clin Pharmacol Ther* 11:460, 1970.

87. Conn RD: Diphenylhydantoin sodium in cardiac arrhythmias. *N Engl J Med* 272:277, 1965.

88. Helfant RH, Scherlag BJ, Damato AN: Protection from digitalis toxicity with the prophylactic use of diphenylhydantoin sodium: an arrhythmic-inotropic dissociation. *Circulation* 36:119, 1967.

89. Turner JRB: Propranolol in the treatment of digitalis-induced and digitalis-resistant tachycardias. *Am J Cardiol* 18:450, 1966.

90. Marcus FI, Gordon AE: Digitalis intoxication. In Mason DT (ed): *Cardiac Emergencies.* Williams & Wilkins, Baltimore, 1978, p. 363.

91. Lown B: Electrical reversion of cardiac arrhythmias. *Br Heart J* 29:469, 1967.

92. Bigger JT Jr, Strauss HC: Digitalis toxicity: Drug interactions promoting toxicity and the management of toxicity. *Sem Drug Treatment* 2:147, 1972.

93. Helfant RH, Scherlag BJ, Damato AN: Diphenylhydantoin prevention of arrhythmias in the digitalis-sensitized dog after direct-current cardioversion. *Circulation* 37:424, 1968.

94. Chou TC: Digitalis-induced arrhythmias. *Mod Treatment* 7:96, 1970.

95. Leon-Sotomayor L, Myers WS, Hyatt KH: Digitalis-induced ventricular asystole treated by an intracardiac pacemaker. *Am J Cardiol* 10:298, 1962.

CHAPTER 21

PERIOPERATIVE CARDIAC REHABILITATION

GENE ROBINSON, M.D.
VICTOR F. FROELICHER JR., M.D.

Despite clinical improvement, psychological problems are common after cardiac surgery, and the rate of returning to work is often less than expected. The effects of exercise training in cardiac rehabilitation programs are presented, and provide an interesting comparison to the changes observed after bypass surgery. Coronary artery bypass surgery (CABS) reduces ischemic symptoms by directly improving myocardial perfusion, whereas exercise training improves functional status predominantly by altering peripheral adaptations, thereby reducing the work of the heart and its oxygen consumption. Despite the apparent beneficial complementary actions of CABS and exercise training, few studies of CABS patients in exercise programs have been performed. The available studies have demonstrated that trained CABS patients achieve equal or greater increases in maximal oxygen consumption (V_{O_2}) max than post-myocardial infarction (MI), trained patients, further improve functional capacity initially improved by surgery, and train safely with no evidence of increased morbidity or mortality. Psychological well-being may also be improved.

Coronary artery disease (CAD) can present as the clinical syndromes of angina pectoris, acute MI, sudden cardiac arrest, and/or ischemic cardiomyopathy. Rehabilitation of persons with CAD may be defined as all efforts designed to restore and maintain the optimal level of physiological, psychosocial, and vocational function in the affected individuals. The most frequent symptom of CAD is angina, and so rehabilitation most commonly includes the control of angina. The two basic modes of therapy are medical and surgical.

If, after careful and intensive medical treatment, the patient believes that the quality of life is so adversely affected that other alternatives must be sought, CABS may be advised. Bypass surgery has become increasingly popular since the saphenous vein procedure began to be widely applied in 1968; approximately 110,000 operations were performed in the United States in 1979 at an average cost of $15,000 per patient.[1] The studies that have examined the added benefits of exercise training after CABS will be reviewed in this chapter, but first some background will be covered.

POSTOPERATIVE ANGINA RELIEF

The symptom of angina pectoris is reported to be relieved in 80 to 90% of patients undergoing surgery for chronic stable angina.[1] The majority of patients have had angina eliminated or reduced, and have improved their functional classification after operation. The mechanism of pain relief has been a controversial subject since the introduction of the procedure.[2–5] Placebo effect,[4] perioperative infarction,[6–9] and interruption of perivascular nerves[4] have all been proposed. Placebo effect would be difficult to prove, as a study design employing sham coronary artery bypass is currently not possible. A perioperative MI could eliminate or reduce the ischemic focus that produced angina. Complicating this possible explanation is the difficulty diagnosing perioperative MI.[10] Perivascular nerves accompanying the coronary arteries may be divided or traumatized during the grafting procedure. This interruption of the pain pathway from the heart might account for postoperative angina relief.

However, the evidence clearly favors increased oxygen delivery to the ischemic myocardium by increased myocardial blood flow as the usual mechanism of angina relief. Other nonspecific factors may possibly contribute.[5] Postoperative angiography has demonstrated more widespread opacification of the coronary system than exists preoperatively, with disappearance of collateral flow. Graft patency after surgery has been related to relief of angina and improved exercise tests.[7,9,11] However, angiography can only assess anatomical changes, not physiological, and provides a crude assessment of perfusion. Patients with all grafts occluded may show improved exercise tests and have no ischemic symptoms.[5,12]

Correction of ST-segment abnormalities in postbypass patients provides indirect evidence of increased perfusion of the formerly ischemic myocardium. Myocardial lactate production at rest and with exercise or atrial pacing has been used as a sensitive metabolic indicator of ischemic myocardium, corrected postoperatively by CABS.

The exercise thallium-scanning technique can demonstrate improved perfusion postoperatively.[13-17] Graft closure or areas of nonoperated disease may be detected by this technique, which has been correlated with blood flow or radiolabeled-carrier particles and angiography. There is little doubt that successful coronary bypass surgery can improve myocardial perfusion.[1]

POSTOPERATIVE PHYSIOLOGICAL CHANGES

As previously mentioned, on postoperative exercise training CABS can result in correction of ST-segment abnormalities and reduced myocardial lactate production. There are many reports of physiological changes after surgery, but few studies have had medical controls. Many compare physiological effects with postoperative coronary angiograms demonstrating patent or occluded grafts.

The physiological parameter most important to the patient's activity status is functional capacity, a measure of the patient's ability to perform physical work. The best noninvasive measure of this parameter is V_{O_2} max, which may be estimated or measured directly during exercise testing. V_{O_2} max can more accurately and objectively determine the degree of hemodynamic impairment than the physician's assessment of functional classification based upon anginal symptoms. Functional capacity has often been measured before and after CABS, and in the vast majority of patients it is significantly increased after surgery, due to relief of angina. In the subset of patients with residual angina, the symptom-limited V_{O_2} max often increases.[18] These results are seen in patients with patent grafts, but also in patients with partial occlusion and areas of residual ischemia. Absence of angina on postoperative exercise testing has even been seen in patients with all grafts occluded angiographically.[2,5] Block et al.[2] found that in 23 patients with all grafts occluded, exercise performance improved in some individuals and was roughly correlated with loss of abnormal ST-segment depression characteristic of ischemia.

Depression of ST segment during exercise testing is the most sensitive EKG indicator of ischemia, and many studies have shown fewer positive tests in postbypass patients. However, one controlled study demonstrated no significant difference in incidence of positive tests in medically and surgically treated patients,[19] and another controlled study revealed significantly more positive tests in post-CABS patients.[5]

In a study by Barry et al.,[20] 38 postbypass patients showed a significant increase in resting heart rate after 1 year. One possible explanation for this result is that preoperative tests were conducted while the subjects were taking beta-blocking drugs, which were discontinued postoperatively. Beta-blocking drugs lower heart rate, but all patients had received no propranolol for 48 hours before preoperative cardiac catheterization. No patients were taking propranolol after surgery. The lower preoperative resting heart rates may be attributable to a persistent negative chronotropic effect lasting greater than 48 hours. It may also be that the increased resting heart rate is simply an unexplained result of bypass surgery.

Rod and colleagues[21] established the feasibility, safety, and the cardiovascular responses to predischarge symptom-limited treadmill testing in patients soon after CABS. They tested 86 men (aged 55 ± 10 years) using a modified Naughton protocol 11 ± 26 days postsurgery. Twenty-four patients were taking propranolol. No major complications occurred during the study, and the main reason for termination of the tests was fatigue (88%). Serial data showed the average heart rate and systolic blood pressure responses to be linear with increasing multiples of resting metabolic equivalents (METs). The average heart rate increment per MET increase in exercise intensity was 6 beat/minute for the no-propranolol group and 4 beat/minute for the propranolol group. The average increase in systolic blood pressure per MET was 7 mm Hg for the no-propranolol group and 5 mm Hg for the propranolol group. In 10 patients, two of whom were taking propranolol, systolic blood pressure did not rise appropriately during graded exercise. Four patients who showed ST-segment changes greater than 2 mm from rest were taking digoxin. The only serious dysrhythmia was ventricular coupling in eight patients. Fewer significant medical problems were revealed during exercise in these surgery patients than has been reported for MI patients. Maximum heart rate with exercise usually increases after bypass surgery. This finding on the treadmill or supine bicycle exercise test is substantiated by atrial pacing studies which increase heart rate to the maximum attainable for that individual or to the "angina threshold."[1]

Studies have shown no significant change in stroke volume after CABS. One study of a single postsurgical individual found an increase in this determination of left ventricular (LV) function,[21] but another study of 30 patients found a significant decrease.[22] The stroke work index was found to increase after bypass surgery in another study.[23] Cardiac output at rest and during exercise has been demonstrated to increase. As cardiac output is the product of heart rate and stroke volume, the increase is apparently related to the increased postoperative heart rates previously described.

LV function assessed by regional wall-motion analysis has improved in most patients studied. An older study of the first 153 cases of saphenous vein surgery performed at Johns Hopkins disagrees,[6] but recent studies show an improvement in regional function at rest[20, 24, 25] and with exercise.

Ejection fraction (EF) at rest and LV end-diastolic pressure after bypass surgery remain unchanged. Others studied radionuclide exercise EFs in 25 medically managed patients and found no changes at 6- and 14-month intervals, but 17 of 23 postbypass patients showed improved EFs with exercise.[8] This response corresponded to the loss of angina with surgery.

The maximal double product, an index of myocardial oxygen consumption calculated from the heart rate and systolic blood pressure at maximal exercise usually increases after CABS. Double product at the point of ST depression and at the onset of angina during exercise testing can also increase. This generally correlates with V_{O_2} max which cannot be measured directly in patients. After bypass surgery, a decreased or below average maximal double product may indicate graft occlusion or poor LV function.[27]

LONG-TERM OUTCOME AFTER CORONARY ARTERY BYPASS SURGERY

Having considered the excellent symptomatic relief and favorable physiological changes resulting from CABS, two questions of utmost concern to the patient should be answered: (a) how long will improvement persist, and (b) does bypass surgery prolong life?

Angina will recur or progress after bypass surgery in about 5% of patients per year.[1] In approximately two-thirds of these patients with recurrent postoperative angina, symptoms are related to closure of the vein graft or progression of the disease in the native circulation. Early patency has been directly correlated with graft flow rate measured at the time of surgery, and long-term vein graft patency may be dependent upon the state of the distal vascular bed at surgery. Saphenous vein grafts to the left anterior descending artery, which usually provides greater runoff, have better patency rates than those attached to the right and circumflex coronary arteries. Vein graft closure or disease progression in the native circulation may be related to persistent elevation of blood lipids or poor control of other risk factors.

The impact of CABS on survival of patients with CAD has been a controversial topic, but two large randomized studies[28, 29] and the report of a National Institutes of Health Consensus-Development Conference[1] have recently summarized the available knowledge.

It is estimated that 5 to 10% of patients undergoing CABS have intraoperative MIs. Hammermeister[30] has concluded that this is not a benign event, as most clinicians and surgeons have thought. He estimated a three-fold increase in risk for death in these patients. Currently, patients who have an intraoperative infarction are not treated in a manner different from other postoperative patients in cardiac rehabilitation.

PSYCHOLOGICAL OUTCOME AFTER CORONARY ARTERY BYPASS SURGERY

Psychological problems are common following cardiac surgery, despite the clinical improvement discussed in previous sections of this review. It is unreasonable to expect cure of chronic depression after bypass surgery, yet the marked symptomatic alleviation may lead the physician and patient to expect this. Several studies have examined

personality and psychologic functioning after open heart surgery.

Frank et al.[31] surveyed 800 patients postoperatively who had had open heart surgery, but no CABS. Two-thirds of the patients reported anxiety, depression, confusion, and feelings of unreality following cardiac surgery. Seventeen percent claimed that psychological factors interfered with their recovery up to 1 year postoperatively, despite improved medical status. In another study of open heart surgery (without CABS), Heller et al.[32] conducted preoperative and 1-year postoperative interviews with patients, and found one-third were still encountering significant psychological hindrance. This subset of patients showed considerable anxiety, depression, somatic preoccupation, social withdrawal, and impaired sexual function. Overall, the study found patients became less self-reliant and more socially constricted after surgery, despite little physical impairment.

Rabiner and Wilner[33] studied 51 CABS patients soon after operation and again at 18 months. Formal psychological impairment was present in 16% of the patients, with depression and/or chronic brain syndrome as the chief disorders. Significantly, the patient's psychopathology in the immediate postoperative period was not predictive of difficulty late in convalescence, but preoperative psychiatric illness was very related to the psychopathology seen at 18-month followup.

Gundle et al.[34] studied 30 patients before and 1 to 2 years after CABS. The average age was 51.4 years. Seventy-seven percent were employed and 73% sexually functional before surgery. One to 2 years after surgery, only 17% were employed and 43% sexually functional. Return to work, as will be discussed in the next section, is dependent on many factors, but evidence of damaged self-image was thought to be prominent in these low-socioeconomic status patients. This damaged self-concept was thought to be reinforced rather than repaired by surgery.

The effect of cardiac rehabilitation on psychological status in medically and surgically treated coronary patients was assessed by Soloff.[35] This study did not evaluate patients preoperatively, but the 27 postoperative bypass surgery patients were found to have less mood disturbance at the beginning of a 6-week exercise program than medically managed patients. The two groups did not differ in the use of denial. Mood improved in both groups after exercise training, and individual mood changes were independent of changes in physical performance assessed by exercise testing.

RETURN TO WORK FOLLOWING CORONARY ARTERY BYPASS SURGERY

Resumption of gainful employment after surgery for coronary artery disease has been widely studied. The number of patients employed postoperatively has been selected as a fairly objective measure of the true functional status of the patient. Theoretically, improvements in symptoms and functional capacity should enable more patients to return to work and, thereby, economically justify surgical treatment of CAD by increasing productivity.[36] The results of nearly every published study assessing the impact of bypass surgery on employment are presented in Tables 21.1 and 21.2. Those studies which demonstrate increased employment postoperatively or greater return to work with surgical therapy compared to medical therapy are listed in Table 21.1. The majority of studies have shown a disappointing retention of or resumption of gainful employment, and are detailed in Table 21.2. A recent supplement to *Circulation* examined the economic, ethical, and social issues in relation to coronary artery bypass surgery.[37]

Johnson and colleagues[56] have reported a study of 2229 consecutive male patients followed for as long as 10 years with a 90% followup. They concentrated on their employment patterns before and after myocardial revascularization surgery. Every living male patient operated on from 1968 to 1978 was surveyed for his pre- and postoperative work status and compared with the United States population as reported by the United States Bureau of Labor Statistics. Comparisons were made on an age-for-age basis and adjustments were made for changes in national employment patterns. Preoperatively, the younger patients had a 10% lower employment rate than the male population at large. Postoperatively, many returned to work, but some who worked preoperatively did not postoperatively. The ability to work full-time with little or no limitation increased 20% postoperatively. The main reason for not working was physical disability, with doctor's advice a distant second. Older patients showed a trend of accelerated retirement after surgery. Of all older subjects, 30% said that the desire to relax was the main reason for not working. Patients with severely impaired LV function did worse, but the improvement was the same as for other patients.

Dimsdale and colleagues[57] studied the clinical history, epidemiological risk factors, psychosocial factors, angiographic findings, and treatment characteristics in relationship

Table 21.1.

Return to Work following CABS: Studies Demonstrating Increased Employment Postoperatively

Reference	No. of Subjects	Mean Postoperative Followup At:	Working	
			Preoperative	Postoperative
36 Crosby et al. (U.S.) 1980	52	6 to 8 weeks	33%	63%
38 Frick et al. (Finland) 1979	50 surgical	2 years	60%	36%
	50 medical		68%	18%
39 Liddle (U.S.) 1981	358	6 months	44%	85%
40 Niles et al. (U.S.) 1980	105	20 months	50%	60%
41 Symmes et al. (Canada) 1978	329	23 months	54%	65%
42 Wallwork et al. (U.K.) 1978	115	16 months	22%	65%
43 Westaby et al. (U.K.) 1979	130	16.5 months	8%	60%

Table 21.2.
Return to Work following CABS: Studies Demonstrating No Clear Increase in Postoperative Employment

Reference	No. of Subjects	Mean Postoperative Followup At	Working	
			Preoperative	Postoperative
44 Anderson et al. (U.S.) 1980	564	1 and 4 years	91%	79% (1 year) 70% (4 years)
45 Barnes et al. (U.S.) 1977	350	1 year	No net improvement; no increase in hours worked	
54 Cannon et al. (U.S.) 1974	400	10 months	(−)	59%
46 Danchin et al. (Canada) 1980	1320	2 and 5 years	84%—12 months preop 66.5%— 6 months preop	66.5% (2 years) 53% (5 years)
47 David (Canada) 1978	500	"Postop"	(−)	62% "active"
48 Dussek et al. (U.K.) 1979	123	1 year	(−)	72%
49 English et al. (U.S.) 1975	110 private patients	26 months	82%	75%
	168 VA patients		44%	32%
50 Fox et al. (U.S.) 1975	32	1 to 4 years	(−)	56%
34 Gundle et al. (U.S.) 1980	30	1 to 2 years	77%	17%
51 Hammermeister et al. (U.S.) 1979	201 medical 1198 surgical	1 year	74% 75%	62% 62%
19 Kloster et al. (U.S.) 1977	49 medical 51 surgical	6 months to 4.5 years	(−) (−)	20% 20%
52 Love (U.S.) 1980	95	15.5 months	64%	54%
53 Rimm et al. (U.S.) 1976	893	14 months (median)	91%	53%

to the work status of 182 men who underwent coronary angiography for evaluation of CAD. Followup at 1 year found 42% of the cohort persistently unemployed or working at a lower level, 40% at the same job, and 19% at a more demanding job. Multiple-regression analysis was used to derive the most important variables predictive of work status. Neither number of vessels diseased nor CABS entered the multiple-regression analysis. Instead, the most important variables, listed in decreasing order of importance, were: age, subsequent cardiac morbid events, past MI, and mood during the followup year. Together, they accounted for 24% of the variance in work status outcome ($p < .001$).

The objective of a recent West German study[58] was to determine the long-term effects of coronary artery bypass graft surgery on exercise capacity and vocational rehabilitation. Four hundred sixty-seven patients who had undergone CABS at age 55 years or younger between 1973 and 1979 responded to a questionnaire inquiring about their present work status. The mean followup was 3.5 years. Exercise capacity improved from 62 watts preoperatively to 96 watts 1 year postoperatively. Five years after surgery, exercise capacity was still markedly improved 85 watts ($p < .0005$). The percentage of patients working from 1 to 4 years after CABS remained between 53 and 56%, and decreased to 47% at 5 years. The percentage of patients able to return to work after surgery was clearly related to postoperative exercise capacity. Only 30% of patients with an exercise capacity of less than 60 watts were working, as opposed to 75% of patients with an exercise capacity greater than 120 watts. The beneficial effect of CABS on exercise capacity was maintained for at least 5 years after surgery. Improved exercise capacity correlated with the return-to-work rate. The percentage of patients with angina pectoris and exercise-induced ST depression increased at a rate of 5%/year. An optimal surgical result with high exercise capacity without angina is a prerequisite for good employability and successful rehabilitation. Nonmedical factors related to the social system, particularly relative to being a blue or white collar worker, also influence the return-to-work rate.[58]

What are the reasons for failure to return to work in apparently symptomatically-improved individuals with demonstrated increased work capacities? Table 21.3 covers many of the factors found to be significant in various studies, showing that predominantly nonmedical reasons govern failure to return to work. Recent work status (e.g., having worked within the period 6 months prior to surgery) consistently favors return to work after surgery. The longer the patient has been unemployed, the less likely the return to work. This association has been used to argue that minimally-incapacitated patients are chosen for surgery, thereby inflating postoperative rates of return to work.

Preoperative predictors of postoperative employment status were studied in 228 patients (aged 25 to 64 years) who underwent cardiac surgery.[59] Of the 150 patients working in the year before surgery, 73% returned to work within 6 months. Of those not so employed, 18% started working. Patients who expected preoperatively to return to work did so at an 82% rate compared with 39% of the others. This was a strong predic-

Table 21.3.
Determinants of Return to Work after CABS

Favoring Factors	Nonpredictive Factors	Deterring Factors
Recent work status (unemployed less than 6 months)	Improvement in symptoms Angina pectoris Dyspnea	↑ Age at surgery ↓ Educational level ↓ Social class scale ↑ Family income
Physician encouragement of prompt return to work	Improvement in exercise tolerance Severity of coronary disease	Vocationally disadvantaged patients Anxiety or depression Physical requirements of job
Rehabilitation program	Completeness of myocardial revascularization	Prior MI Postoperative symptoms with effort (functional class) Angina pectoris, severe Dyspnea Palpitations
Patient's expectation to work Good exercise capacity		Perception of illness as job-related Financial/social/disability compensation Pension and retirement benefits Legislation re: employer liability, health care costs, insurance costs

tor in the multiple-regression analysis. Educational level and family income were stronger predictors than occupation or level of physical exertion required. Rates of return were higher in patients with less severe angina and less fatigue preoperatively, but did not differ significantly by sex, surgical procedure, or duration of illness. Seven variables predicted work status correctly for 86% of persons. These results suggest that determinants of return to work are largely present before surgery, and that patients' attitudes and expectations play an important role.[59]

Physician advice may contribute to the patient's failure to return to work. Many do not make consistent recommendations to patients regarding exercise potential and employability after successful coronary surgery. In a study by David[47] of 500 postbypass males, 62% were working and 38% inactive. Of the men not working, 77.5% were assessed objectively as able to return to work, but 60.6% attributed nonreturn to work to medical advice. Physicians should become aware of the importance of encouraging prompt return to work in their surgically treated patients. Yet it also is the physician's duty to discuss carefully return to work with the patient to ensure that a return to the premorbid, coronary-prone pattern of overly ambitious pursuit of work and high job dissatisfaction does not occur.

Postoperative nonwork income in the form of Workmen's compensation, disability payments, and pensions may deter resumption of employment. Danchin et al.,[46] in a French-Canadian population, found that the majority of patients who did not return to work kept a stable income, and 83% received financial aid from the government. Russell et al.[60] examined variables affecting return to work in a small, randomized study, and found surgical patients could more easily become eligible for disability compensation than medically-treated patients. The most important negative predictor of return to work in this study was nonwork income postoperatively. However, in a followup of 105 CABS patients without medical controls, Niles et al.[40] found that preoperative work status and symptomatic relief were more predictive of return to work than a comparison of preoperative and postoperative means of support.

Postoperative symptoms also deter return to work. Angina and dyspnea after surgery are generally associated with failure to return to work,[41, 44, 45] although two recent studies dispute the importance of angina to postoperative work status.[46, 60] Improvement in symptoms is, therefore, classified as nonpredictive of return to work in Table 21.3, while the presence of symptoms is considered a deterrent. Technical aspects of surgery, such as completeness of revascularization[38] and absence of significant postoperative LV dysfunction[52] have been associated with increased return to work, but are disputed.[59] Many other factors such as age, educational level, social class, prior MI, physical requirements of one's job, and perception of illness as job-related will determine return to work, as summarized in Table 21.3.

In summary, return to work, although widely used as such, is a poor measure of efficacy of therapy, as it depends on too many nonmedical factors. However, the enormous economic cost to society of bypass surgery may require the postoperative return of the majority of individuals to gainful activity to justify the procedure.

As studies have shown disappointing rates of resumption of employment after surgery, there has been increasing interest recently in programs of cardiac rehabilitation involving exercise training and/or vocational rehabilitation.[45] Crosby et al.[36] demonstrated increased employment from 33% preoperatively to 63% postoperatively in two groups of 66 patients. These patients were not involved in a formal cardiac rehabilitation program, but were encouraged to participate in an unsupervised, inexpensive physical rehabilitation program early in the postoperative period. This included simple calisthenics performed at home and a graduated walking regimen; 6 weeks after surgery most patients were walking 2 to 5 miles daily. This encouraging, small study illustrates the possible benefits of exercise training in the postbypass patient, which will be discussed further in the next section.

THE RESPONSE TO AN EXERCISE PROGRAM

Chronic exercise or an exercise program has also been called "training" or "physical conditioning." What is meant is that an individual maintains a regular habit of exercise at levels greater than he or she usually performs. Exercise can be designed for increasing muscular strength or dynamic (aerobic) performance. The type of exercise that results in an increase in muscular strength is isometric exercise or exerting muscular tension with little movement against resistance. Although this results in an increase in muscular mass along with strength, such exercises have little effect on the cardiovascular system. The heart works against a pressure load without much of an increase in cardiac output. Dynamic exercise, also called isotonic or aerobic, involves the rapid movement of large muscle masses that results in the need for the body to respond with increasing ventilation in order to increase oxygen consumption. Such exercise is also called aerobic since it must be performed without accumulating an anaerobic debt. The heart must increase its output and performs flow work rather than pressure work. This is the type of exercise that results in the cardiovascular changes that will be described.

The features of an aerobic exercise program that must be considered include: the mode, duration, intensity, and frequency of exercise. In general, the mode of exercise must involve movement of large masses of muscle. Such exercise includes bicycling, walking, running, and swimming. The exercise should be performed at least three sessions a week and be interspaced throughout the week. Duration should be 30 minutes to 1 hour. Intensity should be 50% or greater of the V_{O_2} max and involve at least 300 k/cal of energy expenditure. The percentage of V_{O_2} max being performed can be approximated from the heart rate and perceived exertion.

The results of such an aerobic exercise program can be grouped as: (a) hemodynamic; (b) morphological; and (c) metabolic. The hemodynamic consequences of an exercise program include a decrease in resting heart rate, a decrease in the heart rate and systolic blood pressure at any matched submaximal workload, an increase in work capacity and V_{O_2} max and a faster recovery from an exercise bout. Whether these changes are due to peripheral or to central adaptations has been argued, but they are probably due to both. Peripheral adaptations are more important in older individuals and in patients with heart or lung disease, while central changes are probably more of a factor in younger individuals. Central hemodynamic changes that have been observed in some instances include enhanced cardiac function and cardiac output.

The morphological changes that occur with an exercise program are clearly age-related. These changes occur most definitely in younger individuals, and may not occur in older individuals. The exact age at which the response to chronic exercise is altered is uncertain, but it would seem to be in the early 30s. Morphological changes include an increase in myocardial mass and LV end-diastolic volume. Paralleling these changes are increases in coronary artery size and in the myocardial capillary-to-fiber ratio. These changes are clearly beneficial, making it possible for the heart to function better and be better perfused during any stress. In older individuals, there might even be a decrease in myocardial mass that still results in an improvement in capillary-to-muscle fiber ratio, but no change in coronary artery size.

In patients with CAD, training is usually associated with increased tissue oxygen extraction. The major cause of the increased oxygen extraction is the augmentation of oxidative metabolic capacity in the skeletal muscles of trained subjects. Mitochondrial volume and oxidative energy stores of glycogen and triglycerides all increase in trained skeletal muscle, and lower blood lactate levels are observed in response to exercise. Whether parallel changes occur in the human myocardium is unknown. A light increase in hemoglobin concentration and arterial oxygen saturation is observed in some patients after exercise training.

Increased oxygen extraction from the perfusion blood permits a lower blood flow per unit of tissue, particularly at submaximal levels of exercise. Thus, peripheral oxygenation of skeletal muscles can be maintained with the same or lower cardiac output. The trained individual is able to respond to exertion without taxing the circulation and possibly compromising myocardial oxygen needs.

The most easily measured change observed in cardiac performance is the slowing of resting or submaximal exercise heart rate. This effect is universally observed with an adequate training program. Elevated resting heart rates are seen in patients soon after bypass surgery, as previously discussed. This may be a result of deconditioning after surgery. At the maximal or symptom-limited exercise level, the heart rate is usually not altered by aerobic conditioning programs, but has been reported to increase in certain patients limited by angina.

Exercise training affects not only the cardiovascular system; very important strengthening of the musculoskeletal system also occurs. Patients with CAD sufficiently severe to warrant CABS often have changes in the peripheral musculature caused by disuse. After CABS, the patient may experience further degeneration of the skeletal muscles as a result of prolonged bed rest. Low back pain from the immobility in the operating room and restricted activity, and pain of the sternum and chest wall from the surgical manipulation and forced coughing contribute to the deconditioning. Pain from the saphenous vein graft extraction site in the leg is common and leads to more inactivity. These musculoskeletal problems may be deleterious to the morale of the patient after surgery and, if not managed properly by postoperative exercise and early ambulation, may become sources of chronic disability. Chest wall pain due to the incision and splitting of the sternum may simulate angina and complicate the subsequent management of the patient. Postoperative exercises directed toward optimal flexibility, strength, muscle coordination and joint mobility may effectively control chest wall pain and other postsurgical problems.

THE EFFECTS OF BED REST

There are definite hemodynamic alterations due to deconditioning and more noticeably with bed rest. Young men maintained at bed rest for 3 weeks demonstrated a 20 to 25% decrease in V_{O_2} max.[61] Other than decreased functional capacity, prolonged bed rest results in orthostatic hypotension and venous thrombosis by a loss of blood volume, plasma loss exceeding red blood cell mass loss. Pulmonary function is decreased, and the patient can be in negative nitrogen and calcium balance.[62] Naturally, these effects can be avoided by early ambulation postoperatively.

The question has been raised as to whether the deleterious hemodynamic effects of bed rest, including decreased work tolerance, are due to inactivity or to the loss of the upright exposure to gravity. There are at least four reasons supporting the concept that much of these alterations are due to loss of the upright exposure to gravity: (a) supine exercise does not prevent the deconditioning effects of being in bed[63]; (b) there is both less and a slower decline in V_{O_2} max with chair rest than with bed rest[64]; (c) there is a greater decrease in the V_{O_2} max after a period of bed rest measured during upright exercise versus supine exercise[65]; (d) a lower body positive pressure device decreases the deconditioning effect of bed rest.[66] Perhaps intermittent exposure to gravitational stress during the bed rest stage of hospital convalescence from surgery or MI may obviate much of the deterioration in cardiovascular performance that can follow these events. Previous efforts to limit the decrease in capacity after MI or surgery have emphasized low level exercise training, but these data suggest that simple exposure to gravitational stress substantially accomplishes this purpose.

A continued program of exercise training results in strength and muscular endurance, which maintain proper muscle tone and protect against injury and low back pain. Flexibility exercises are important for similar reasons and should be practiced often, as reduced flexibility can lead to poor posture, fatigue, and injury. An endurance activity such as jogging in a program of exercise training can reduce the flexibility of the extensor muscles of the hip, leg, and ankle. Proper stretching exercises for these areas can prevent low back, hamstring, or calf muscle problems.

STUDIES OF THE USE OF EXERCISE TRAINING FOR CORONARY ARTERY BYPASS SURGERY PATIENTS

Cardiac rehabilitation programs emphasizing exercise training were originally conceived as an adjunctive therapy in the medical management of patients with chronic angina or following MI. Rehabilitation programs have expanded their scope to include patients treated with CABS, due to the large numbers of these patients and a theoretically excellent potential for rehabilitation. Bypass surgery patients have generally received the same rehabilitative efforts that medically-managed patients with CAD have. However, less than 120 surgical patients in a total of six studies have been studied in postoperative exercise programs.

Adams and colleagues[67] were the first to study training in bypass patients. They entered four male surgical patients into a training program with 45 sedentary normal males and 11 men with a history of prior MI training on their own. They found that after 3 months of walking and jogging at least 3 days a week, 40 minutes a day, at a heart rate of 75 to 85% of maximum, the bypass patients had functional capacities equal to the trained infarction patients, and had shown an 11% increase in V_{O_2} max. The sedentary normal men out-performed both groups, however. The heart rate response in later work stages increased 4 to 6 beat/minute after training in the surgical patients. No submaximal workload V_{O_2} changes were seen in these four subjects.

Oldridge and colleagues[68] conducted a study of the effects of bypass surgery and an exercise program of 32 months' duration. Twenty-one patients with angina were given maximal treadmill tests 1 week prior to CABS and again 16 weeks after surgery. Six of these patients then entered a program

of 45 to 60 minutes of exercise, 3 times a week, at heart rates achieved at 65 to 75% of their postoperative functional capacity. A control group of six subjects from the remaining group of bypass patients was chosen. These men were matched "as closely as possible" (details not provided) to the exercising patients. The control group patients had only participated in sporadic physical activities such as tennis or walking since surgery. Treadmill tests were then carried out on the conditioned subjects 32 months after training began, and 28 to 34 months after surgery in the control group. No significant change in resting heart rate or blood pressure was found in either group. Treadmill V_{O_2} max increased significantly by 28% in the conditioned group, with only a 3% increase observed in the unconditioned group during this same time period. The conditioned group had been tested previously after 4 months of conditioning, and by that time 90% of the total improvement in functional capacity observed at the end of 32 months had already occurred ($p <$ .005). Maximal rate pressure product (RPP, an indicator of myocardial V_{O_2}) was the same for the two groups at the end of the study, but the increase in the conditioned group RPP was due primarily to a higher heart rate. Submaximal workload RPP was decreased after 4 and 32 months in the conditioned patients, and was significantly lower than in the nonconditioned group at 32 months.

Soloff[35] conducted a nonrandomized, noncontrolled study of the effect of cardiovascular rehabilitation on mood and physical performance in 27 surgically treated and 18 postinfarction medically-managed patients. The postbypass patients significantly improved V_{O_2} max and maximum heart rate after an inpatient program of bedside exercise and early ambulation, followed by 6 weeks of EKG-monitored, 3 times weekly directed calisthenics, and 20-minute stationary bicycle rides at a heart rate determined from hospital discharge low-level exercise testing.

In Ireland, Horgan and colleagues[69] trained 51 patients three times a week, in a program which began 8 to 10 weeks after

CABS. These patients exercised for 16 minutes each session at a heart rate equal to 85% of their postoperative maximum. After 8 weeks of conditioning, duration of exercise and maximum workload were found to be significantly increased. Similar results were seen in a group of 57 postinfarction patients trained with the surgically treated group.

Hartung and Rangel[70] studied 10 CABS patients who began 3 to 6 months of three times a week, 20- to 40-minute sessions of walking, jogging, or stationary cycling at an intensity of 70 to 85% of maximum heart rate beginning an average of 10 months after surgery. V_{O_2} max had increased significantly at the conclusion of the study in the trained postbypass patients, with no significant changes in the other parameters studied. Improved V_{O_2} max was also seen in 24 postinfarction patients and 16 patients with positive exercise tests or multiple risk factors for CAD. No significant difference was found among the three groups in any of the variables evaluated, indicating a fairly uniform response to this exercise program in surgically and medically treated patients.

To assess the benefits of regular participation in a medically supervised cardiac rehabilitation program, 22 patients who had undergone coronary artery bypass (two groups of 11 each) were studied retrospectively.[71] Group 1 (mean age 53 years) was currently enrolled in the rehabilitation program. Group 2 (mean age 56 years) had begun, but had discontinued the program. The stated reasons for discontinuation were not medical. There was no difference in entry exercise tests, and presurgical catheterization data in both groups were comparable. Mean peak V_{O_2} by modified Douglas bag technique, heart rate × systolic blood pressure product, and treadmill duration time were recorded in a single testing period. Results revealed that Group 1 had higher peak V_{O_2} (30 ml/kg/min) than Group 2 (24 ml/kg/min) ($p < .005$) and greater treadmill time (11 min) than Group 2 (8 min) ($p < .01$). Nine of 11 subjects in Group 1 were fully employed versus four of 11 in Group 2 ($p < .01$). One of 11 subjects in Group 1 had been rehospitalized versus five

in Group 2. No one in Group 1 smoked, although four of the 11 subjects in Group 2 did smoke. The authors concluded that the coronary artery bypass patients in their rehabilitation program had greater peak V_{O_2} and treadmill test time, smoked less, were less often rehospitalized, and were more often fully employed than those who were not in such programs.

In a study testing the relationship between ratings of perceived exertion and heart rate, Gutmann et al.[72] have also provided information on the conditioning of postbypass surgery patients. Twenty patients (each averaging 4.2 bypass grafts) completed the inpatient cardiac rehabilitation program at Mount Sinai Medical Center, and entered the Phase II outpatient program immediately after hospital discharge. At 2 weeks after surgery, they received a moderate level treadmill test with a specified end-point of 6 to 7 METs, an increase in heart rate 30 beat/minute above standing resting heart rate, or signs and symptoms contraindicating further testing. Thirteen of the 20 patients were stopped after they reached the heart rate-MET criteria. Eight weeks after surgery, and following participation in three supervised aerobic exercise sessions per week, a symptom-limited treadmill test was administered. Submaximal parameters appeared to improve, but the two tests were not comparable and there were no controls.

Another report by the same group documented the hemodynamic, electrocardiographic, perceptual responses and medical problems associated with range of motion, exercise, and ambulation begun within 24 hours after CABS.[73] Twenty-four male patients without surgical complications received daily treatment during an average of 11 ± 3 days of hospitalization after surgery. Resting and peak exercise heart rate, immediate postexercise systolic blood pressure, and rating of perceived exertion using the Borg scale were obtained for range of motion, exercise ambulation, and stair climbing. On the first treatment day, the average patient completed five repetitions of range of motion exercises with active assistance and walked 133 ± 59 feet. Heart rate increased 5 ± 4 and 13 ± 12 beat/minute over rest for range of motion and ambulation, respectively, and systolic blood pressure increased less than 5 mm Hg over resting values for both range of motion and ambulation. By the final treatment day, all patients completed 15 repetitions of active-resistive range of motion exercise, had averaged 23 ± 9 minutes of treadmill ambulation at the speed of 1.7 mph, and had climbed 15 stairs. Heart rate increased 13 ± 6 and 11 ± 5 beat/minute over rest for range of motion and ambulation including stair climbing, respectively. Systolic blood pressure increased an average 4, 15, and 44 mm Hg for range of motion, ambulation, and stair climbing, respectively. Perceived exertion from the third to the final treatment day was from 10 to 13 (light to somewhat difficult) for all three modes of exercise. Medical problems occurred frequently throughout the 11-day treatment period, but were not serious. Ventricular dysrhythmias were exerted by 70% of patients and dyspnea was reported by 54%. They concluded that the hemodynamic and perceptual responses of CABS patients to early exercise and ambulation were moderate and not too fatiguing. Patients tolerated the rehabilitation program and did not exhibit serious medical problems.

In a prospective study, 521 consecutive patients who underwent CABS at their institution from 1978 to 1980 were referred for cardiac rehabilitation.[74] All patients who participated in this project were ambulatory and could perform activities conducted in their inpatient exercise center. This study was designed to see if low-level exercise could be performed safely after CABS, what medical problems would occur, how many problems would require intervention, what the electrocardiographic and hemodynamic postoperative responses were, and whether daily supervised, monitored exercise sessions would improve patient surveillance. Their program began as soon as 12 hours after surgery. The most common medical problems were ventricular dysrhythmias, hypotension, and angina pectoris. Heart rate and systolic blood pressure were only moderately elevated at the 2-MET level of activity which they used. Though they detected more ventricular dysrhythmias than were recognized previously, few of these required treatment. The duration of exercise was markedly increased from the first to the last day, while the intensity was augmented more moderately. Four percent of their patients developed angina, but they were complicated patients often having second or third bypass procedures. Ten percent of the patients exhibited systolic blood pressure drop, but rarely was this symptomatic. However, because some patients dropped their blood pressure during stair climbing, they have become more careful with monitoring blood pressure during stair climbing. The average total energy expenditure per session increased three-fold from 20 to 60 kcal in the first to the last session in the Inpatient Exercise Center. Ventricular dysrhythmias were first documented in 22% of the patients in the Inpatient Exercise Center. Just before hospital discharge, the average CABS patient increased his heart rate only 33 beat/minute over resting levels during a symptom-limited progressive treadmill test. The perceived exertion was 16.5 (very difficult) and a perceived exertion of 13 (somewhat difficult) corresponded to a heart rate that exceeded rest by 20 beat/minute. Because of these results, the upper limit for the increase in heart rates during inpatient exercise programs has been lowered from 30 to 20 beat/minute. Nearly 10% of the patients exhibited either orthostatic or exercise-induced hypotension, and so criteria for hypotension were developed. If patients exhibited a 10- to 20-mm Hg drop in systolic blood pressure in the absence of symptoms, the medical director should be consulted. If an asymptomatic patient exhibits a drop in systolic blood pressure greater than 20 mm Hg, the patient is not exercised. Symptomatic hypotension is considered an absolute contraindication to exercise. Hypotension was observed particularly more often after stair climbing than after treadmill ambulation. Therefore, blood pressures are now measured after six stairs have been completed. It is important that patients not stand motionless while blood pressure measurements are made. The specific causes of the orthostatic exertional hypotension observed were not clear. Of this population, 14% (14 patients) reported lightheadedness, 14% reported incisional discomfort, 3% reported claudication, and 4% reported angina pectoris. Forty patients exhibited hypotension, but only 11 required medical intervention. Hypertension occurred in only three patients, and in two of these it was exercise-induced. In short, this one study presents more data on exercising patients post-CABS than any previous report. Regarding safety, Pollock's group[74] has exercised more than 1300 surgical patients, representing approximately 1900 patient-hours of treadmill and bicycle ergometer exercise with no resulting morbidity or deaths. Other hours of ambulation in the cardiovascular ICU and the wards have been completed without any serious incidents.

The studies cited, although limited by methodology, patient numbers, and highly variable details of the rehabilitation programs employed, demonstrate several important points regarding the exercise training of CABS patients.

1. Early ambulation and routine immediate postoperative exercises for CABS can be accomplished safely. The Appendix contains exercises modified from Pollock's program that have been used successfully at our hospital.
2. Exercise-trained CABS patients achieve equal or greater increases in V_{O_2} max than post-MI patients trained in a similar exercise program.
3. Functional capacity and other indicators of cardiac performance are usually improved after surgery in CAD patients, and can increase further after exercise training.
4. CABS patients enter exercise training programs with less mood disturbance than MI patients and may, therefore, have improved participation and better compliance than medically managed patients.
5. Properly supervised and progressive exercise training of the CABS patient is safe. No studies have shown increased morbidity or mortality in CABS patients participating in cardiac rehabilitation programs. In fact, the program appears to be helpful in identifying medical problems.

References

1. Frye RL, Frommer PL: Consensus development conference on coronary artery bypass surgery: Medical and scientific aspects. *Circulation* (Suppl 2) 65:II1, 1982.
2. Block TA, Murray JA, English MT: Improvement in exercise performance after unsuccessful myocardial revascularization. *Am J Cardiol* 40:673, 1977.
3. Frick MH: An appraisal of symptom relief after coronary bypass grafting. *Postgrad Med J* 52:765, 1976.
4. Miller DW Jr, Dodge HT: Benefits of coronary artery bypass surgery. *Arch Intern Med* 137:1439, 1977.
5. Mnayer M, Chahine RA, Raither AE: Mechanisms of angina relief in patients after coronary artery bypass surgery. *Br Heart J* 39:605, 1977.
6. Achuff SC, Griffith LSC, Conti CR, et al: The "angina producing" myocardial segment: An approach to the interpretation of results of coronary bypass surgery. *Am J Cardiol* 36:723, 1975.
7. Bartel AG, Behar VS, Peter RH, et al: Exercise stress testing in evaluation of aortocoronary bypass surgery. *Circulation* 48:141, 1973.
8. Kent KM, Borer JS, Green MV, et al: Effects of coronary artery bypass on global and regional left ventricular function during exercise. *N Engl J Med* 298:1434, 1978.
9. Nitter-Hauge S: Exercise ECG in evaluation of aortocoronary bypass surgery; report on 66 patients. *Eur J Cardiol* 9:191, 1979.
10. Moore CH, Gordon FT, Allums JA, et al: Diagnosis of perioperative myocardial infarction after coronary artery bypass. *Ann Thorac Surg* 24:323, 1977.
11. Siegel W, Lim JS, Proudfit WL, et al: Spectrum of exercise test and angiographic correlations in myocardial revascularization surgery. *Circulation* (Suppl 1)51–52:I156, 1975.
12. McConahay DR, Valdes M, McCallister BD, et al: Accuracy of treadmill testing in assessment of direct myocardial revascularization. *Circulation* 56:548, 1977.
13. Greenberg BH, Hart R, Botvinich EC, et al: Thallium-201 myocardial perfusion scintigraphy to evaluate patients after coronary bypass surgery. *Am J Cardiol* 42:167, 1978.
14. Kolibash AJ, Call TD, Bush CA, et al: Myocardial perfusion as an indicator of graft patency after coronary artery bypass surgery. *Circulation* 61:882, 1980.
15. Kostuk WJ, Deatrich D, Chamberlain MJ: Noninvasive assessment of patients following aortocoronary bypass surgery. *Can J Surg* 21:104, 1978.
16. Ritchie JL, Narahara KA, Trobaugh GB, et al: Thallium-201 myocardial imaging before and after coronary revascularization: Assessment of regional

myocardial blood flow and graft patency. *Circulation* 56:830, 1977.

17. Verani MS, Marchus ML, Spoto G, et al: Thallium-201 myocardial perfusion scintigrams in the evaluation of aortocoronary saphenous bypass surgery. *J Nucl Med* 19:765, 1978.

18. Guiney TE, Rubenstein JJ, Sanders CA, et al: Functional evaluation of coronary bypass surgery by exercise testing and O₂ consumption. *Circulation* (Suppl 3)48:141, 1973.

19. Kloster FE, Kremkau EL, Rahimtoola SH, et al: Prospective randomized study of coronary bypass surgery for chronic stable angina. *Cardiovasc Clin* 8:145, 1977.

20. Barry WH, Pfeifer JF, Lipton MJ, et al: Effects of coronary artery bypass grafting on resting and exercise hemodynamics in patients with stable angina pectoris: A prospective, randomized study. *Am J Cardiol* 37:823, 1976.

21. Rod JL, Squires RW, Pollock ML, et al: Symptom-linked graded exercise testing soon after myocardial revascularization surgery. *J Cardiac Rehab* 2:199, 1982.

22. Brundage BH, Anderson WT, Davia JE, et al: Determinants of left ventricle function following aortocoronary bypass surgery. *Am Heart J* 93:687, 1977.

23. Carlens P, Landon C, Pehrsson K: Left ventricle pump function before and after aortocoronary bypass surgery. *Scand J Thorac Caridovasc Surg* 14:191, 1980.

24. Kolibash AJ, Goodenow JS, Bush CA, et al: Improvement of myocardial perfusion and left ventricle function after coronary artery bypass graft in patients with unstable angina. *Circulation* 59:66, 1979.

25. Kir LM, Dinsmore R, Vexendis M, et al: Effects of coronary bypass grafting on resting left ventricle contraction in patients studied 1–2 years after operation. *Am J Cardiol* 44:601, 1979.

26. Kent KM, Borer JS, Green MV, et al: Letter to the Editor. *N Engl J Med* 299:956, 1978.

27. Merrill AJ Jr, Thomas C, Schechter E, et al: Coronary bypass surgery: Value of maximal exercise testing in assessment of results. *Circulation* (Suppl 1)51–52:I173, 1975.

28. Varnauskas E, European Coronary Surgery Study Group: Prospective randomized study of coronary artery bypass surgery in stable angina pectoris. *Lancet* 2:491, 1982.

29. Murphy ML, Hultgren HN, Detre K, et al: Treatment of chronic stable angina: A preliminary report of survival data of the randomized VA cooperative study. *N Engl J Med* 297:621, 1977.

30. Hammermeister KE: Myocardial infarction during coronary artery bypass surgery—not a benign event. *Int J Cardiol* 2:516, 1983.

31. Frank KA, Heller SS, Kornfeld D: A survey of adjustment to cardiac surgery. *Arch Intern Med* 130:735, 1972.

32. Heller S, Frank K, Kornfeld D, et al: Psychological outcomes following coronary open-heart surgery. *Arch Intern Med* 135:908, 1974.

33. Rabiner CJ, Wilner AE: Psychopathology observed on followup after coronary bypass surgery. *J Nerv Ment Dis* 163:295, 1976.

34. Gundle MJ, Reeves BR, Tate S, et al: Psychosocial outcome after coronary artery surgery. *Am J Psychiatry* 137:1591, 1980.

35. Soloff PH: Medically and surgically treated coronary patients in cardiovascular rehabilitation: A comparative study. *Int J Psychiatry Med* 9:93, 1978.

36. Crosby IK, Wellons HA Jr, Martin RP, et al: Employability—A new indication for aneurysmectomy and coronary revascularization. *Circulation* (Suppl 2)62:I79, 1980.

37. Eliastam M, Gastel B: Technology assessment forum on coronary artery bypass surgery: Economic, ethical, and social issues. *Circulation* (Suppl 3)66:III-1, 1982.

38. Frick MH, Harjola PT, Valley M: Work status after coronary bypass surgery. A prospective randomized study with ergometric and angiographic correlations. *Acta Med Scand* 206:61, 1979.

39. Liddle JV: Presidential address. Perspectives in coronary artery surgery. *J Thorac Cardiovasc Surg* 81:1, 1981.

40. Niles NW II, VanderSalm TJ, Cutler BS: Return to work after coronary artery bypass operation. *J Thorac Cardiovasc Surg* 79:916, 1980.

41. Symmes JC, Lenkei SC, Berman ND: Influence of aortocoronary bypass surgery on employment. *Can Med Assoc J* 118:268, 1978.

42. Wallwork J, Potter B, Caves PK: Return to work after coronary surgery for angina. *Br Med J* 2(6153):1680, 1978.

43. Westaby S, Sapsford RN, Bentall HH: Return to work and quality of life after surgery for coronary artery disease. *Br Med J* 2(6197):1028, 1979.

44. Anderson AJ, Barboriak JJ, Hoffman RG, et al: Retention or resumption of employment after aortocoronary bypass operation. *JAMA* 243:543, 1980.

45. Barnes GK, Ray MJ, Oberman A, et al: Changes in working status of patients following coronary bypass surgery. *JAMA* 238:1259, 1977.

46. Danchin N, David P, Robert P: Changes in work status in a French-Canadian population after aortocoronary bypass surgery. *Arch Mal Coeur* 73:585, 1980.

47. David P: Contributing factors preventing return to work of cardiac surgery patients. *Cleve Clin Q* 45:177, 1978.

48. Dussek JE, Thompson HT, Williams BT: Return to work after coronary artery surgery for angina. *Br Med J* 1(6167):890, 1979.

49. English MT, Logan GA, Eyer KM, et al: Employment following coronary artery surgery. (Abstr) *Circulation* (Suppl 2)51–52:144, 1975.

50. Fox HE, May IA, Ecker RR: Long term functional results of surgery for coronary artery disease in patients with poor ventricular function. *J Thorac Cardiovasc Surg* 70:1064, 1975.

51. Hammermeister KE, DeRouen TA, English MT, et al: Effect of surgical *vs.* medical therapy on return to work in patients with coronary artery disease. *Am J Cardiol* 44:105, 1979.

52. Love JW: Employment status after coronary bypass operations and some cost considerations. *J Thorac Cardiovasc Surg* 80:68, 1980.

53. Rimm AA, Barboriak JJ, Anderson AJ, et al: Changes in occupation after aortocoronary vein-bypass operation. *JAMA* 236:361, 1976.

54. Cannon DS, Miller DC, Shumway NE, et al: The long-term follow-up of patients undergoing saphenous vein bypass surgery. *Circulation* 49:77, 1974.

55. Lawrie GM, Morris GC, Howell JF, et al: Results of coronary bypass more than five years after operation in 434 patients. Clinical, treadmill exercise and angiographic correlations. *Am J Cardiol* 40:665, 1977.

56. Johnson WD, Kayser KL, Pedraza PM, et al: Employment patterns in males before and after myocardial revascularization surgery. *Circulation* 65:1086, 1982.

57. Dimsdale JE, Hackett TP, Hutter Am Jr, et al: The association of clinical, psychosocial, and angiographic variables with work status in patients with coronary artery disease. *J Psychosom Res* 26:215, 1982.

58. Gohlke H, Schnellbacher K, Samek L, et al: Long-term improvement of exercise tolerance and vocational rehabilitation after bypass surgery: A five-year follow-up. *J Cardiac Rehab* 2:531, 1982.

59. Stanton BA, Jenkins CD, Denlinger P, et al: Predictors of employment status after cardiac surgery. *JAMA* 249:907, 1983.

60. Russell RO, Wayne JB, Kronenfeld J, et al: Surgical *vs.* medical therapy for treatment of unstable angina: Changes in work status and family income. *Am J Cardiol* 45:134, 1980.

61. Saltin B, Blomquist G, Mitchell JH, et al: Response to exercise after bedrest and after training. *Circulation* (Suppl 7)38:I78, 1968.

62. Leon AS, Blackburn H: Exercise rehabilitation of the coronary heart disease patient. *Geriatrics* 32:66, 1977.

63. Stremel RW, Convertino VA, Bernauer EM, Greenleaf JE: Cardiorespiratory deconditioning with static and dynamic leg exercise during bed rest. *Appl Physiol* 41:905, 1976.

64. Lamb LE, Stevens PM, Johnson RL: Hypokinesi secondary to chair rest from 4 to 10 days. *Aerospac Med* 36:755, 1965.

65. Convertino VA, Hung J, Goldwater D, DeBusk RF: Cardiovascular responses to exercise in middle-aged men following ten days of bed rest. *Circulation* 65:134, 1982.

66. Convertino VA, Sandler H, Webb P: The effect of an elastic reverse gradient garment on the cardiorespiratory deconditioning following 15 days bed rest. Reprints of Annual Scientific Meeting Aerospace Medical Association, Washington, DC, 1978, pp. 148–149.

67. Adams WC, McHenry MM, Bernauer EM: Long term physiologic adaptations to exercise with special reference to performance and cardiorespiratory function in health and disease. *Am J Cardiol* 33:765, 1974.

68. Oldridge NB, Nagle FJ, Balke B, et al: Aortocoronary bypass surgery: Effects of surgery and 32 months of physical conditioning on treadmill performance. *Arch Phys Med Rehabil* 59:268, 1978.

69. Horgan JH, Teo KK, Murren KM, et al: The response to exercise training and vocational counselling in post-myocardial infarction and coronary artery bypass surgery patients. *Irish Med J* 73:463, 1980.

70. Hartung GH, Rangel R: Exercise training in post-myocardial infarction patients: Comparison of results with high risk coronary and post-bypass patients. *Arch Phys Med Rehabil* 62:147, 1981.

71. Waites TF, Watt EW, Fletcher GF: Comparative functional and physiologic status of active and dropout coronary bypass patients of a rehabilitation program. *Am J Cardiol* 51:1087, 1983.

72. Gutmann MC, Squires RW, Pollock ML, et al: Perceived exertion-heart rate relationship during exercise testing and training in cardiac patients. *J Cardiac Rehab* 1:52, 1981.

73. Silvidi GE, Squires RW, Pollock ML, et al: Hemodynamic responses and medical problems associated with early exercise and ambulation in coronary artery bypass graft surgery patients. *J Cardiac Rehab* 2:355, 1982.

74. Dion WF, Grevenow P, Pollock ML, et al: Medical problems and physiologic responses during supervised inpatient cardiac rehabilitation: The patient after coronary artery bypass grafting. *J Cardiac Rehab* 2:248, 1982.

APPENDIX

DEEP BREATHING

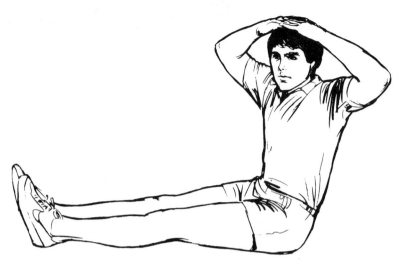

Repeat exercise:

Step 1–10 times

Directions: While sitting up in bed, lock hands on top of head and extend elbows out to sides. Take a slow, deep breath. Repeat 10 times. Do <u>not</u> breathe rapidly or hold your breath.

NECK CIRCLES

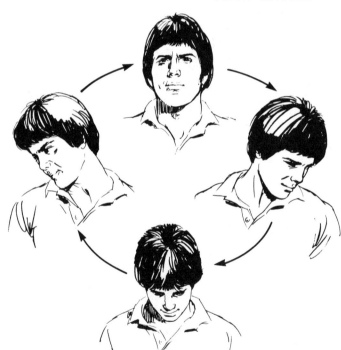

Repeat exercise:

Step 1 (A.M. & P.M.)—3 times
Step 2—5 times
Step 3—5 times
Step 4—5 to 10 times
Step 5—10 times
Step 6—10 times
Step 7—15 times
Step 8—15 times
Step 9—15 times

Directions: Slowly bend head to the right, then back, then to your left, and then forward. Leave your shoulders relaxed. Repeat the circle three times in each direction for Step 1.

Appendix Figure 1

SCAPULAR ELEVATION-DEPRESSION

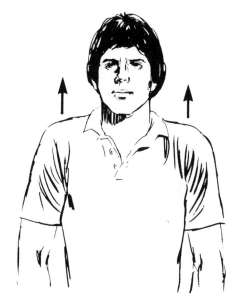

Repeat exercise:

Step 1 (A.M. & P.M.)—3 times
Step 2—5 times
Step 3—5 times
Step 4—5 to 10 times
Step 5—10 times
Step 6—10 times
Step 7—15 times
Step 8—15 times
Step 9—15 times

Directions: Keep back straight and hold arms at sides of body. Shrug shoulders up and then relax, letting shoulders fall. Repeat three times for Step 1.

SCAPULAR RETRACTION-PROTRACTION

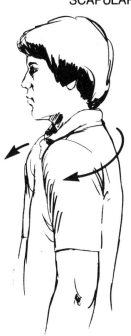

Repeat exercise:

Step 1 (A.M. & P.M.)—3 times
Step 2—5 times
Step 3—5 times
Step 4—5 to 10 times
Step 5—10 times
Step 6—10 times
Step 7—15 times
Step 8—15 times
Step 9—15 times

Directions: Keep back straight and hold arms at sides of body. Pull shoulders forward and in toward midline of body. Relax. Do not hold shoulders forward for a prolonged period of time. Return to starting position. Repeat three times for Step 1.

Appendix Figure 2

ELBOW-ABDUCTION-ADDUCTION

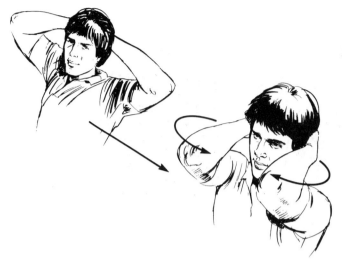

Repeat exercise:

Step 1 (A.M. & P.M.)—3 times
Step 2—5 times
Step 3—5 times
Step 4—5 to 10 times
Step 5—10 times
Step 6—10 times
Step 7—15 times
Step 8—15 times
Step 9—15 times

Directions: With hands locked behind the head, bring elbows together in front of you. Do not hold your breath. Return to starting position. Repeat three times for Step 1.

KNEE TO CHEST AND EXTENSION

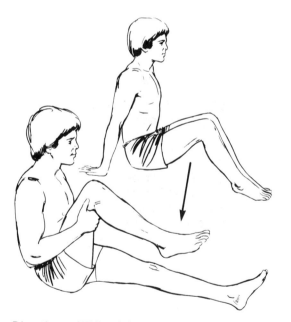

Repeat exercise:

Step 1 (A.M. & P.M.)—3 times
Step 2—5 times
Step 3—5 times
Step 4—5 to 10 times

Directions: While sitting up in bed or in a chair, bring one knee up toward your chest as far as you can. Do not hold your breath or hold your knee flexed for a prolonged period of time. Return to starting position. Repeat three times for Step 1.

Appendix Figure 3

ACTIVE ANKLE CIRCLES

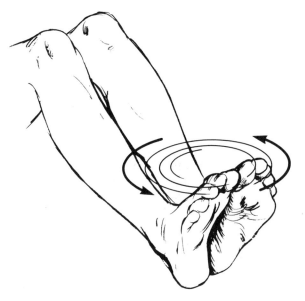

Repeat exercise:

Step 1 (A.M. & P.M.)—3 times
Step 2—5 times
Step 3—5 times
Step 4—5 to 10 times

Directions: While sitting up in bed or in a chair with your feet together, twist your feet to the right, forward, left, then back. Repeat three times in each direction for Step 1.

STANDING TRUNK LATERAL BENDING AND ROTATION

(Trunk Twisters)

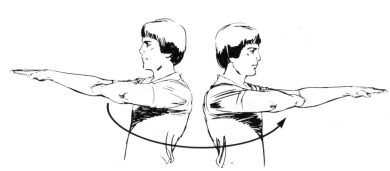

Repeat exercise:

Step 3—3 times
Step 4—5 to 10 times
Step 5—10 times
Step 6—10 times
Step 7—15 times
Step 8—15 times
Step 9—15 times

Directions: Stand with arms extended out to sides at shoulder level. Swing arms at shoulder level while bending and rotating at waist, left to right, then right to left. Keep arms relaxed and breathe regularly. Return to starting position. Begin this exercise on Step 3, repeating three times.

Appendix Figure 4

WALL STRETCH

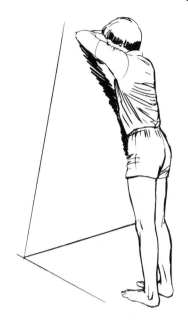

Repeat exercise:

Step 5—15 seconds
Step 6—30 seconds
Step 7—30 seconds
Step 8—30 seconds
Step 9—30 seconds

Directions: Stand arm's length away from a wall with feet less than shoulder width apart, toes turned slightly inward. Lean against the wall on your forearms, resting your head on your forearms, and slowly move your hips forward, keeping your back straight, holding your heels on the floor. You should feel a stretch in the back of your legs. Hold this position for 15 seconds (Step 5).

ARM CIRCLES

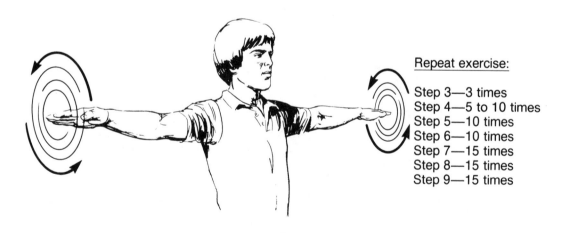

Repeat exercise:

Step 3—3 times
Step 4—5 to 10 times
Step 5—10 times
Step 6—10 times
Step 7—15 times
Step 8—15 times
Step 9—15 times

Directions: Stand with arms extended out to sides at shoulder level. Make small circles and gradually increase their size, then reverse direction. Begin this exercise on Step 3, repeating three times.

Appendix Figure 5

HAMSTRING STRETCH

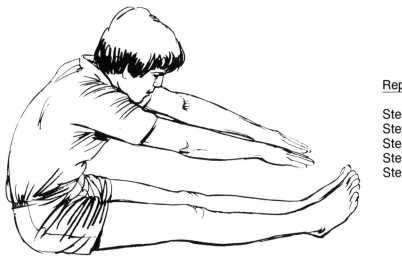

Repeat exercise:

Step 5—15 seconds
Step 6—30 seconds
Step 7—30 seconds
Step 8—30 seconds
Step 9—30 seconds

Directions: Sitting in a chair with feet propped up or sitting on the floor with legs extended in front of you, slowly reach your hands toward your feet and hold for 15 seconds (Step 5). Do not bounce or hold your breath.

MARCHING

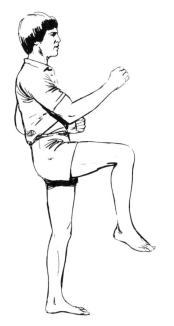

Repeat exercise:

Step 5—10 times
Step 6—10 times
Step 7—15 times
Step 8—15 times
Step 9—15 times

Directions: March in place, swinging your arms forward and lifting your knees as high as you can. Repeat lifting each knee 10 times for Steps 5 and 6.

Appendix Figure 6

INDEX

Page numbers in *italics* denote figures; those followed by "*t*" or "*f*" denote tables or footnotes, respectively.

Acetylstrophathidin, 42
Adenosine triphosphate, in myocardial ischemia, 85
Afterload, 143, 145
    in management of impaired myocardial performance, 154
Afterload mismatch, 159–160
    and aortic stenosis, 164*f*, 165
    and chronic mitral regurgitation, 162–165
    framework using end-systolic relations, 160–162
    in basal state, 160
    in chronic myocardial disease, 160
    in heart failure, 165–167
        correction, 167–168
    in normal heart, 159
Air embolism
    coronary, 128
    in surgery, 230
Alpha-adrenergic agonists, for pregnant patient, 21–22
Amrinone, 239, 244
Anasarca, 3
Anemia, 152–153
Anesthesia
    and coronary artery spasm, 134
    and myocardial oxygenation, 92
    circulatory depressant effects, digitalis to counteract, 247–248
    for coronary bypass, in patients with recent acute myocardial infarction, 172
    for pregnant patient, 20, 27
    in coronary artery disease
        cardiac catheterization data, 90–91
        monitoring, 91
        physical examination, 90
        preoperative evaluation, 89
        risks, 213
        technique, 94–96
    teratogenic effects, 25
Anesthesia-drug interaction, 89–90
Anesthetics
    and coronary artery disease, 92–93
    pharmacology, 92–94
    volatile, 94–96, *see also specific anesthetic*
        hemodynamic effects, 92*t*
Angina, 37
    after bypass surgery, 257
    and carotid sinus pressure, 36
    and hypertension, 40
    postinfarction, 57, 176–177
    postoperative relief, 254–255
    Prinzmetal's, 39
    relief, 39
    unstable, 57, 111, 133, 173
        risk of coronary spasm with, 132
    variant, 133
Angiocardiography, in differential diagnosis of pericardial disease, 9–10
Angiography
    and coronary spasm, 133
    assessment of myocardial perfusion, 255
    in detection of coronary artery disease in surgical patients, 214
Angioplasty, percutaneous transluminal coronary, with vascular surgery, 214, 215
Anoxia, metabolic consequences, 99
Antiarrhythmic drugs, as adjuvants to defibrillatory efforts, 128
Anticoagulants
    and anesthesia, 90
    for pregnant patient, 24
Antidiuretic hormone, 32–33, 42
Antihypertensives
    and anesthesia, 90
    for pregnant patient, 24–25
Aorta, occlusion, 2
Aortic aneurysm
    abdominal, operative mortality, 214, 215
    monitoring, in labor, 19–20
Aortic arch, barosensitive region, 30–31
Aortic crossclamping, duration
    and myocardial damage, 230, 231*t*
    and perioperative myocardial infarction, 108*t*, 109*t*
Aortic stenosis, monitoring, in labor, 19–20
Aortic valve
    disease, 150–151
        effect on cardiac resuscitation, 123
    incompetence, 123
    insufficiency, 150–151
    mechanical, stuck, 129
    obstruction, 208
    regurgitation, 123, 160, 162
    stenosis, 150, 151, 159–160, 163, 164*f*
        afterload mismatch and, 165
        cardiac receptor function in, 42–43
Aortocaval compression, by pregnant uterus, in

cardiac surgery, 27
Aortocoronary bypass, 135
Arfonad, 154
Arrhythmias, 32, *see also specific arrhythmia*
  after coronary bypass following myocardial infarction, 173–175
  associated with digitalis toxicity, 249–250
  diagnosis, carotid sinus pressure in, 36
  in pregnancy, 18
  postoperative
    management, electrodes used in, 180
    and prophylactic digitalization, 245–246
  role of cardiac receptors in, 41–42
Arterial baroreceptors
  anatomy, 30–31
  function
    in congestive heart failure, 35
    in coronary artery disease, 36
    in hypertension, 34
    in shock, 35–36
  orthostatic function, 31
Arterial desaturation, 153f
Arteriolar tone
  in adults, 219–220
  in children, 220–221, 223f
  pulmonary, with cardiopulmonary bypass, 219
  systemic, with cardiopulmonary bypass, 217–218
Ascites, 4
Asystole
  refractory to pacing, 126–127
  terminal, 127
Atenolol, 89
Atherosclerosis, 38
Atrial electrogram, 180, 181, 182f
Atrial fibrillation, 41, 145
  diagnosis and treatment, 181–183
  in constrictive pericarditis, 4
Atrial flutter, 36
  diagnosis, 183
  Type I, 183
    atrial pacing to interrupt, 196
    treatment, 183–186, 187f
  Type II, 183
Atrial pacing, 183–190, 196
  continuous rapid, to precipitate and sustain atrial fibrillation, 193, 194f
  rapid, to produce 2:1 atrioventricular conduction, 193–194, 195f
Atrial receptors, 32
  Type A, 32
  Type B, 32
Atrial reflexes, 32–33
Atrial septal defect, 15
Atrial tachycardia, *see also* Paroxysmal atrial tachycardia
  ectopic (nonparoxysmal)

atrial pacing to interrupt, 196
  diagnosis, 190, 191f
  treatment, 190–191, 192f
Atropine, 38
  in treatment of digitalis cardiotoxicity, 251
Automaticity, disturbances, 122
Automatic tachycardias
  atrioventricular junctional, treatment, 192–193
  sinus and AV junctional, diagnosis, 191–192
Autonomic nervous system, in heart disease, 35

Bainbridge reflex, 32
Baroreceptors, *see* Arterial baroreceptors
Bed rest, effects, 263–264
Beta-adrenergic agonists, 134
  for pregnant patient, 22
Beta-adrenergic blockers, 215
  and anesthesia, 89–90
Biomedicus pump, *see* Rotor impeller pump
Bladder pump, 66–68
Blood, oxygen content, in management of impaired myocardial performance, 152–153
Blood pressure
  arterial
    interpretation, 140–141
    monitoring, 151
  bedside measurement, interpretation, 140–143
  diastolic, determination, 140f
  interpretation, 143–145
  regulation, 30
  systolic, determination, 140f
Blood substitutes, synthetic, 104–105
Bradyarrhythmias, and myocardial infarction, 40
Bradycardia, postoperative, diagnosis and treatment, 181
Bradykinin, 34, 40–41
Bretylium, 128

Calcium
  in cardioplegic solution, 100
  in contractile mechanism, 232–233
Calcium antagonists, 108, 215
Calcium channel blockers, 97, 134
  and anesthesia, 90
  effect on abnormalities of diastolic function, 211–212
  in cardioplegic solution, 100–101
Calcium chloride, in cardiac resuscitation, 126
Carbon dioxide, 40
Cardiac arrest, IABP for, 58
Cardiac cachexia, 3
Cardiac catheterization, 114, 177
  after acute myocardial infarction, 171–172
  IABP with, 57
  in constrictive pericarditis, 6
  in differential diagnosis of pericardial disease, 9–10

Cardiac filling, *see also* Rapid filling; Slow filling
    effect of pericardium, 206
Cardiac fossa, 3
Cardiac hypertrophy, and diastolic function, 200
Cardiac index, pre- and postoperative, effects of
    preload elevation, afterload reduction,
    and preload restoration, 220–221, 223*f*
Cardiac muscle, *see* Muscle
Cardiac output, *see also* Low output syndrome
  adequacy, clinical evaluation and interpreta-
    tion, 140
  clinical assessment, 143–148
  determinants, 143
    in management of impaired cardiac per-
    formance, 153–154
  inadequate, postoperative, 139
  inotropic drugs and, 235
  measurement, 139–140
    interpretation, 140–143
  postoperative, 230
    improved, by increased preload, 153*f*
  regulation, 222*f*
  relation to venous return, 167*f*
  signs for estimating, 231
Cardiac receptors
  anatomy, 30–31
  function
    in aortic stenosis, 42–43
    in congestive heart failure, 42
    in ischemic heart disease, 38–41
      clinical studies, 39–40
    in production of arrhythmias, 41–42
    Type B, 41, 42
Cardiac rehabilitation, perioperative, 254–269
Cardiac surgery, in pregnancy, 25–27
Cardiac tamponade, 12–13, 139, 145, 147, 205
  atypical features, in postoperative patients, 12–
    13
  classical, 12
  delayed, 12
  diagnosis, 13
  treatment, 13
Cardiogenic shock, 39, 51–52, 56–57, 68, 75, 76,
    170, 230
Cardiomyopathy, hypertrophic, 208, 209, 211–
    212
Cardioplegia, 98, 128
  basic physiological principles, 98–99
  chemical, 98
  cold blood system, 101–103
    additives, 102*t*
    operative mortality with, 104
  crystalloid vs. blood, 100*t*
  hypothermic, 98–100, 108–109
  intermittent perfusion in, 99
  secondary, 108
  solutions, 99–101

  buffer, 100
  calcium antagonists in, 100–101
  calcium in, 100
  magnesium in, 100
  oncotic pressure, 100
  osmolarity, 100
  oxygen in, 100
  potassium in, 99
  substrate enhancement, 108
  warm, 104
  warm induction, 108
Cardiopulmonary bypass, 97
  degrees, and infarct size, in animals, 65*f*
  hypertension and, 40
  in management of impaired myocardial per-
    formance, 157
  myocardial failure with, 56
  physiological changes with, 217–219
  postbypass period, 95–96
  pregnant patient, in, 26–27
    fetal oxygenation in, 26, 27
  prolonged, 76
  reduced oxygen consumption in, 64–65
  sedation on, 95
  termination, 95
  transition to intensive care unit after, 96
  use of vasodilators on, 226–227
  weaning from, 56, 60, 63, 68, 74, 85
Cardioversion, in treatment of digitalis cardiotox-
    icity, 251
Carotid endarterectomy, operative mortality, 214
Carotid sinus
  barosensitive region, 30–31
  hypersensitive reflex, 37
  hypersensitive syndrome, 37–38
  hypotension, effect on cardiac output, 31
  pressure, 38
    dangers, 37
    in angina, 36
    in diagnosis of arrhythmias, 36
    technique of applying, 37
Catecholamines
  in congestive heart failure, 35
  inotropic effect, 232–233
Chamber, passive properties, 201
Chamber compliance, 202, 203
  definition, 200–201
  effect of pericardium, 206
Chamber stiffness, 202, 203
  definition, 201
Chest radiogram
  in pericardial disease, 8
  in pregnancy, 18
  in tricuspid incompetence, 9
Chloride, in reanimation of heart, 125
Citrate toxicity, 146
CK MB, in diagnosis of perioperative myocardial

infarction, 110–112
Clonidine, for pregnant patient, 24
Coarctation of aorta, 19
Cobe roller pump, 70
Cold-spot imaging, 113
Computerized tomography
  in cardiac tamponade, 13
  in diagnosis of constrictive pericarditis, 5–6
  in pericardial disease, 8
Concentric tube pump, 81–82
  removal, 81
Conduction disturbances, 122
Congestive heart failure, 241, 245–246
  arterial baroreceptor function in, 35
  cardiac receptor function in, 42
Constrictive pericarditis
  classicial chronic tuberculous, 3, 4, 6
  differential diagnosis, 4
  occult, 3, 6–8
    diagnosis, 7
    fluid challenge in, 7–8
    pressure tracings in, 7
  overt, postoperative, 8–10
    differential diagnosis, 8–10
  postoperative, 3–8
    cardiac catheterization for, 6
    causes, 3
    clincal signs, 3–4
    diagnosis, 3
    laboratory findings, 4–5
    pressure tracings in, 6–7
  resemblance to acute volume overload, 211
Contractility, in impaired myocardial perform-
    ance, 155
Cooperative Coronary Artery Surgery study, 214
Coronary arterial system, normal physiology,
    131–132
Coronary artery, occlusion, 38–39
Coronary artery bypass, 91, 113–114, 254
  after acute myocardial infarction, 170–179
    actuarial survival, 175–176
    criteria for operation, 171
    hospital morbidity and mortality, 172–175
    late follow-up, 175
    operation, 172
    patient selection, 177
    perioperative complications, 173–175, 178
  after failure of percutaneous coronary angio-
    plasty, 174f, 175
  exercise training after, studies of, 264–267
  in presence of vascular disease, 215–216
  long-term outcome, 256–257
  postoperative physiological changes, 255–256
  prior to other surgery, morbidity and mortality,
    215
  psychological outcome, 257–258
  return to work after, 258–261

determinants, 260–261
  survival, 257
Coronary artery disease, 254
  anesthetic considerations, 89–96
  baroreceptor function in, 36
  exercise training with, 262–263
  noncardiac surgery and, 213–216
  in patients with recent acute myocardial in-
    farction, 172
  rehabilitation, 254
Coronary artery spasm
  and anesthesia, 134
  diagnosis, 132–133
  electrocardiogram findings, 133
  factors in, 132t
  operation with, 134–136
  treatment, 133–134
Cor pulmonale, 207
Coumadin, for pregnant patient, 24
Counterpulsation, 51–52, see also Intra-aortic
    balloon pumping in management of im-
    paired myocardial performance, 156–157
Creatine phosphokinase, 110

Decompression, 122
Diastole
  definition, 200
  pressure-volume relationship in, determinants,
    201–208
Diastolic function, in hypertrophied states, 200
Diastolic pressure time index, 149
Diazepam, 95, 172, 250
Diazoxide, 90
Dibenzyline, 154
Digitalis, 38, 42, 168, 239
  and cardiac performance, 243–245
  cardiotoxicity, 249–251
    diagnosis, by serum concentration assay,
      250
    factors enhancing, 250
    management, 250–251
  effect on carotid sinus reflex, 36
  effect on contractile mechanism, 233f
  for pregnant patient, 23–24
  interaction with baroreceptors, 35
  perioperative usefulness, 244–245
  positive inotropic action, 243
  presurgical withdrawal, 248–249
  role in heart failure, 241–245
  toxicity
    arrhythmias associated with, 249–250
    carotid sinus pressure in diagnosis, 36
    systemic manifestations, 249t
Digitalization
  preoperative, dose, 248
  prophylactic, 245–248
    for prevention of cardiac complication after

thoracic surgery, 245–246
in prevention of supraventricular tachyarrthy-
mias, 246–248
Digital subtraction ventriculography, 117
Digitoxin, 241
for pregnant patient, 23
Digoxin, 241
for pregnant patient, 23
in cardiac resuscitation, 125
Diphenylhydantoin
before cardioversion, 251
in treatment of digitalis cardiotoxicity, 250
Diuretics, and cardiac performance, 242, 244
Dobutamine, 95, 168, 234, 244
and dopamine, after coronary artery bypass,
comparison, 235–236
clinical indications for, 237f
in low output syndrome, 238
in management of impaired myocardial performance, 156
inotropic effect, 232–233
relative potency, 233t
structure, 233t
Dopamine, 95, 168, 234, 244
and dobutamine, after coronary artery bypass,
comparison, 235–236
and systemic hemodynamics in children, 221,
226
clinical indications for, 237t
compared to isuprel, after cardiopulmonary
bypass, 236
for pregnant patient, 22t, 23
in low output syndrome, 237–238
in management of impaired myocardial performance, 156
inotropic effect, 232–233
relative potency, 233t
structure, 233t
Dressler's syndrome, 11
Ductus arteriosus, patent, 15
Dyspnea, clinical significance, 208

Echocardiography
in cardiac tamponade, 12, 13
in diagnosis of constrictive pericarditis, 4–5
in evaluation of myocardial performance, 116–
117
in pericardial disease, 8
intra-operative hand-held, 116f
in tricuspid incompetence, 9
of postoperative patients, 10–11
Edema, 4
in pregnancy, 18
Ejection fraction, 90–91
after mitral valve replacement, 163f
and mitral regurgitation, 164f

determination, 114–116
in perioperative myocardial infarction, 117
Electrocardiogram
in diagnosis of perioperative myocardial infarction, 109–110
in pericardial disease, 8
in pregnancy, 16
in tricuspid incompetence, 9
Emboli, see also Air embolism
pulmonary, 68
End-diastolic pressure, as index of myocardial
function, 91
Endocarditis, bacterial, 15
End-systolic volume
determinant of diastolic pressure and volume,
206
determinants, 206
effect of heart rate on, 208
Enflurane, 94
hemodynamic effects, 92t
Ephedrine, for pregnant patient, 22t, 23
Epinephrine, 95, 128
clinical indications for, 237t
for pregnant patient, 22t, 23
in cardiac resuscitation, 126
in low output syndrome, 238
in management of impaired myocardial performance, 156
inotropic effect, 232–233
relative potency, 233t
structure, 233t
Ergot, effects on cardiovascular system, 19
Estrogen, cardiovascular changes caused by, 17
Ethanol, for pregnant patient, 27
Excitability, abnormal, 122
Exercise
aerobic, 262
dynamic, 262
Exercise capacity, and rehabilitation after coronary artery bypass, 259–260
Exercise training
after coronary artery bypass, 261
response to, 262–263
studies of, 264–267
exercises, 271–276
in cardiac rehabilitation, 254
Extracorporeal circulation, 63
in management of impaired myocardial performance, 157
Extrasystole
diagnosis, 197–198
treatment, 198

Fentanyl, 92–95
hemodynamic effects, 92t
Fetal heart rate, in hypoxia and acidosis, 26
Fetal monitoring, in patients requiring cardiopul-

monary bypass, 26–27
Fick equation, 139
Filling volume, as index of preload, 209
Fluid challenge, 7–8
Fluorocarbons, 104–105
Frank-Starling curves, 234
Frank-Starling relation, shift in, with alterations
    in diastolic function, 208–209

Glyceryl trinitrate
  and myocardial function, 223–225
  and venous tone, 222
  mode of action, 226
Gott shunt, 69
Guanethidine, 90

Halothane, 93–95, 247
  for pregnant patient, 27
  hemodynamic effects, 92t
Heart, see also Ventricle(s)
  as pump, 219–223
  disease
    congenital, 15
    in pregnancy, see Pregnancy, cardiac disease
    in
  energy consumption
    determinants, 63–64
    relationship to wall tension, 64–65
  oxygen demand, estimation, 150
  oxygen supply, 148–150
  pressure overload, pericardial function in, 2
  reanimation, 122–130
    blood gases, 124–125
    perfusion hemodynamics, 124
    pH in, 125
  volume overload, pericardial function in, 2
Heart block, 36
Heart failure
  afterload mismatch in, 165–167
    correction, 167–168
  definition, 241
  relation between cardiac output and venous
    return in, 166f
  treatment, 241
Heart rate
  abnormalities, 143–145
  and vasodilators, 224–225
  as extrinsic determinant of pressure and vol-
    ume during diastole, 208
  effects on disease states, 152
  increasing, to improve output in failing heart,
    154–155
Heart sounds, in pregnancy, 18
Heart transplant, IABP for circulatory support in,
    58–59
Heparin, for pregnant patient, 24
Heparin-bonded tubing, 69
High-risk cardiac patients, requiring noncardiac
    surgery, IABP for, 58

Hydralazine, 90, 168, 217, 219
  and cardiac output, 222f
  for pregnant patient, 24–25
Hydrogen ions, 40
Hypertension, 38, 150, 152, 162
  after coronary artery surgery, 218
  and myocardial infarction, 41
  arterial baroreceptor function in, 34
  in angina, 40
  postbypass, 40
  pulmonary venous, 208
  systemic, 208
Hypotension
  in pregnancy, 18
  presurgical, 150, 151
Hypothermia
  effect on myocardial oxygen consumption, 99
  in cardioplegia, 99–100
Hypovolemia, 145–147, 205
Hypoxia, 41
  metabolic consequences, 99

Idiopathic hypertrophic subaortic stenosis, 15
Impeller pump, 80–81, see also Rotor impeller
    pump removal, 81
Indomethacin, 41
Inotropic drugs
  clinical indications for, 237t
  effects on contractile mechanism, 232–234
  for coronary bypass patients with recent acute
    myocardial infarction, 172–174
  general policies in use of, 238–239
  perioperative uses, 230–240
  positive, 235
  postoperative, conditions commonly requiring,
    231t
  therapy, physiology, 234–235
  use after coronary bypass, 177–178
Intra-aortic balloon
  designs, 53
  in cardiac resuscitation, 127
  long sheath-dilator combination for, 53–54
  percutaneous implantation, 52, 75–76
    complications, 55
    experience with, 54–56
    technique, 52–53
  removal, 53
Intra-aortic balloon pumping, 51–52, 74, 177,
    178, 236, 238
  after coronary bypass following myocardial
    infarction, 173–175
  for cardiac arrest, 58
  for circulatory support in heart transplant, 58–
    59
  compared to extracorporeal ventricular sup-
    port, 66
  complications, 59–60
  contraindication, 68

dependency on, 86
for coronary bypass patients with recent acute myocardial infarction, 172
for myocardial contusion, 58
for support during weaning from cardiopulmonary bypass, 63
in community hospital, 58–59
indications, 52, 60, 75
in management of impaired myocardial performance, 156–157
perioperative, 56
preoperative, 57
Ischemia, 132, 133, *see also* Myocardial ischemia
depression of ST segment as indicator, 255
in coronary disease, 150–151
management
postoperative considerations, 152
preoperative considerations, 151–152
metabolic consequences, 99
postinfarction, 176–177
subendocardial, 152
Ischemic heart disease, 208
cardiac receptor function in, 38–41
cardiac reflexes in, potential chemical mediators, 40–41
Isoflurane, hemodynamic effects, 92t
Isoproterenol, 64, 147
in low output syndrome, 237
in management of impaired myocardial performance, 155, 156f
inotropic effect, 232–233
in pregnant patient, 22t
relative potency, 233t
structure, 233t
Isuprel, 134, 234
clinical indications for, 237t
compared to dopamine, after cardiopulmonary bypass, 236

Jugular venous pressure, in constrictive pericarditis, 3–4

Labetolol, 133
Labor
blood volume changes in, 19
cardiac output in, 16, 18–19
in cardiac patient, 18–20
major risk periods, for cardiac patient, 19–20
premature, and cardiac surgery, 25
Lactate, 40
Lactic dehydrogenase, 110
La Place relation, 203
Left bundle branch block, 36
Left ventricle, *see also* Ventricular bypass
afterload, response to changes in, 160–162
compliance, 141, 142f
diastolic function, alterations in, clinical significance, 208–209

failure, 75, 76, 85, 146f, 170, 217
and response to vasodilator therapy, 219–220
function
after acute myocardial infarction, 171–172
after coronary artery bypass, 256
and vasodilators, 219–221, 222f
effect of revascularization after myocardial infarction, 178
scintigraphic evaluation, 114–116
hypertrophy, 209
alterations in diastolic function in, 209–212
forms, 209–211
intact, determinants of diastolic pressure and volume
extrinsic, 201, 206–208
intrinsic, 201–206
relationship, 201–208
overdistension, 122–123
passive pressure-volume relation, 202–204
effect of pericardium, 206
recovery, 84–85
right ventricular diastolic pressure acting on, 207
venting, 101, 122
Left ventricular assistance, 83–84
device, 82, *see also* Concentric tube pump
indications for, 76
positioning, 81–82
requirements for, 74–75
Left ventricular balloon pumping, combined with IABP, 63
Left ventricular volume, determination, 140f
Levarteranol, 64
Lidocaine, 128
before cardioversion, 251
for pregnant patient, 21
in treatment of digitalis cardiotoxicity, 250
Lorazepam, 95
Low output syndrome, 56, 74
diagnosis, 230–231
first- and second-line agents for, 236–238
postbypass, treatment options, 239
typical patient, 232
Lungs, and heart, interplay, 207

Magnesium
in cardioplegic solution, 100
in reanimation of heart, 125
Magnesium sulfate
effects on cardiovascular system, 19
for pregnant patient, 27
Mediastinum, as external restraint upon heart, 3
Medtronic pump, *see* Rotor impeller pump
Metaraminol, for pregnant patient, 22t, 23
Methoxamine, in pregnant patient, 22t
Methyldopa, 38
for pregnant patient, 24

Metoprolol, 89
Mitral valve
  incompetence, pericardial restraint function in, 2
  insufficiency, 150–151
  regurgitation, 160, 162
    and afterload mismatch, 162–165
  stenosis, 15
    surgical correction, in pregnant patient, 25–26
Morphine, 92–96, 146, 172
  hemodynamic effects, 92t
Muscle
  blood contained in, 207–208
  compliance, definition, 201
  creep, 205
  elastance, 201
  erectile property, 208
  passive properties, 201
  stiffness, 209
    calculation, 203
    definition, 201
    related to chamber stiffness or compliance, 204
    strain component, calculation, 203–204
  strain, definition, 201
  stress, definition, 201
  stress relaxation, 205
Myocardial contusion, IABP therapy, 58
Myocardial disease, 8, 10
Myocardial dysfunction, physiological abnormalities related to, 230
Myocardial failure, 139, 147–148
Myocardial function, effect of vasodilators, 223–226
Myocardial imaging, infarct-avid, 112–113
Myocardial infarction, 10, 11, 36, 39, 40, 133
  acute
    clinical course, 170
    clinical profile of patient population, 171
  acute evolving anterior, 174f, 175
  angina after, 57
  clinical course, 176
  during coronary arteriography, 57
  extension, 176
  incidence, 51, 175
  intraoperative, 230, 257
  management, 175–178
  morbidity, 176
  mortality, 176
  pain following, 176
  perioperative, 107–121, 255
    clinical associations, 107–108
    clinical presentation, 108
    diagnostic techniques, 109–117
    effect of myocardial protection, 108–109
    incidence, 107

mortality, 117
prognosis, 117
under general anesthesia, mortality, 213–214
Myocardial ischemia, 34, 38–39, 84–85, 152
  and cell death, 107
  biochemistry, 85
  blood flow to, effect of vasodilators, 223–224, 225f
  caused by postoperative hypertension, 154f
  during coronary arteriography, 57
  intra-aortic balloon counterpulsation for, 54
Myocardial necrosis, 107
  acute, 110
  intervals during perioperative period for occurrence, 108t
  in open heart procedures, 230
  postoperative, 110
Myocardial performance
  assessment, 145–146
  impaired, management, 152–157
Myocardial perfusion imaging, 113–115
Myocardial relaxation, quantification, 204–205
Myocardial scintigram, 111f, 113
  preoperative, 112
Myocardium
  contractility, 143
  damage, 230
  intramyocardial compressive forces, 148f
  intraoperative protection, 97–106
    conduct of operation, 103–104
    effect on perioperative myocardial infarction, 108–109
    historical review, 98
    left ventricular venting, 101
    venous decompression, 101
  left ventricular, viscous resistance to stretch, 205
  oxygen consumption, 64–65, 150
    after coronary artery bypass, 256
    effect of hypothermia, 99
  oxygen demand and supply
    and vasodilators, 223–226
    with cardiopulmonary bypass, 218–219
  perfusion, by coronary bypass surgery, 255
  perioperative injury, 75
  perioperative protection, 75, 97, 123
  restrictive disease, 10
  viscous behavior, 205

Narcotics, 92, 95
Nifedipine, 90, 134
Nitroglycerin, 95, 97, 134, 217, 244
  and cardiac output, 222f
  and myocardial function, 225f
  and venous tone, 221–222
  in cardioplegic solution, 101
  indications for, 226

for pregnant patient, 25
ST-segment improvement from, 224f
Nitroprusside, 95, 166, 217, 238, 244
  afterload reduction by, 154f
  and arteriolar tone, 220, 221f
    in children, 220–221, 223f
  and myocardial function, 223, 225f
  and pulmonary vascular resistance, 226
  and systemic hemodynamics in children, 221, 226
  and venous tone, 222
  for pregnant patient, 25
  indications for, 226
  mode of action, 225–226
  ST-segment improvement from, 224f
Nitrous oxide, 172
  in postbypass period, 95–96
Nodal rhythm, 145
Norepinephrine
  clinical indications for, 237t
  in congestive heart failure, 35
  in low output syndrome, 238
  in management of impaired myocardial performance, 155–156
  inotropic effect, 232–233
  in pregnant patient, 22t
  relative potency, 233
  structure, 233
Nuclear magnetic resonance, 117

Open heart surgery
  cardiopulmonary bypass for, in pregnant patient, 26–27
  IABP with, 56
  personality and psychologic function after, 257
Organ hypoperfusion, 146
Oxygen, in cardioplegic solution, 100
Oxygen poisoning, 124
Oxytocin, effects on cardiovascular system, 19

Pacemaker, demand, 38
Pain
  cardiac, 39, see also Angina
  ventricular fibers signalling, 34
Papaverine, 134
Paroxysmal atrial tachycardia, 36, 186–190
  atrial pacing to interrupt, 196
  diagnosis, 186–188
  treatment, 188–190
Pericardial disease, overt, postoperative, treatment, 10
Pericardial effusion, postoperative, 11
Pericardial friction rubs, 10, 11
Pericardial knock, 8
Pericardial reserve volume, 1
Pericardiectomy, 10
Pericarditis, see also Constrictive pericarditis

acute, 10–11
Pericardium
  and diastolic ventricular interaction, 207
  effect on cardiac function, 1
  in acute cardiac dilation, 1–3
  influence on passive pressure-volume relation in left ventricle, 206
  intracardiac filling pressure borne by, 2
  response to chronic volume overload, 211
  response to stretch, 1
  restraining force on filling, 206
Peripheral vascular disease, surgery for, combined with coronary bypass, 215
Phentolamine, 134
Phenylephrine, in pregnant patient, 22t
Pleural effusion, 13
Positive airway pressure, 207
Postpartum
  cardiac output, 20
  risk factors for cardiac patient, 20
Postpericardiotomy syndrome, 8, 11–12
  etiology, 11
  symptoms and signs, 11
  treatment, 11–12
Potassium, 40
  effect on AV conduction, 251
  imbalance, detected during cardiac resuscitation, treatment, 125
  in cardioplegia solution, 99
  in reanimation of heart, 125
  in treatment of digitalis cardiotoxicity, 250, 251
Practolol, 89
Prazosin, 220
  and cardiac output, 222f
Prednisone, therapy, of postpericardiotomy syndrome, 12
Pre-eclampsia, 24–25
Pregnancy, see also Labor
  anatomical changes, 16
  anticoagulant therapy in, 24
  antihypertensive therapy in, 24–25
  blood volume changes, 16
  cardiac disease in, 15–29
    diagnostic features, 18
    etiology, 15
    incidence, 15
    maternal mortality, 15
  cardiac output, 16
  cardiac surgery during, 25–27
  cardiovascular alterations of, 15–18
    clinical findings, 18
  hemodynamic alterations, 16–18
  pharmacological considerations in, 20–25
  respiratory changes, 18
  supine syndrome in, 18
  systemic vascular resistance in, 16
  vascular pressure changes in, 16–17

vascular volume changes, 16
vena caval compression in, 17–18
Preload, 143, 144f, 145
in management of impaired myocardial performance, 153
Preload reserve, analyzed at sarcomere level, 160–161
Procainamide, in treatment of digitalis cardiotoxicity, 251
Propranolol, 38, 97
and anesthesia, 89
fetal and neonatal effects, 20–21
for pregnant patient, 20–21
in treatment of digitalis cardiotoxicity, 251
Prostacyclin, 41
Prostaglandins, 34, 40–41
Prostigmine sulphate, 128
Proximal aortocoronary anastamosis, open technique, 103–105
Pseudopericardium, 6
Pulmonary arterioles, in children, after cardiac surgery, 219
Pulmonary artery, occlusion, 2
Pulmonary artery catheter, for patient monitoring in anesthesia, 91
Pulmonary hypertension, primary, monitoring, in labor, 20
Pulmonary vascular resistance
in children, 226
increase, after cardiac surgery, 219
Pulsatile flow, 66
Pulsus paradoxus, 12–13
Pumps, *see also* specific pump
for extracorporeal circulatory support
indications for, 68
types, 66–68
for ventricular assistance, types, 77–84

Quinidine, 250
Q waves
after coronary bypass after myocardial infarction, 173–175
in open heart surgery, 109–110
in perioperative myocardial infarction, 117

Radionucleotide study, in pericardial disease, 8
Rapid filling, 202, 205
Reserpine, 90
Restrictive cardiomyopathy, 10
Rheumatic fever, 15
Rheumatic valvular disease, surgical correction, in pregnancy, 25–26
Right-to-left shunt, monitoring, in labor, 19–20
Right ventricle
failure, 75–76, 85–86
overdistention, 124
postoperative infarction, 10

Right ventricular assist device, 82
indications for, 76
Roller pump, 66–68, 77–80
cannulae, 77–80
removal, 79
Rotor impeller pump, 66–68, 70

Sac pump, 82–84, *see also* Bladder pump
Saphenous vein graft, late spasm in, 135–136
Septal hypertrophy, 15
Serotonin, 41
Serum enzymes and isoenzymes, in diagnosis of perioperative myocardial infarction, 110–112
Serum glutamic oxaloacetic transaminase, 110
Shock, *see also* Cardiogenic shock
baroreceptor function in, 35–36
Sinus tachycardia, 36
Slow filling, 202–203
Sodium, in reanimation of heart, 125
Sodium nitroprusside, *see* Nitroprusside
Stellate ganglia, removal, 39
Steroids, therapy, of postpericardiotomy syndrome, 12
Stone heart, 127
Stroke volume
after coronary artery bypass, 256
determinants, 143
with cardiopulmonary bypass, 217–218
Subendocardium
ischemia, 148
left ventricular, 148
area for potential blood supply to, 149f
necrosis, 147–148, 155
oxygen supply, 149–150
Supraventricular tachyarrhythmias
desirable, pacing to produce, 193–194
diagnosis and treatment, 181–194
postoperative
prevention, 246–248
risk, 248
with thoracic surgery, 245–246
Syncope, 37–38, 42–43
Systemic blood flow, total, left ventricular contribution to, 84

Tachycardia, 150, 152
Technetium-99m glucoheptonate, in diagnosis of myocardial infarction, 112
Technetium-99m pyrophosphate, in diagnosis of myocardial infarction, 112
Tension time index, 149f, 150
Thallium-201, in detection of myocardial infarction, 113–115
Thallium-scanning, assessment of myocardial perfusion, 255
Thiazide diuretics, for pregnant patient, 24

Thiopental, 247
Thoracic surgery, prophylactic digitalization with, 245–246
Tissue oxygen supply, 139
Tolazoline, 226
Treadmill testing, predischarge, in coronary by-pass patients. 257
Tricuspid valve
  incompetence, 8, 9
  regurgitation, 9–10
  stenosis, 9
Trimethaphan, 219

Uteroplacental perfusion, effects of drugs, 21–25
Uterus
  response to beta-adrenergic substances, 22
  suppressants, 27

Valsalva maneuver, in cardiac patient, 20
  during labor, 19
Vascular surgery, 213
  cardiac-related morbidity and mortality, 214
Vasoactive drugs, for pregnant patient, 21–24
Vasodilator therapy
  and cardiac performance, 242–243, 244
  effect, 217
  in surgical patients, 217
  perioperative, 219–229
  response to, 165–166
  use on bypass, 226–227
Vena cava, compression, in pregnancy, 17–18
Venous bed, pressure-volume characteristics, 141–142
Venous pressure, 141–143
  central, 141–142
  pulmonary, 141–143
Venous return
  and response to vasodilators, 165–167
  relation to cardiac output, 167f
  role in afterload reduction therapy, 166–167
Venous tone
  after cardiopulmonary bypass, 218
  and vasodilators, 221–223
Ventricle(s), *see also* Left ventricle; Right ventricle
  chemosensitive receptors in, 34
  compliance, 141–142, 143
  fiber stretch, 143, 145, *see also* Preload
  function, effects of digitalis, 243–244
  interaction, 207
    diastolic, 207
    in presence of pericardium, 3
  mechanosensitive receptors in, 33–34
  vulnerability to ischemic injury, 150
Ventricular assist devices, 74–88
  biventricular, 82
  cannulation technique, 76–77

clinical results with, 77t
complications, 86
contraindications, 76
preparation for implantation, 76–77
problems, 85–86
sepsis with, 86
weaning process, 84
Ventricular bypass
  biventricular, 71
  left, 68–71
  right, 71
  types, 68–71
Ventricular contraction, sustained, 127
Ventricular failure, *see also* Left ventricle; Right ventricle
  and decision to use assist pump, 75–77
  conventional therapy, 75–76
  etiology, 75
Ventricular fibrillation
  postoperative, 108
  prolonged, consequences, 99
  recurring, 128–129
  resistant to electroshock, 127–128
Ventricular irritability, postinfarction, 57–58
Ventricular pacing, 196
Ventricular power failure, 68
Ventricular receptors, 33
Ventricular reflexes, 33–34
Ventricular septal defect, 15
Ventricular suction, 205
Ventricular support
  extracorporeal, 66
  methods, 63
Ventricular tachycardia, 108
  diagnosis, 194–196
  treatment, 196, 197f
Verapamil, 134, 248, 250
Vo₂ max, 255
  in exercise-trained coronary artery bypass patients, 265, 267
Volume overload, 2
  acute, 211
Volume replacement, 146, 147

Wall stress, 160
  calculation, 203
Wire electrodes, epicardial
  diagnostic uses, 180
  in management of perioperative arrhythmias, 180
  in pacing, 180, 183–186
  uses, 180–181
  ventricular, 181

Xylocaine, in cardioplegic solution, 101